Introduction to

Physical Education and Sport Science

Robert C. France, MS, RSMT, CSMT

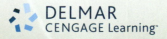
DELMAR
CENGAGE Learning™

Australia • Brazil • Japan • Korea • Mexico • Singapore • Spain • United Kingdom • United States

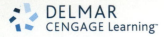

Introduction to Physical Education and Sport Science
Robert C. France

Vice President, Career and Professional Editorial: Dave Garza

Director of Learning Solutions: Matthew Kane

Acquisitions Editor: Matthew Seeley

Managing Editor: Marah Bellegarde

Senior Product Manager: Debra Myette-Flis

Editorial Assistant: Megan Tarquinio

Vice President, Career and Professional Marketing: Jennifer McAvey

Senior Marketing Manager: Kristin McNary

Marketing Coordinator: Erika Ropitzky

Production Director: Carolyn S. Miller

Content Project Manager: Kenneth McGrath

For product information and technology assistance, contact us at **Professional & Career Group Customer Support, 1-800-648-7450**

For permission to use material from this text or product, submit all requests online at **www.cengage.com/permissions.** Further permissions questions can be e-mailed to **permissionrequest@cengage.com**

Library of Congress Control Number: 2008930301

ISBN-13: 978-1-418-05529-5

ISBN-10: 1-4180-5529-8

Delmar
5 Maxwell Drive
Clifton Park, NY 12065-2919
USA

Cengage Learning products are represented in Canada by Nelson Education, Ltd.

For your lifelong learning solutions, visit **delmar.cengage.com**

Visit our corporate website at **cengage.com**

Notice to the Reader

Publisher does not warrant or guarantee any of the products described herein or perform any independent analysis in connection with any of the product information contained herein. Publisher does not assume, and expressly disclaims, any obligation to obtain and include information other than that provided to it by the manufacturer. The reader is expressly warned to consider and adopt all safety precautions that might be indicated by the activities described herein and to avoid all potential hazards. By following the instructions contained herein, the reader willingly assumes all risks in connection with such instructions. The publisher makes no representations or warranties of any kind, including but not limited to, the warranties of fitness for particular purpose or merchantability, nor are any such representations implied with respect to the material set forth herein, and the publisher takes no responsibility with respect to such material. The publisher shall not be liable for any special, consequential, or exemplary damages resulting, in whole or part, from the readers' use of, or reliance upon, this material.

Printed in Canada
1 2 3 4 5 6 7 12 11 10 09 08

Contents

UNIT 2 Exercise and Movement

UNIT 3 Adaptive Physical Education

UNIT 4 Coaching: The Challenges and the Benefits

UNIT 6 Opportunities and Challenges in Physical Education and Exercise Science

Preface

Introduction to Physical Education and Sport Science was written for individuals with a passion for fitness and a desire to engage others in the current methodology of physical education and sport science, and for those who desire a basis of knowledge of physical education and sport science. This textbook was developed to encompass a wide range of topics, and give the physical education student a solid historical background of one of the most important fields of study. *Introduction to Physical Education and Sport Science* was also designed to use as a reference long into one's physical education and coaching career.

The timing of *Introduction to Physical Education and Sport Science* is critical, and couldn't have come along at a more important time in our history. Our nation has developed an "appetite" for inactivity and an ever-growing desire to be a spectator society. Obesity levels, and the health concerns that go along with them, are at an all-time high. The trend for the immediate future is not so bright.

This textbook will give the physical education student, health professional, and everyone in the fitness and health industry the background, perspective, and tools necessary to engage the youth of America in making better decisions about their free time. It is my sincere belief that knowledge will help precipitate change, and that motivated and informed individuals can change the national consciousness on physical education, health, and recreational choices.

Introduction to Physical Education and Sport Science is organized into six distinct units. Unit 1 gives both a historical perspective of physical education and sport science and a look at physical education in the twenty-first century. Unit 2 delves into exercise and movement. Sport kinesiology, emergency preparedness, prehabilitation and preseason conditioning are covered in Unit 2. Adaptive Physical Education is the topic of Unit 3, which will give students knowledge and perspective in working with athletes of varying abilities. Unit 4 covers all aspects of coaching. Many physical education students will make coaching part of their career. Understanding the different aspects of coaching will be critical in ensuring success. Just like coaching will be a natural progression for many physical education students, athletic administration and management will be as well. Unit 5 will engage students in learning about careers in athletic administration and facility management. Students will also gain a strong understanding of Title IX and how this monumental piece of legislation has affected all aspects of athletics. Tournaments and brackets are covered in the last chapter of Unit 5. The sixth and final unit, Opportunities and Challenges in Physical Education and Exercise Science, covers the future of sport, career perspectives, fitness after retirement.

Finally, two appendixes are included that will greatly benefit students of Physical Education and Sport Science. Appendix 1, titled: Dimensions of Athletic Facilities and Arenas, has been a constant source of information throughout my career as a physical educator. This information will keep Introduction to Physical Education and Sport Science close at all times. Appendix 2, titled: Organizations, Periodicals, and the Internet, gives the learner a resource for finding information on different organizations dealing with physical education, health, fitness, recreation, and sport science.

How to Use This Book

Many features of *Introduction to Physical Education and Sport Science* are designed specifically to enhance comprehension.

Objectives: Objectives begin each chapter and set the stage for content the learner is expected to obtain from the chapter.

Key Terms: Key terms are defined within the chapter and highlighted in Green.

Key Concepts: Key concepts are presented in boxes throughout the chapters. These correspond directly to the objectives presented in the beginning of each chapter. The key concepts highlight the important material the learner needs to obtain from the chapter.

Case Studies: Case studies help learners apply key concepts from the chapter to the real world.

Chapter Summary: The chapter summary emphasizes the main points of the chapter.

Review Questions: Review questions assess learners' comprehension of the chapter material.

Projects and Activities: The Projects and Activities section provides hands-on assignments that emphasize key concepts from the chapter.

Website Resources: The Website Resources section encourages learners to further research chapter topics.

The Instructor Resources

ISBN 1-4180-5532-8

The Instructor Resources is a robust, computerized tool for your instructional needs. A must-have for all instructors, this comprehensive and convenient CD-ROM contains:

- **The Instructor's Manual** is designed to help you with lesson preparation and performance assessment. It includes answers to review exercises in the text

- **Exam View® Computerized Testbank** contains over five hundred questions. You can add these questions to your own questions to create review materials or tests.

- **PowerPoint® Presentations** designed to aid you in planning your class presentations. If a learner misses a class, a printout of the slides for a lecture makes a helpful review page.

About the Author

Robert C. France majored in physical education at Pacific Lutheran University and is a certified and registered sports medicine trainer in the state of Washington. His vast knowledge of physical education, sports medicine, and fitness training comes from his extensive training at some of the finest universities across the United States and Europe. His training as an emergency medical technician has helped him to design disaster preparedness programs and assist in their implementation. Registered as an advanced instructor with the National Safety Council, Robert has instructed hundreds of individuals at the high school, college, and professional level in first aid and CPR.

Robert's unique three-year high school sports medicine curriculum has been recognized nationally for its excellence and preparation of students in the fields of sports medicine and athletic training. Students graduating from his program are now physicians, physical therapists, and athletic trainers throughout the United States. He has helped dozens of high schools across the country design and implement similar sports medicine programs. His first textbook, *Introduction to Sports Medicine and Athletic Training*, published by Delmar-Cengage Learning, is one of the leading sports medicine and athletic training textbooks in the United States today.

Robert has lectured throughout the United States and in Europe. In 1996 he was selected as a member of the medical staff for the Olympic Games in Atlanta, Georgia. National Sports Medicine Trainer of the Year and Teacher of the Year are just two of the many awards he has received. His teaching and coaching background includes 31 years of teaching at the secondary level, coaching several sports, and many years as an athletic director. Robert currently serves as a national consultant on physical education, fitness, and high school sports medicine programs.

Acknowledgments

Writing a textbook is one of the most difficult and enjoyable tasks I have ever attempted. From conception to the finished product, this book has taken more than two years. Thousands of hours of research and hard work have gone into the writing, rewriting, and rewriting again of this manuscript. Needless to say, it would not have been possible without the unique skills and assistance of many people. I would like to sincerely thank the following individuals for their time and expertise in assisting me in the writing of this textbook:

A special "thank you" to my wife Carla for her patience and support during the long process of writing this book. It probably seemed like an eternity that I spent in my office conducting research and writing. She was always very positive and supportive—a writer's dream!

This textbook would have never been published if it wasn't for Matt Seeley, Acquisitions Editor. I sincerely thank him for his insights, his willingness to take a chance on a new direction in Physical Education textbooks, and his always positive feedback. I would also like to acknowledge Debra Myette-Flis, Senior Product Manager, for her attention to detail, suggestions, and occasional extension on my deadlines. She is definitely one of the finest in her field and I was very fortunate to have her work on this project. I would also like to thank everyone at Delmar–Cengage Learning for their hard work on this project.

Additional thanks go to dozens of experts in the fields of physical education, sport science, fitness, athletics, and sports medicine for their insights and assistance throughout this process.

Lastly, I would like to thank my parents, Richard and Carole, for instilling in me the work ethic and the desire to always do my best.

Robert C. France

Reviewers

Terri Pearson-Bloom, MEd
Instructor
Physical Education
Solano Community College
Fairfield, California

Sarah A. Manspeaker, MSEd, ATC
Instructor
Assistant Athletic Trainer
Sports Medicine Department
Marietta College
Mariettta, Ohio

Mark Lafferty, PhD, MEd
Exercise Science Program Coordinator
Delaware Technical and Community College
Wilmington, Delaware

Lori Dewald, EdD, ATC, CHES
Assistant Professor
Department of Health, Physical Education,
    and Human Performance
Salisbury University
Salisbury, Maryland

Lisa T. Petruzzi, MEd, VATL, ATC
H/PE/SpEd Biology Instructor, Athletic Trainer
Fairfax County Public Schools
Fairfax, Virginia

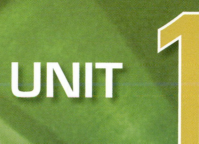

UNIT 1

Physical Education and Exercise Science

History and Development of Physical Education and Exercise Science

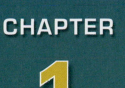

Objectives

Upon completion of this chapter, the reader should be able to:

- Explain the progression of physical education and sport science from the classical era to modern times.

- Explain the historical reasons for the early promotion of physical activity.

- Explain how America's physical education movement was born.

- Describe the importance of physical education and fitness training following World War I.

- Describe the presidential initiatives that promoted physical education and health

Key Terms

Exercise physiology

Galen

Herodicus

Hippocrates

Hua T'o

Olympic Games

President's Council on Physical Fitness and Sports

Tai chi chu'an

Yoga

Physical Education and Sport Science

• KEY CONCEPT •

During the height of the Athenian era, the body was valued equally with the mind and spirit.

Physical education and the science of athletic performance can trace their roots to long before ancient Greek culture ever began to glorify the human body and athletic prowess (Figure 1-1). Expanding our knowledge of personal well-being and athletic performance has been humanity's quest for centuries. When we study, train, and conceive of new programs and practices to motivate today's students and athletes, we build on the knowledge and traditions of the past.

At one time in Western civilization, during the height of the Athenian era in ancient Greece, sport was considered an essential element of the arts and humanities (Figure 1-2). The enriched, fulfilled person was one who continually strove for an integrated balance of physical, mental, and spiritual excellence. The body was valued equally with the mind and spirit.

Society today focuses on physical performance and the condition of one's body. More so than in any other time in history, athletics and exercise occupy a role in the forefront of the American lifestyle, as well as that of the world at large. Today, physically active members of society come in all ages and fitness levels, and are both male and female. If a person aims to get and remain in shape, strenuous exercise and athletic participation are rarely absent from that individual's weekly regimen.

Modern competitive sports have gone above and beyond the athletic activities of the past in terms of their business value, the physical ability

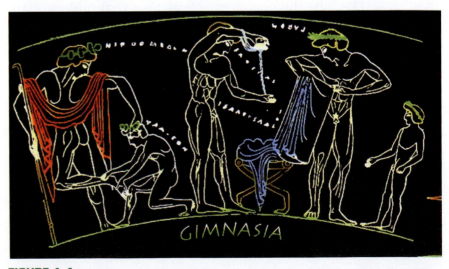

FIGURE 1–1
Ancient physical education (Reprinted with permission of Hogar de los Planetarios Portatiles)

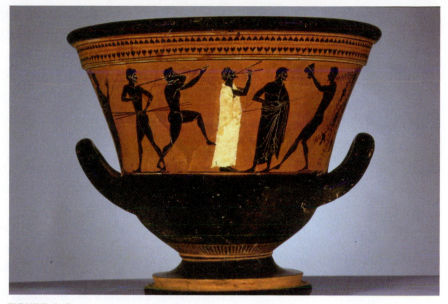

FIGURE 1–2

Excellence and the Competitive Spirit. When the Persian military officer Tigranes, "heard that the prize was not money but a crown [of olive], he could not hold his peace, but cried, 'Good heavens, Mardonius, what kind of men are these that you have pitted us against? It is not for money they contend but for glory of achievement!'"
Herodotus, *Histories*, 8.26.3
Toledo 1963.26, Attic black figure calyx krater
Side B: Athletes and trainers
(The Rycroft Painter, *Calyx Krater, Side B, Athletes and trainers*, about 520-510 BC, Toledo Museum of Art, Purchased with funds from the Libbey Endowment, Gift of Edward Drummond Libbey, 1963.26. Reprinted with permission from the Toledo Museum of Art.)

of the athletes, and the level of importance that is placed on success. In major professional sports, athletes are often multimillion-dollar commodities and any hindrance to their performance is a hindrance to the "industry." Amateur athletes from 14–23 years old are also placing enormous emphasis on their ability to compete and perform.

Yet, despite society's fixation on fitness and the heavy emphasis placed on athletic competition, physical education and sports have been cut back dramatically in the American secondary education curriculum. The prevailing rationale is that core academics are more important to students' development and academic success than physical education and sports programs. As the call for national educational reform is touted in media circles, physical educators have been forced to justify the necessity of conditioning the body along with the mind.

For physical education and sport to assume a more integral and respected position in our nation's secondary schools once again, we need to reassess our priorities with regard to the value of fitness. In so doing, we can ascertain the best possible path to personal enlightenment, educational reform, and social transformation in this era of revision of our scholastic practices and national health initiatives.

Sport in the Ancient World

The exercise boom is not just a fad; it is a return to 'natural' activity—the kind for which our bodies are engineered and which facilitates the proper function of our biochemistry and physiology. Viewed through the perspective of evolutionary time, sedentary existence, possible for great numbers of people only during the last century, represents a transient, unnatural aberration. (Eaton, Shostak, Konner, 1988, p. 168)

This chapter examines the historical development of physical activity as a means of improving health among entire populations, and traces this evolution from prehistoric society to modern America. We will look at societies including ancient Greece and Rome, China, India, Africa, and pre-colonial America.

Archaeologists working in conjunction with medical anthropologists have established that through the beginning of the Industrial Revolution, our ancestors incorporated strenuous physical activity into their daily lives for purposes beyond that of daily subsistence. Physical activity was enjoyed throughout everyday prehistoric life as an integral component of religious, social, and cultural expression. Observations of intact preindustrial societies confirm that physical capability was not just a grim necessity for success at gathering food and providing shelter and safety.

Food supplies for the most part were plentiful, allowing ample time for both rest and recreational physical endeavors. This natural cycle of intermittent activity was likely the norm for most prehistoric societies. Food gathering typically required one- or two-day periods of intense and strenuous exertion; followed by one- or two-day periods of rest and celebration. These days of rest, however, still involved the physical rigor associated with 6- to 20-mile round-trip treks to other villages for the purposes of seeing relatives and friends and trading with other clans or communities.

The Neolithic Agricultural Revolution (approx. 10,000 BCE) allowed more people to live in larger group settings and cities. The resultant specialization of occupations reduced the number and intensity of work-related physical activities. Various healers and philosophers began to stress that long life and health depended on preventing illnesses through proper diet, nutrition, and physical activity. Such broad prescriptions for health, including exercise recommendations, long predated the increasingly specific guidelines of classical Greek philosophy and medicine.

In both India and China during this period, the linking of exercise and health led to the development of a medical subspecialty that today would find its equivalent in sports medicine.

In ancient China, as early as 3,000 BC, the classic *Yellow Emperor's Book of Internal Medicine* first put forth the principles that existing in harmony with the world was the key to preventing illness, and that such prevention was essential to long life. These principles grew into the central concepts of the Chinese philosophy known as Taoism, which promotes the achievement of longevity through simple living. These concepts have guided Chinese culture through the present day. **Tai chi chu'an**, an exercise system that teaches graceful movements, began as early as 200 BC with the teachings of **Hua T'o** and has recently been shown to decrease the incidence of falls in elderly Americans (Figure 1-3).

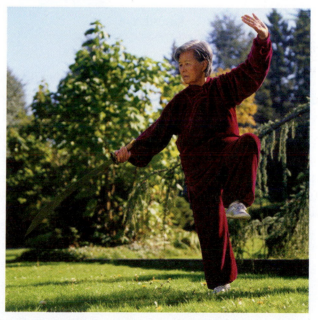

FIGURE 1–3
T'ai Chi training is intended to teach awareness of one's own balance and what affects it, awareness of the same in others, an appreciation of the practical value in one's ability to moderate extremes of behavior and attitude at both mental and physical levels. (Courtesy of Photodisc)

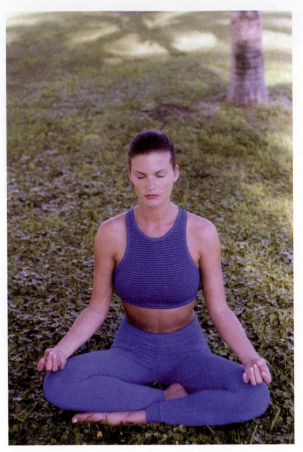

FIGURE 1–4
Yoga (Courtesy of Photodisc)

In India, proper diet and physical activity were known to be essential principles of daily living. The *Ayur Veda*, a collection of health and medical concepts orally transmitted as early as 3,000 BC, developed into **yoga**, a philosophy that included a comprehensive and elaborate series of stretches and postures (Figure 1-4). Yogic principles asserted that physical suppleness, proper breathing, and diet were essential for controlling the mind and emotions and were prerequisites for religious experience.

Although they were less directly concerned with health than with social and religious attainment, other ancient non–Greco-Roman cultures likewise placed value on physical activity. In Africa, systems of flexibility, agility, and endurance training not only represented the essence of martial arts capability but also served as an integral component of religious rituals and daily life. The Samburu and the Masai of Kenya still esteem running as a virtue indicative of great prowess, associated with manhood and social stature.

Similarly, in American Indian cultures, running featured prominently in the important activities of life. Long before the Europeans invaded, Indians ran for purposes of communication, warfare, and hunting. Running was also a means for diverse American Indian cultures to act out their myths and thereby construct a tangible link between themselves and both the physical and metaphysical realms. Even today, the Tarahumarahe of northern Mexico play a version of kickball that involves entire villages for days at a time.

Western Historical Perspectives

> **• KEY CONCEPT •**
>
> The Greeks viewed great athletic achievement as representing both spiritual and physical strength rivaling that of the gods.

The ancient Greek ideals of exercise and health have influenced the attitudes of modern Western culture toward physical activity. The Greeks viewed great athletic achievement as representing both spiritual and physical strength rivaling that of the gods. In the classical-era **Olympic Games**, the Greeks viewed the winners as men who had the character and physical prowess to accomplish feats beyond the capability of most mortals. Although participants in the modern Olympic Games are no longer believed to compete with the gods, today's athletes inspire others to be physically active and to realize their potential, an inspiration as important for modern peoples as it was for the ancient Greeks.

Ancient Promotion of Physical Activity for Health

Throughout much of recorded Western history, philosophers, scientists, physicians, and educators have promoted the idea that being physically active contributes to better health, improved physical functioning, and increased longevity. Although some of these claims were based on personal opinions or clinical judgment, others were the result of systematic observation. Among the ancient Greeks, the recognition that proper amounts of physical activity are necessary for healthy living dates back to at least the fifth century BC. The lessons found in the "laws of health" taught during the ancient period sound familiar to us today: breathe fresh air; eat proper foods; drink the right beverages; take plenty of exercise; get the proper amount of sleep; and account for an individual's emotions when analyzing his or her overall well-being.

Western historians agree that the close connection between exercise and medicine dates back to three Greek physicians: **Herodicus** (480 BC), **Hippocrates** (460–377 BC), and **Galen** (129–199 AD). The first to study therapeutic gymnastics, or gymnastic medicine as it was often called, was the Greek physician and former exercise instructor Herodicus. His dual expertise united the gymnastic with the medical art, thereby preparing the way for subsequent Greek study of the health benefits of physical activity.

Although Hippocrates is generally known as the father of preventive medicine, most historians credit Herodicus as the influence behind Hippocrates' interest in the hygienic uses of exercise and diet. *Regimen*, the longer of Hippocrates' two works dealing with hygiene, was probably written sometime around 400 BC. In Book l, he writes:

> *Eating alone will not keep a man well; he must also take exercise. For food and exercise, while possessing opposite qualities, yet work together to produce health. For it is the nature of exercise to use up material, but of food and drink to make good deficiencies. And it is necessary, as it appears, to discern the power of various exercises, both natural exercises and artificial, to know which of them tends to increase flesh and which to lessen it; and not only this, but also to proportion exercise to bulk of food, to the constitution of the patient, to the age of the individual, to the season of the year, to the changes in the winds, to the situation of the region in which the patient resides, and to the constitution of the year.*

Hippocrates had a major influence on the career of Claudius Galenus, or Galen, the Greek physician who wrote numerous works of great importance to medical history during the second century (Figure 1-5).

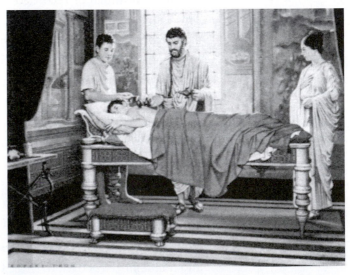

FIGURE 1–5
Claudius Galenus (Galen) was one of the first physicians to use dissections to understand how the body works. (Courtesy of Parke-Davis & Company, copyright 1957.)

Of these works, his book entitled *On Hygiene* contains the most information on the healthfulness of exercise. In one passage he states:

> The uses of exercise, I think, are twofold, one for the evacuation of the excrements, the other for the production of good condition of the firm parts of the body. For since vigorous motion is exercise, it must needs be that only these three things result from it in the exercising body: hardness of the organs from mutual attrition, increase of the intrinsic warmth, and accelerated movement of respiration. These are followed by all the other individual benefits which accrue to the body from exercise; from hardness of the organs, both insensitivity and strength for function; from warmth, both strong attraction for things to be eliminated, readier metabolism, and better nutrition and diffusion of all substances, whereby it results that solids are softened, liquids diluted, and ducts dilated. And from the vigorous movement of respiration the ducts must be purged and the excrements evacuated.

The classical notion that one could improve one's health through one's own actions—for example, by eating properly and getting enough sleep and exercise—proved highly influential in the development of medical theory over the centuries.

The practitioners of classical medicine had made it clear to physicians and the lay public alike that responsibility for disease and health was not the province of the gods. Each person, either independently or in counsel with a physician, had a moral duty to attain and preserve his or her health. When the Middle Ages gave way to the Renaissance with its individualistic perspective and its recovery of classical humanistic influences, this notion of personal responsibility acquired even greater emphasis. Early vestiges of a self-help movement arose in Western Europe in the sixteenth century. As that century progressed, laws of bodily health were expressed as valued prescriptions.

The leading medical schools of the time—at Salerno, Padua, and Bologna—taught hygiene as part of their students' general instruction in the theory and practice of medicine. The works of Hippocrates and Galen dominated a system in which the ultimate goal was the ability to practice medicine in the manner of the ancient physicians. Hippocrates' *Regimen* also figured prominently during the Renaissance in the genre of preventive hygiene literature that sought to address the attainment of an increased lifespan through healthy habits. Central to this body of medical texts was the belief that persons who desired to live a temperate life, especially by reforming habits of diet and exercise, could significantly extend their longevity. Beginning with the writings of Luigi Cornaro in 1558, the classic Greek preventive hygiene tradition attracted increasing attention from those wishing to live longer and healthier lives. Cristobal Mendez, who received his medical training at the University of Salamanca, was the author of the first printed book devoted to exercise, *Book of Bodily Exercise*, published in 1553. His novel and comprehensive ideas preceded and anticipated developments in exercise physiology and sports medicine often thought to be unique to the early twentieth century. The book consists of four treatises that cover such topics as the effects of exercise on the body and on the mind. Mendez believed, as the humoral theorists did, that the physician had to clear away excess moisture in the body. Then, after explaining the ill effects of vomiting, bloodletting, purging, sweating, and urination, he noted that "exercise was invented and used to clean the body when it was too full of harmful things."

Did You Know?

Ancient physicians utilized phlebotomy, or bloodletting—the practice of draining some of the patient's blood—to release "evil humors" thought to be responsible for causing diseases (Figure 1-6). Bloodletting came to the United States on the *Mayflower*. The practice achieved great popularity in the eighteenth and early nineteenth centuries. The first U.S. president, George Washington, died from a throat infection in 1799 after being drained of nine pints of blood within 24 hours. Typically, one to four pints of blood were drained and the blood was caught in a shallow bowl. When the patient became faint, the treatment was stopped. Bleeding by multiple incisions over large areas of a patient's body was often encouraged. By the end of the nineteenth century, phlebotomy was generally viewed as quackery and its practice became outdated.

It cleans without any of the above-mentioned inconvenience and is accompanied by pleasure and joy. If we use exercise under the conditions which we will describe, it deserves lofty praise as a blessed medicine that must be kept in high esteem.

These were the words of Hieronymus Mercurialis, who in 1569 published *The Art of Gymnastics among the Ancients* in Venice. Mercurialis quoted Galen extensively and provided a descriptive compilation of ancient material from nearly two hundred works by Greek and Roman authors. He established the following general exercise principles: that

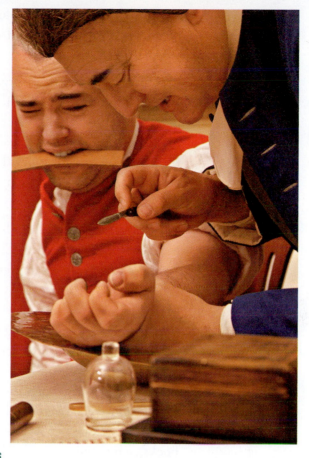

FIGURE 1–6
Bloodletting (in modern medicine referred to as phlebotomy) was a popular medical practice from antiquity up to the late nineteenth century, involving the withdrawal of often considerable quantities of blood from a patient in the hopeful belief that this would cure or prevent a great many illnesses and diseases. (Reprinted with permission from The Colonial Williamsburg Foundation)

people who are ill should not be given exercise that might aggravate existing conditions; that special exercises should be prescribed on an individual basis for convalescent, weak, and older patients; that people who lead sedentary lives urgently need exercise; that each exercise should preserve the individual's existing healthy state; that exercise should not disturb the harmony among the principal bodily systems, known as *humors*; that exercise should be suited to each part of the body; and that all healthy people should exercise regularly.

Although Galen's theory of medicine was displaced by new ideas, particularly through the study of anatomy and physiology, the Greek principles of hygiene and maintaining a healthy regimen continued to flourish in eighteenth-century Europe. For some eighteenth-century physicians, such nonintervention tactics were practical alternatives to traditional medical therapies that employed bloodletting and heavy dosing with compounds of mercury and drugs, resulting in a cure that was often worse than the disease.

One such physician, George Cheyne, published his *Essay of Health and Long Life* in London in 1724. By 1745, it had gone through ten editions and various translations. Cheyne recommended walking as the "most natural" and "most useful" exercise but considered riding on horseback as the "most manly" and "most healthy." He also advocated exercises in the open air, such as tennis and dancing, and recommended cold baths and the use of a "flesh brush" to promote perspiration and improve circulation.

John Wesley's *Primitive Physic*, first published in 1747, was influenced to a large degree by George Cheyne. In his preface, Wesley noted that "the power of exercise, both to preserve and restore health, is greater than can well be conceived; especially in those who add temperance thereto." William Buchan's classic *Domestic Medicine*, written in 1769, prescribed a proper regimen for improving individual and family health. The book contained rules for the healthy and the sick and stressed the importance of exercise for good health of both children and adults. During the nineteenth century, both the classical Greek tradition and the general hygiene movement were finding their way into the United States through American editions of Western European medical treatises or through books on hygiene written by American physicians.

Early vestiges of a self-help movement had arisen in Western Europe in the sixteenth century. Classical Greek preventive hygiene remained a part of formal Western European medical training through the eighteenth century and continued to inform American health reform literature for most of the nineteenth century. Both the classical Greek tradition and the contemporary hygiene movement were spreading their influence in the United States during this period through American editions of Western European medical treatises or through books on hygiene written by American physicians.

In the nineteenth century, an effort was made to popularize the classical Greek laws of health and emphasize each person's responsibility for the maintenance and balance of his or her own health. Writers who addressed the importance of health reform on a personal basis thus wrote about self-improvement, self-regulation, and self-management. If people ate too much, slept too long, or did not get enough exercise, they could only blame themselves for illness. By the same token, through the right practices they could determine and maintain their own good health.

A. F. M. Willich's *Lectures on Diet and Regimen* (1801) emphasized the necessity of exercise within the bounds of moderation. He included information on specific exercises, the proper times for exercise, and the duration of exercise. According to Willich, the essential advantages of exercise included increased bodily strength, improved circulation of the blood and all other bodily fluids, aid in the elimination of secretions and excretions, assistance in clearing and refining the blood, and removal of obstructions.

John Gunn's classic, *Domestic Medicine, Or Poor Man's Friend*, was first published in 1830. The section entitled "Exercise" recommends temperance, exercise, and rest and emphasizes his value of natural over traditional medical treatment. Gunn also urged exercise for women and claimed that all of the "diseases of delicate women" like "hysterics and hypochondria, arise from want of due exercise in the open, mild, and pure air."

In an interesting statement for the 1830s, Gunn recommended a universal training system:

> *The advantages of the training systems are not confined to pedestrians or walkers, or to pugilists or boxers alone; or to horses which are trained for the chase and the race track; they extend to man in all conditions; and were training introduced into the United States, and made use of by physicians in many cases instead of medical drugs, the beneficial consequences in the cure of many diseases would be very great indeed.*

> • **KEY CONCEPT** •
>
> If people ate too much, slept too long, or did not get enough exercise, they could only blame themselves for illness.

Associating Physical Inactivity with Disease

Throughout history, numerous health professionals have observed that sedentary people appear to suffer from more maladies than active people. An early example is found in the writings of English physician Thomas Cogan, author of *The Haven of Health* published in 1584. He recommended his book to students who, because of their sedentary ways, were believed to be most susceptible to sickness.

In his 1713 book *Diseases of Workers*, Bernardino Ramazzini, an Italian physician considered the father of occupational medicine, offered his views on the association between chronic inactivity and poor health. In the chapter entitled "Sedentary Workers and Their Diseases," Ramazzini notes that "those who sit at their work and are therefore called 'chair workers,' such as cobblers and tailors, suffer from their own particular diseases." He concludes that "these workers suffer from general ill-health and an excessive accumulation of unwholesome humors caused by their sedentary life," and he urges them to at least exercise on holidays, "so to some extent counteract the harm done by many days of sedentary life."

Shadrach Ricketson, a New York physician, wrote the first American text on hygiene and preventive medicine. In his 1806 book *Means of Preserving Health and Preventing Diseases*, Ricketson explains, "[A] certain proportion of exercise is not much less essential to a healthy or vigorous constitution, than drink, food, and sleep; for we see that people, whose inclination, situation, or employment does not admit of exercise, soon become pale, feeble, and disordered." He also notes that "exercise promotes the circulation of the blood, assists digestion, and encourages perspiration."

America and the Physical Education Movement

The exercise movement found further expression in nineteenth century America through a new literature devoted to "physical education." In the early part of the century, many physicians began using the term in journal articles, speeches, and book titles to describe the task of teaching children the ancient Greek laws of health. As A. F. M. Willich explained in his *Lectures on Diet and Regimen* (1801), "by *physical education* is meant the bodily treatment of children; the term *physical* being applied in opposition to *moral*." In the section entitled "On the Physical Education of Children," he proceeds to discuss stomach ailments, bathing, fresh air, exercise, dress, and diseases of the skin, among other topics. Physical education, then, implied not merely exercising one's body but also becoming educated about one's body.

These authors were joined by a number of early nineteenth-century educators. For example, an article entitled "Progress of Physical Education" (1826), which appeared in the first issue of *American Journal of Education*, declared:

> [T]he time we hope is near, when there will be no literary institution unprovided with the proper means to healthful exercise and innocent recreation, and when literary men shall cease to be distinguished by a pallid countenance and a wasted body.

Both William Russell, who was the journal's editor, and Boston educator William Fowler voiced their belief that girls as well as boys should have ample outdoor exercise.

Knowledge of one's body was deemed crucial for the development of a well-educated, healthy individual by several physicians who dedicated their careers to the modern physical education movement. Charles Caldwell held a prominent position in Lexington, Kentucky's Transylvania University Medical Department. Although he wrote on a variety of medical topics, his *Thoughts on Physical Education* (1834) gained him national recognition. Caldwell defines physical education as:

> …that scheme of training, which contributes most effectually to the development, health, and perfection of living matter. As applied to man, it is that scheme that raises his whole system to its summit of perfection. Physical education, then, in its philosophy and practice, is of great compass. If complete, it would be tantamount to an entire system of hygiene. It would embrace everything that, by bearing in any way on the human body, might injure or benefit it in its health, vigor, and fitness for action. (p. 28)

● KEY CONCEPT ●

The exercise movement found further expression in nineteenth-century America through a new literature devoted to "physical education."

During the first half of the nineteenth century, systems of gymnastic and calisthenic exercise that had been developed abroad were imported to the United States. The most influential were exercises advanced by Per Henrik Ling in Sweden in the early 1800s and the "German system" of gymnastic and apparatus exercises, based on the work of Johan Christoph Gutsmuths and Friedrich Ludwig Jahn. Americans like Catharine Beecher (1856) and Dioclesian Lewis (1883) devised their own extensive systems of calisthenic exercises intended to benefit both women and men. By the 1870s, American physicians and educators were frequently discussing exercise and health. As evidence of this trend, physical training in relation to health was a regular topic in the *Boston Medical and Surgical Journal* from the 1880s to the early 1900s.

Early Fitness Testing

Physical fitness testing as a component of physical education began with the extensive anthropometric documentation—or measurements of the body—undertaken by Edward Hitchcock in 1861 at Amherst College. By the 1880s, Dudley Sargent at Harvard University was also recording the bodily measurements of college students and promoting strength testing. During the early 1900s, the focus on measuring body parts shifted to tests of vital working capacity. These tests included measures of blood pressure, pulse rate, and fatigue. As early as 1905, C. Ward Crampton, former director of physical training and hygiene in New York City, published the article "A Test of Condition" in the journal *Medical News*. Attempts to assess physical fitness constituted a significant portion of the work of turn-of-the-century physical educators, many of whom were physicians.

Physical Education and Fitness after World War I

Allegations that American servicemen during World War I were inadequately fit to serve their country helped shift the emphasis of physical education from health-related exercise to physical performance-based outcomes. Public concern stimulated legislators to make physical education a required subject in schools. However, the financial constraints of the Great Depression had a negative effect on education in general, and physical education suffered as well during the period from 1929 to the late 1930s. At the same time, the combination of increased leisure time for many Americans and a growing national interest in college and high school sports shifted the emphasis on physical education away from the earlier aim of enhancing performance and health to a new focus on sports-related skills and the worthy use of leisure time.

"Physical efficiency" was a term widely used in the literature of the 1930s. Another term, "physical condition," also found its way into research reports. In 1936, Arthur Steinhaus published one of the earliest articles on "physical fitness" in the *Journal of Health, Physical Education, and Recreation*. In 1938, C. H. McCloy's article "Physical Fitness and Citizenship" appeared in the same journal.

As the United States entered World War II, the federal government showed increasing interest in physical education, especially in the area of physical fitness testing and preparedness. In October 1940, President Franklin D. Roosevelt named John Kelly, a former Olympic rower, to the new position of national director of physical training. The following year, Fiorella La Guardia, the mayor of New York City and the director of civilian defense for the Federal Security Agency, appointed Kelly as his assistant in charge of physical fitness. He appointed tennis star Alice Marble to promote physical fitness among females.

In 1943, Arthur Steinhaus chaired a committee appointed by the board of directors of the American Medical Association to review the nature and role of exercise in physical fitness. A. H. Steinhaus and C. Ward Crampton chaired a committee on physical fitness under the direction of the Federal Security Agency. Crampton and his seventy-three–member advisory council were in charge of developing physical fitness in the civilian population.

In 1941, Morris Fishbein, editor of the *Journal of the American Medical Association*, stated that "from the point of view of physical fitness we are a far better nation now than we were in 1917," but he cautioned Americans not to believe "we have attained an optimum in physical fitness." He realized the magnitude of the fitness problem when he noted that the poor results of physical examinations reported by the Selective Service Board (the draft board) were "a challenge to the medical profession, to the social scientists, the physical educators, the public health officials, and all those concerned in the United States with the physical improvement of our population." The goals most frequently cited for physical education between 1941 and 1945 were resistance to disease, muscular strength and endurance, cardiorespiratory endurance, muscular growth, flexibility, speed, agility, balance, and accuracy.

The Emergence of the Science of Physical Education

After World War II, a continuing public interest in physical fitness convinced key members of the medical profession and the American Medical Association to persist in the study of exercise. Much of this interest can be attributed to the pioneering work of Thomas K. Cureton, Jr., and his Physical Fitness Research Laboratory at the University of Illinois. Cardiologists, health education specialists, and physicians who practiced preventive medicine were becoming aware of the contributions of exercise to the overall health and efficiency of the heart and circulatory system. In 1946, the American Medical Association's Bureau of Health Education designed and organized the Health and Fitness Program to provide assistance to local organizations throughout the nation in the development of satisfactory health education programs. This program provided an important link between physical educators, physicians, and physiologists.

The event that attracted the most public attention to physical fitness, including that of President Dwight D. Eisenhower, was the publication of the article "Muscular Fitness and Health" in the December 1953 issue of the *Journal of Health, Physical Education, and Recreation*. The authors, Hans Kraus and Ruth Hirschland of the Institute of Physical Medicine and Rehabilitation at the New York University Bellevue Medical Center, stated that 56.6 percent of the American schoolchildren tested "failed to meet even a minimum standard required for health." When this rate was compared with the 8.3 percent failure rate for European children, a call for reform went out. Kraus and Hirschland labeled the lack of sufficient exercise "a serious deficiency comparable with vitamin deficiency" and declared "an urgent need" for its remedy.

John Kelly, the former national director of physical fitness during World War II, notified Pennsylvania Senator James Duff of these startling test results. Duff, in turn, brought the research to the attention of President Eisenhower, who invited several athletes and exercise experts to a meeting in 1955 to examine this issue in more depth. The President's Conference on Fitness of American Youth, held in June 1956, was attended by 150 leaders from government, physical education, medical, public health, sports, civic, and recreational organizations. This meeting eventually led to the establishment of the President's Council on Youth Fitness and the President's Citizens Advisory Committee on the Fitness of American Youth.

When John F. Kennedy became president in 1961, one of his first official actions was to convene a conference on the physical fitness of young people. In 1963, the President's Council on Youth Fitness was renamed the President's Council on Physical Fitness. In 1968, the word "sports" was added to the name, making it the **President's Council on Physical Fitness and Sports (PCPFS)**. The PCPFS was charged with promoting physical activity, fitness, and sports for Americans of all ages.

During the 1960s, a number of educational and public health organizations published articles and statements on the importance of fitness for children and youths. The American Association for Health, Physical Education, and Recreation (AAHPER) expanded its physical fitness-testing program to include college-aged men and women. The association developed new norms from data collected from more than 11,000 boys and girls ages 10–17 years. The AAHPER also joined with the President's Council on Physical Fitness to conduct the AAHPER Youth Fitness Test, which offered motivational awards to participants. In 1966, President Lyndon B. Johnson's newly created Presidential Physical Fitness Award was incorporated into the program.

In the mid-1970s, the perceived need to promote health benefits generated from physical fitness rather than concentrate exclusively on athletic performance began to reemerge in professional circles. In 1975, the AAHPER stated it was time to differentiate physical fitness related to health from performance related to athletic ability. Accordingly, the AAHPER commissioned the development of the Health-Related Physical Fitness Test. This movement in the development of youth fitness paralleled the evolution of the "aerobics" movement, which promoted endurance-based exercise for the general public.

Exercise Physiology Research and Health

The study of **exercise physiology** began in France, when Antoine Lavoisier in 1777 (Figure 1-7) and Pierre de Laplace in 1780 developed techniques to measure oxygen uptake and carbon dioxide production at rest and during exercise. During the 1800s, European scientists used and advanced these procedures to study the body's metabolic responses to exercise. The first major application of this research involved human subjects. *The Influence of the Labour of the Tread-wheel over Respiration and Pulsation, and Its Relation to the Waste of the System, and the Dietary (Sic) of The Prisoners,*

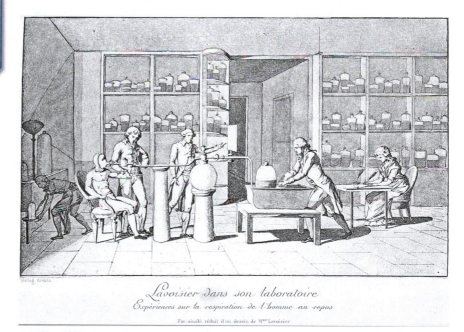

Lavoisier dans son laboratoire
Expériences sur la respiration de l'homme au repos
Fac-simile réduit d'un dessin de Mme Lavoisier

FIGURE 1–7

French chemist Antoine Lavoisier is considered the founder of modern chemistry. He found that the amount of matter before a chemical reaction is equal to the amount of matter afterwards, even though the matter may change form. Lavoisier also experimented with the role of oxygen in combustion and respiration in both plants and animals. (Courtesy of Chemical Heritage Foundation)

Edward Smith's 1857 study of the effects of "assignment to hard labor" on prisoners in London, was designed to determine whether hard manual labor negatively affected the health and welfare of the prisoners and whether it should be considered cruel and unusual punishment.

William Byford published "On the Physiology of Exercise" in the *American Journal of Medical Sciences* in 1855, and Edward Mussey Hartwell, a leading physical educator, wrote a two-part article, "On the Physiology of Exercise," for the *Boston Medical and Surgical Journal* in 1887. The first important book on the subject, George Kolb's *Beitrage zur Physiologie Maximaler Muskelarbeit Besonders des Modernen Sports*, was published in 1887. The following year, Fernand Lagrange's *Physiology of Bodily Exercise* was published in France.

From the early 1900s to the early 1920s, several further works on exercise physiology appeared. George Fitz, who had established a physiology of exercise laboratory during the early 1890s, published his *Principles of Physiology and Hygiene* in 1908. R. Tait McKenzie's *Exercise in Education and Medicine* (1909) was followed by Francis Benedict and Edward Cathcart's *Muscular Work, a Metabolic Study with Special Reference to the Efficiency of the Human Body as a Machine* (1913). The next year, a professor of physiology at the University of London, F. A. Bainbridge, published the second edition of Physiology of Muscular Exercise.

In 1923 Archibald Hill was appointed Joddrell Professor of Physiology at University College, London. In Hill, the physiology of exercise acquired one of its most respected researchers and staunchest supporters. Hill had won the Nobel Prize in Medicine and Physiology in 1922. "The Physiological Basis of Athletic Records," Hill's 1925 address, to the British Association for the Advancement of Science, appeared in both *The Lancet* and *Scientific Monthly* in 1925. In 1926, he published his landmark book *Muscular Activity*. The following year, Hill published *Living Machinery*, which was largely based on his lectures before audiences at the Lowell Institute in Boston and the Baker Laboratory of Chemistry in Ithaca, New York.

Several leading physiologists besides Hill were interested in the human body's response to exercise and environmental stressors, especially activities involving endurance, strength, altitude, heat, and cold. Consequently, they studied soldiers, athletes, aviators, and mountain climbers, whom they considered the best subjects for the purposes of acquiring data.

In the early twentieth century, American research on exercise was centered in the Boston area, first at the Carnegie Nutrition Laboratory and later at the Harvard Fatigue Laboratory, which was established under the leadership of Lawrence Henderson in 1927. That year, Henderson and his colleagues first demonstrated that endurance exercise training improved the efficiency of the cardiovascular system by increasing stroke volume and decreasing resting heart rate. Two years later, E. C. Schneider and G. C. Ring published the results of a twelve-week endurance training program, demonstrating a 24 percent increase in crest load of oxygen (maximal oxygen uptake) in the individual who undertook the program.

Over the next fifteen years, a limited number of exercise training studies were published that evaluated the correspondence between an individual's maximal oxygen uptake or endurance performance capacity and exercise training. However, none of these early studies compared the effects of different types, intensities, durations, or frequencies of exercise on performance capacity or health-related outcomes.

Activities surrounding World War II, such as combat training and observations of pilot fatigue, greatly influenced the exercise physiology research, and several laboratories, including the Harvard Fatigue Laboratory, began directing their efforts toward topics of importance to the military.

The other national concern that created much interest among physiologists was the fear that American children were less fit than their European counterparts. Research was directed toward the concept of fitness in growth and development, ways to measure fitness, and the various components of fitness.

Major advances were also made in the 1940s and 1950s in developing the components of physical fitness and determining the effects of endurance and strength training on measures of performance and physiologic function, especially adaptations of the cardiovascular and metabolic systems. Also investigated were the effects of exercise training on health-related outcomes, such as cholesterol metabolism.

Starting in the late 1950s and continuing through the 1970s, a rapidly increasing number of published studies evaluated or compared different components of endurance-oriented exercise training regimens. Other researchers began to evaluate the effects of different modes and durations of endurance-type training on physiologic and performance measures.

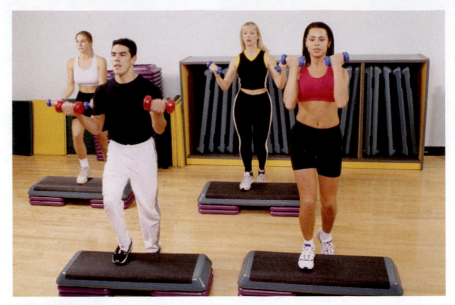

FIGURE 1-8
Modern Exercise (Courtesy of Photodisc)

In 1957, M. J. Karvonen and his colleagues published a landmark paper, "The Effect of Training on Heart Rate," that introduced the concept of using "percent maximal heart rate reserve" to calculate or express exercise training intensity. This was one of the first studies designed to compare the effects of two different exercise intensities on cardiorespiratory responses. Over the next twenty years, numerous investigators documented the effects of different exercise training regimens on a variety of health-related outcomes among healthy men and women, and among persons under medical care. Many of these studies evaluated the effects of endurance or aerobic exercise training on cardiorespiratory capacity (Figure 1-8). The American College of Sports Medicine (1975, 1978) and the American Heart Association (1975) further refined the results of this research.

Over the past two decades, experts from numerous disciplines have determined that exercise training substantially enhances physical performance and have begun to establish the characteristics of the exercise required to produce specific health benefits. Behavioral scientists have begun to evaluate what determines physical activity habits among different segments of the population and are developing strategies to increase physical activity among sedentary individuals.

> **● KEY CONCEPT ●**
>
> Over the past two decades, experts from numerous disciplines have determined that exercise training substantially enhances physical performance.

Chapter Summary

The assertion that frequent participation in physical activity contributes to better health has been a recurring theme in medicine and education throughout much of Western history. Early observations and case studies suggesting that a sedentary life was not healthy have been supported by rigorous scientific investigation over the past century. In recent decades, a number of experimental and clinical specialties have contributed substantially to an emerging field that may accurately be described as exercise science. This field includes disciplines ranging from exercise physiology and biomechanics to physical activity epidemiology, exercise psychology, clinical sports medicine, and preventive medicine.

Numerous expert panels, committees, and conferences have convened over the years to evaluate the evidence relating physical activity and health. These gatherings have laid a solid foundation for the current consensus that, for optimal health, people of all ages should be physically active as many days of the week as possible.

Chapter Review Questions

1. What role did sport and physical fitness play in ancient Greece?

2. Has today's focus on physical fitness changed much from that of ancient times? If so, how?

3. What role do physical education and fitness play in today's schools? Has the emphasis on them changed in the past several years?

4. Explain the historical development of physical activity in ancient China and India.

5. How does the development of physical fitness in ancient China and India compare with origins of fitness in Africa and the American Indian cultures?

6. Explain what is meant by the term classical medicine.

7. When did the belief in preventive hygiene gain acceptance?

8. What was Bernardino Ramazzini's view on activity and physical fitness?

9. Summarize America's early physical fitness and education movement.

10. What is "extensive anthropometric documentation"?

11. How did the United States respond to the allegations that servicemen's fitness levels were inadequate for the demands of service during World War I?

12. What was Thomas K. Cureton, Jr.'s role in the development of sport science?

13. When did the President's Council on Physical Fitness and Sports originate? Who founded it?

14. What is the purpose of exercise physiology?

15. How has exercise training substantially enhanced physical performance over the past two decades?

Projects and Activities

1. Select a country (other than the United States), and research the historical development of physical fitness within that country. Write a short paper in which you show a linear progression up to modern times.

2. There have been many initiatives and programs set up over the past several decades aimed at combating the lack of youth fitness in the United States. Have they been a success or a failure? Carefully explain your answer, and be sure to back it up with evidence. Now share your vision of how you would address this situation.

3. Many books have been written on the subject of the ancient and modern Olympic Games. Research this topic and then discuss what you feel are the major differences between the two. Have the Olympic Games kept, lost, or changed their focus?

4. Read and write a report on Claudius Galenus's book *On Hygiene*.

5. Create a timeline of the important events in the history of physical education and exercise science explained in this chapter.

Physical Education in the Twenty-First Century

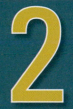

Objectives

Upon completion of this chapter, the reader should be able to:

- Explain how changes in physical education are essential to the future of the nation's health.
- Define the types of goals and standards that are required in building a comprehensive health and physical education program.
- Explain new trends in physical education and health education.
- State the major points of the *Shape of the Nation Report*.
- Explain the national physical education standards.

Key Terms

Exercise science

Healthy People 2010

National standards

Physical education

Shape of the Nation Report

Physical Education in the Twenty-First Century

As described in Chapter 1, **physical education** has been evolving for thousands of years. Physical educators will be challenged in the years ahead to re-create a discipline that is taking a back seat to other, more traditional curricula. During these "back to basics" times, there will be an opportunity to reinvent what physical education is, and the future it holds for today's youth. There will also be a reawakening of priorities associated with fitness and health. America has cut back on physical education courses, and America's school districts are accepting waivers for physical education courses. No wonder that there has been a direct correlation between the epidemic of obesity in today's society and the lack of emphasis on a healthy lifestyle and daily fitness.

Defining a Focus

As the nation moves forward into the twenty-first century, a tremendous opportunity exists to enhance our health and well-being. Much of that opportunity lies in our ability to address the growing health challenges that are facing children and youth. Although progress is being made, poor physical fitness, violence, lack of proper nutrition, communicable diseases, and alcohol, tobacco, and other drug use continue to plague our society and, most notably, our youth.

> **• KEY CONCEPT •**
>
> Comprehensive physical development and health programs offer great potential for enhancing students' minds and bodies.

Comprehensive physical development and health programs offer great potential for enhancing students' minds and bodies. Extensive research connects the ability to learn with good health. Healthy minds and bodies are basic to academic success and, in later life, enhance the ability to contribute to a productive work environment (Figure 2-1).

The benefits of comprehensive health and physical education include promoting a healthy generation of students who are able to achieve their highest potential; reversing the trend toward deteriorating health and physical fitness among youth; and helping to lower the cost of health care in the United States.

The goals and standards for physical development and health foster workplace skills, including identifying short- and long-term goals, utilizing technology, following directions, and working cooperatively with others. Problem solving, communication, responsible decision making, and team-building skills are major items of emphasis.

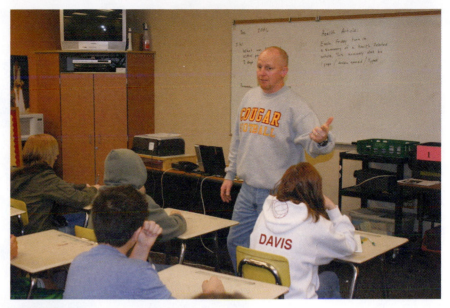

FIGURE 2–1
Health and fitness education plays a vital role in having students understand their bodies and the proper choices that need to taken to remain healthy.

Technology and Physical Education Programs

• KEY CONCEPT •

In Minneapolis, the online physical education curriculum has been developed using national and district standards.

School districts across the country are finding creative ways for students to fulfill their physical education requirements. Even though it may be a little early to say the trend is sweeping the nation, online physical education programs are gaining popularity. Jan Braaten, curriculum coordinator for physical education and health for the Minneapolis Public Schools (MPS), explained why her district began offering online physical education classes in spring 2005. "Things have changed in the twenty-first century in many ways, and one change is the wide variety of options and lifestyles for our students," Braaten said. "We still think it is a great benefit for our students to participate in a traditional physical education course. The online courses are really there to fill a niche for certain populations of our students and to allow them to benefit from what we have to teach."

Students who wish to free up their schedule for advanced placement classes, as well as teen mothers, multisport athletes, and students with medical problems, benefit from the flexibility of the online physical education class, Braaten said.

In Minneapolis, the online physical education curriculum has been developed using national and district standards. Once students obtain a medical waiver from a doctor, they meet face-to-face with their instructor

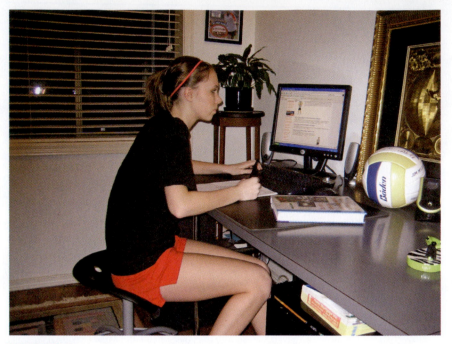

FIGURE 2–2
Ashley files workout reports from her computer at home.

to establish their baseline fitness level. Braaten said after students have completed these initial tasks, they receive a heart rate monitor and begin progressing through a variety of physical education modules. "Each module has a sport/activity journal piece," Braaten explained. "This is the 'meat' of the course, because we want our students to engage in vigorous physical activity three times a week for a minimum of 30 minutes. In the sport/activity journal, students will record their activity, their heart rate, their perceived exertion rate, and other aspects of a good workout (Figure 2-2). The sport/activity journal must be signed off on by a parent, coach, trainer, or other adult."

Over the past year, MPS has accommodated more than three hundred students with its online physical education offerings. Kathy Burns, an MPS spokesperson, noted demand is up, too. "The online learning coordinator indicated that she has more requests than they can accommodate as the class has become very popular and in demand within our district," Burns said. "She also reports other school districts are asking if their students can participate as well." Burns said growing media attention in the past few months has drawn requests for information about online physical education classes from around the United States and as far away as Australia.

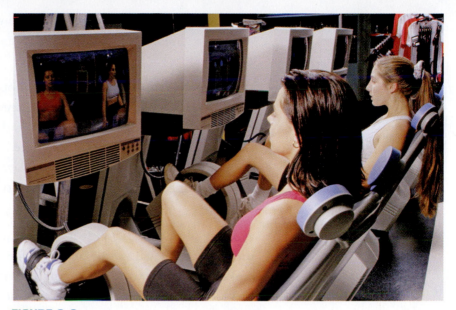

FIGURE 2-3
Exercise science is driving the resurgence of physical education programs today.

Exercise Science

There has been considerable interest in the inclusion of **exercise science** within the physical education curriculum. Exercise science is designed to address student needs and future trends. These classes can offer a balance between classroom information and laboratory experiences. Students have the chance to understand, practice, and compare results utilizing a variety of tests. These tests could include body composition, VO_2 max, lactate levels, anaerobic power, blood pressure and heart rate responses to exercise, as well as other exercise parameters. An interdisciplinary approach that links biology, physical education, and other subjects brings greater understanding and promotes collegiality across various disciplines (Figure 2-3).

Transforming the "Now" into the "Future" in the Public School System

Schools have enormous potential for helping students develop the knowledge and skills they need to be healthy and to achieve academically. As rapidly changing and evolving disciplines, health education and physical education must look and be different than the old "gym class." Health education and physical education are separate disciplines, each with a distinct body of knowledge and skills; however, the two disciplines complement and reinforce each other to support a healthy lifestyle.

Health education and physical education programs promote each student's optimum physical, mental, emotional, and social development. Effective programs are grounded in scientific research and public health knowledge. They are student-centered and utilize multiple learning theories and models to support and promote health-enhancing behaviors. As a result, students are empowered to develop and demonstrate increasingly sophisticated knowledge, skills, attitudes, and practices.

These programs provide cognitive content and learning experiences in a variety of physical activity areas: basic movement skills such as team, dual, and individual sports; physical fitness and exercise science; rhythm and dance; and lifetime recreational activities. These activities are linked to health concepts and skills, such as healthy eating, safety, and stress management. Additionally, effective programs consider children's changing physical capabilities based on their developmental status, previous experiences, skill level, body size, body type, and age and are culturally, ethnically, and gender sensitive.

Health education and physical education programs must also address and integrate the full range of health problems and issues that impact the quality of life. Unfortunately, quality classroom instruction is not enough. School policies and procedures must support and reinforce classroom instruction. Health messages must be clear and consistent. Students must be given every opportunity to engage in healthful behaviors in the classroom, and cafeteria, as well as in the gym on the playground.

Quality programs incorporate technology and encourage students to research and use valid and reliable sources of health information. For example, using heart rate monitors (Figure 2-4) makes aerobic exercise safer and more productive by helping the teacher and student individualize participation in physical activity.

As a form of authentic assessment, heart-rate monitors enhance interdisciplinary technological instruction while allowing for a more objective estimation of a student's effort and individual progress. Students are able to set goals, monitor performance, and experience real gains in fitness status.

The best programs are student-centered and interactive. Teachers should encourage classroom discussion, research, modeling, and skill practice. Skilled health teachers address social influences on behavior and strengthen individual and group norms that support health-enhancing

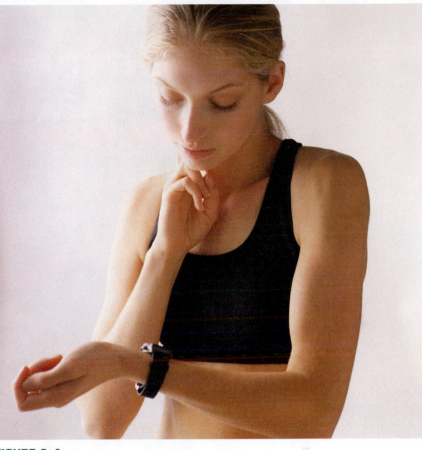

FIGURE 2-4
Fine-tuning an individual's workout will allow for greater gains in fitness. (Courtesy of Photodisc)

behaviors. Students discuss issues that have real application to their lives with assessments that are authentic and contextual. Teachers who are well-versed in current health issues and resources challenge students to take responsibility for their own health. Providing information is not enough. Information must be coupled with skill development and practice in order to have any impact on behavior. As a result, students are progressively prepared and empowered to use higher-level thinking skills to address a myriad of wellness issues, now and throughout their lifetime.

The *Shape of the Nation Report*

Since 1987 the National Association for Sport & Physical Education (NASPE) has been producing the *Shape of the Nation Report* (Figure 2-5) every few years. This report, aimed at both the profession and the public,

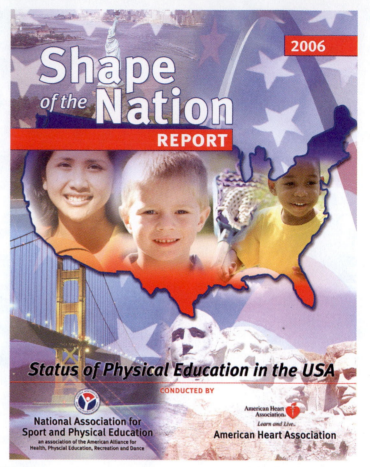

FIGURE 2–5
Shape of the Nation (*Shape of the Nation Report (2006)* reprinted with permission from the National Association for Sport and Physical Education (NASPE).

summarizes information regarding the status of physical education in the American educational system. The challenges reported in the 1987 survey continue to date. There is no federal law that requires physical education to be provided to students in the American education system, nor any incentives for offering physical education programs. States may set some general or minimum requirements, but individual school districts provide specific direction and may exceed the minimum recommendations. Many states delegate responsibility for all content taught in schools to local school districts.

The latest survey, conducted in 2006, as well as the 1997 survey report that most states do not live up to the calls to action in the landmark 1996 Surgeon General's Report. This report, titled *Physical Activity and Health*, as well as the Centers for Disease Control and Prevention *Guidelines for Schools and Community Programs to Promote Lifelong Physical Activity*

Among Young People, both recommend that daily physical education should be required for all students in kindergarten through twelfth grade.

The importance of physical education in promoting the health of young people has been an important component of the health objectives for the nation since 1990. The Office of Disease Prevention and Health Promotion, U.S. Department of Health and Human Services provides a framework for prevention for the nation. This framework, called *Healthy People 2010*, is a statement of national health objectives designed to identify the most significant preventable threats to health and to establish national goals to reduce these threats. *Healthy People 2010* includes three objectives related to school physical education: increase the proportion of the nation's public and private schools that require daily physical education for all students, increase the proportion of adolescents who participate in daily school physical education, and increase the proportion of adolescents who spend at least 50 percent of school physical education class time being physically active.

Another call for daily physical education came in November 2000. In *Report to the President: Promoting Better Health for Young People through Physical Activity and Sports,* Health and Human Services Secretary Donna Shalala and Education Secretary Richard Riley wrote, "Our nation's young people are, in large measure, inactive, unfit, and increasingly overweight. This report should stimulate action to make sure that daily physical activity for young people becomes the norm in our nation."

The 2000 *Shape of the Nation Report* also includes important related information from the latest *School Health Policies and Programs Study 2000* and the *Youth Risk Behavior Surveillance* (1999). The development of this report was made possible by a grant from the American Alliance for Health, Physical Education, Recreation and Dance (AAHPERD). The purpose of the *Shape of the Nation Report* is to determine the

- Mandate for and availability of physical education programs at each level (elementary, middle, and high school) in each state
- Qualifications of those teaching physical education
- Existence of curricular standards for physical education
- Class size
- Accountability criteria for student achievement

Through this report, NASPE brings attention to the importance of quality, daily physical education programs for all school-age children by

---

• KEY CONCEPT •

Healthy People 2010 includes three objectives related to school physical education: increase the proportion of the nation's public and private schools that require daily physical education for all students, increase the proportion of adolescents who participate in daily school physical education, and increase the proportion of adolescents who spend at least 50 percent of school physical education class time being physically active.

• KEY CONCEPT •

"Our nation's young people are, in large measure, inactive, unfit, and increasingly overweight."

providing information about the current status of physical education in each state. The status of physical education is particularly relevant at this time of growing concern about reduced levels of physical activity and increased levels of obesity, diabetes, and related health problems for all age groups.

During the spring of 2001, NASPE sent a questionnaire to the physical education directors and consultants in all fifty state departments of education (SDEs) and the department of education of the District of Columbia. The survey requested information about the mandate for physical education at the elementary, middle, and high school levels; state standards; assessment of student learning; acceptance of substitutions for physical education; time allocations; licensing requirements for teachers of physical education; and current issues and concerns. Follow-up phone calls achieved a complete response by all fifty states and the District of Columbia. Dr. Marian Kneer, a NASPE past president, reviewed and compiled the information provided. The summary information compiled for each state was returned to the respective state department of education representatives for confirmation of content.

Results of the 2001 NASPE Questionnaire

Fifteen years after the U.S. Congress passed Resolution 97 encouraging state and local governments and local educational agencies to provide high-quality daily physical education programs for all children in kindergarten through grade twelve, and ten years after *Goals 2000* called for inclusion of physical education as an integral component of all school programs, little progress has been made. Most states are not living up to the recommendations of multiple reports and recommendations from the federal government and other national organizations. That is the major finding of the *Shape of the Nation Report (2006)* issued by the National Association for Sport & Physical Education.

Unfortunately this does not represent dramatic change from the previous survey. It indicates that most states, in the face of the growing crisis in childhood obesity, Type II diabetes, and increasing sedentary lifestyles, have taken no action to provide adequate health and physical education. Since the last report there has been a greater emphasis on standards-based reform. The establishment of standards for what "students shall know and be able to do" has occurred across most states and in most cases has or will include physical education. However, there has been significant pressure on school leaders to demonstrate increased achievement of recently developed standards in academic areas, particularly reading and

> **• KEY CONCEPT •**
>
> Most states are not living up to the recommendations of multiple reports and recommendations from the federal government and other national organizations.

math. As states develop or select standardized tests to hold schools and students accountable, content that is not tested becomes lower in priority. Several states have called for standards for learning in physical education but do not hold students or schools accountable for achievement of the standards. However, in several states, state tests are being developed for health and physical education.

Another general area of impact on physical education is local control of education. States that establish standards or very broad guidelines for curriculum content defer specific decisions regarding time, allocations, class size and accountability for physical education to local school districts or even individual schools.

Highlights of the *Shape of the Nation Report*, Produced by the National Association for Sport & Physical Education

Mandate for and Availability of Physical Education

In many states, the legislated mandate requires only that physical education be provided, while local districts provide the content and format guidelines. At the elementary school level, state-mandated requirements for physical education time range from 30–150 minutes per week. (NASPE recommends 150 minutes per week.)

At the middle school level, physical education time requirements range from 80–275 minutes per week. (NASPE recommends 225 minutes per week.)

The majority of high school students take physical education for only one year between 9th and 12th grades. The time requirements range from no time specified to 225 minutes a week. (NASPE recommends 225 minutes per week.)

Qualifications of Those Teaching Physical Education

Certified physical education specialists are the only professionals that should be teaching physical education in the school system. Most states do not require physical education classes to be taught by certified specialists. In some states the individual school districts either set or may add to the state requirement for maintaining teacher certification. The majority of states require five or six credit hours every five or six years to maintain teacher certification in physical education or any other area of teacher licensure.

Existence of Curricular Standards

Most states are in the process of developing physical education standards. In the states that have standards for physical education, over 80 percent of standards are based on NASPE's *national standards for physical education.*

Class Size

Across all education levels nearly 80 percent of the states allow a teacher student ratio of 1:30 in physical education classes. Class size for physical education should be the same as for any other subject. Large classes put students at greater risk of injury and reduce learning and teacher feedback. Nearly 25 percent of the states report that they have no regulations for class size.

Accountability for Student Achievement

Physical education is being measured by state-approved assessments in several states. More states are developing assessments to coincide with national standards. It is important that all states require stringent assessment of approved state standards. Mandated standards and assessments will help force implementation of modern physical education methodology and increase accountability to the public. If physical education is to survive into the next century, it will be paramount that the old "PE" be replaced with a true physical education curriculum, taught by professionals devoted to reinventing the discipline.

> ● **KEY CONCEPT** ●
>
> If physical education is to survive into the next century, it will be paramount that the old "PE" be replaced with a true physical education curriculum, taught by professionals devoted to reinventing the discipline.

Recommendations for Action

The National Association for Sport & Physical Education strongly recommends that elementary school students have a minimum of 60 minutes of moderate and vigorous activity every day, while middle and high school students should have a minimum of 30 minutes each day. To achieve that level of activity, NASPE recommends that schools across the country make physical education instruction the cornerstone of a systematic physical activity promotion in school that also includes recess, after-school clubs, intramural sports, and competitive athletics. The co-curricular opportunities must be designed to attract all students, especially those not interested in traditional athletic programs.

Physical education is a planned instructional program with specific objectives. As an essential part of the total curriculum, physical education programs increase all students' physical competence, health-related fitness, responsibility, and enjoyment of physical activity so that they can establish physical activity as a natural part of everyday life.

For elementary school students, recess provides an opportunity for needed physical activity. Unstructured time also contributes to creativity, cooperation, and learning about social interaction. Children learn how to cooperate, compete constructively, assume leader/follower roles, and resolve conflicts by interacting in play. Play is an essential element of children's social development.

In addition to providing quality physical education programs and recess, NASPE recommends that schools, after-school programs, and recreation programs provide varied programs to meet the physical activity interests of all children. Coaches and staff need to receive the specialized training needed to provide developmentally appropriate, safe, and enjoyable activities.

Communities need to develop and promote the use of safe, well-maintained and close-to-home sidewalks, bike paths, trails, and recreation facilities.

Parents need to become more effective advocates for quality physical education programs and physical activities. Most important of all, parents need to set a good example by being active themselves.

In summary, the National Association for Sport and Physical Education (NASPE) recommends the following:

- All students, including those with special needs, should receive quality physical education as an integral part of K–12 education.

- Elementary school children should receive a minimum of 150 minutes per week of instruction in physical education; middle and high school students should receive a minimum of 225 minutes per week of instruction in physical education.

- All states should develop standards for physical education that reflect the *National Standards*.

- All should states set minimum standards for achievement in physical education.

- Meeting standards in physical education should be a requirement for graduation.

- Other courses and activities that include physical activity should not be substituted for instructional physical education.

- Physical activity in addition to physical education needs to be incorporated into the school day through recess at the elementary level, physical activity breaks, physical activity clubs, special family fitness events, and other activities.

- Teachers who are specially prepared and licensed in physical education should deliver physical education instruction at all levels.

National Physical Education Standards

A framework of **national standards** has been developed by the National Association for Sport and Physical Education. The national content standards define what a student should know and be able to do as a result of a quality physical education program. They provide a framework for developing realistic and achievable expectations for student performance at every grade level. These expectations are the first step in designing an instructionally aligned program. National standards provide guidance for developing state and local standards. Others have revised their existing standards and curricula to align with the national standards.

The presence of national standards demonstrates that physical education has academic standing equal to that of other subject areas. Standards describe achievement, show that knowledge and skills matter, and confirm that mere willing participation is not the same as education. In short, national physical education standards bring accountability and rigor to the profession.

Standards alone, however, will not ensure a quality program. Although many programs are using the standards to create innovative, coherent, learning-focused programs, the field of physical education, like any other field, is driven as much by tradition as by innovation. Age-old, ineffective practices include militaristic calisthenics, "one size fits all" games, sports for large groups regardless of individual ability, team-sport–dominated programs that focus more on keeping students busy than on increasing student learning, and grading on "dressing out" and participation rather than achievement of important learning outcomes. Such practices lead many students to dislike physical education and physical activity.

Students are often minimally active during physical education class time. A variety of practices create this problem. Many physical education programs limit physical activity, for example through having students wait for or using too much time for roll call. Far too many middle and high school physical education classes focus heavily on team sports, which, if taught in a large-group format, do not necessarily allow all students to achieve moderate levels of physical activity during class time. In addition, programs using a multi-activity format in which students go through activity units of one, two, or three weeks do not provide adequate time for many students to gain a confidence-building level of competence in any activity. Physical education instructors that continue to provide a smorgasbord curriculum, while expecting meaningful learning outcomes, are often unsuccessful.

Teachers must carefully select and sequence content, align instructional methods with learning goals, and create meaningful assessments of physical activity. In programs in which learning skills, fitness concepts, and lifetime physical activities (such as individual and dual sports and adventure selections) are priorities, students are much more likely to be active.

Activities That Promote Learning

Elementary physical education programs should focus on helping students develop as skillful movers. The curriculum should integrate health and fitness concepts and activities into educational games, educational gymnastics, and educational dance. To be successful in lifetime physical activity, children need to develop knowledge and skills in several forms of activity.

Teachers that are well prepared know how to create developmentally appropriate programs that emphasize individual skill and fitness concept learning while maximizing the activity of all students in learning activities. They do not use whole-class games, such as kickball, dodge ball, or team sports, just to keep kids busy; instead, they link activities to desired learning outcomes. They design assessments so that students can demonstrate what they know and what they can do with what they know in authentic, developmentally appropriate ways (Figure 2-6).

In middle and high school, students should continue to hone skills and integrate health and fitness concepts. The curriculum should begin a clear transition in content selection toward lifetime activities. Examples include individual or dual activities such as golf or tennis, recreational and outdoor adventure activities, and fitness activities such as walking or in-line skating. Again, content selection and progression should be developmentally appropriate, emphasizing small teams, cooperative activities, and learning centers or stations, and teachers should maximize activity time for all students. If students do not have adequate skills, high-level competitive activities are inappropriate. To experience most of the health benefits of physical activity, individuals do not have to participate at high levels of energy expenditure. Rather, teachers should provide students with activity choices.

Once teachers devise a carefully crafted curriculum, they need to choose instructional methods that effectively implement the curriculum.

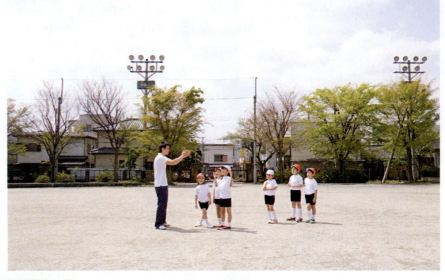

FIGURE 2–6
Teachers create developmentally appropriate programs that maximize the activity of all students in learning activities. (Courtesy of Getty Images)

They can use the following ways to create congruent, engaging instructional practice.

- Each lesson should have a clear instructional purpose. Often, physical education programs focus more on an activity as an end in itself.

- Teachers need to teach toward learning, not just organize for participation. Students need to learn important knowledge, life skills, and movement skills and abilities through proper progressions. Though participation is important, it is a means to accomplish learning outcomes.

- Content selection, management protocols, and instruction should aim toward increasing activity and learning engagement time. Breaking the group into small teams, providing equipment for all students, offering choices of activities with different levels of difficulty and intensity, and minimizing waiting are some ways to increase physical activity engagement time.

- Teachers should remediate if needed. When students do not learn or continue to struggle with accomplishing tasks, they need to provide special assistance. Just having students participate in an activity does not ensure learning. Again, if a teacher's goal is for all students to learn and to enjoy physical activity, he or she needs to attend to their progress and their success.

Chapter Summary

Physical education, fitness, and health education are evolving slowly as mandates from the federal, state, and local governments begin to shape the future of physical education as we know it today. Local school boards are exerting numerous pressures on schools to scale back or eliminate physical education in place of more traditional curricular courses.

If physical education is to survive it must revive. Revival in physical education will require that it be broken down into its constituent parts and be re-created in a proactive, science-based approach. National standards need to be enacted throughout the United States. Programs need to focus on creating innovative, coherent, learning-focused programs designed to promote lifetime fitness and good health.

Unless physical educators get the public behind their efforts to create a more comprehensive curriculum and fitness program, childhood obesity and declining health will become a long-term crisis of national proportions.

Chapter Review Questions

1. How does an online physical education program fulfill students' physical education requirements? How does the curriculum differ from traditional programs?

2. Define "exercise science."

3. In your opinion, what is the future of physical education programs in public schools?

4. Compare and contrast the *Shape of the Nation Report* with the *Healthy People 2010* framework.

5. What does the acronym AAHPERD stand for? What is the purpose of this organization?

6. What are the recommended class size requirements proposed in the *Shape of the Nation Report*? Focus on the final recommendations of this study.

7. Describe the national standards that have been developed by the National Association for Sport & Physical Education. Why are national standards necessary?

8. What are the differences between elementary and secondary physical education programs?

9. What is meant by "developmentally appropriate physical education programs"?

10. How do physical education instructors measure success vis-à-vis their students?

Projects and Activities

1. Select a high school of your choice and research which physical education standards they have enacted. Contact a physical education instructor at this school and ask them if these standards are followed, and if the school supports these standards with adequate staffing and student contact time.

2. Read the entire text of the *Healthy People 2010* report. Write a summary of what you have learned and the impact this report can have on the health and fitness of today's youth.

3. Volunteer for a week at a local elementary school during their physical education classes. Keep a detailed journal of what you observe.

4. On the Internet, go to the website of your state's superintendent of public instruction. What are your state's standards for physical fitness and health education for elementary, middle, and high school? How does they compare with your answer to Question 1 above?

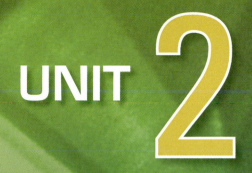

UNIT 2

Exercise and Movement

Kinesiology

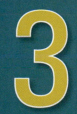

CHAPTER 3

Objectives

Upon completion of this chapter, the reader should be able to:

- Explain the study of kinesiology.
- Define the articular system and describe its importance to movement.
- Define the three classifications of joints.
- State the six types of diarthrosis joints.
- Define the 18 different movements of synovial joints.
- Explain the three anatomical planes and their importance to medicine.
- Explain the concept of open and closed kinematic chains.

Key Terms

Abduction	Condyle	Gliding joint	Pronation
Adduction	Condyloid	Gomphosis	Protraction
Amphiarthroses	(ellipsoidal) joint	Hinge joint	Retraction
Arthrology	Convex	Hyperextension	Rotation
Articular cartilage	Coronal plane	Inversion	Saddle joint
Articular system	Depression	Joint articulation	Sagittal plane
Axial plane	Diarthroses	Joint cavity	Supination
Ball-and-socket	Dorsiflexion	Kinesiology	Sutures
joint	Elevation	Open kinematic	Synarthroses
Circumduction	Eversion	chain	Syndesmoses
Closed kinematic	Extension	Opposition	Synovial fluid
chain	Fibrocartilage	Pivot joint	Synovial joint
Concave	Flexion	Plantar flexion	Synovial membrane

Kinesiology

Kinesiology is the multidisciplinary study of physical activity or movement; it encompasses anatomy, biomechanics, physiology, and psychomotor behavior, as well as various social and cultural factors. The study of kinesiology focuses on exercise stress, movement efficiency, and fitness.

The term is fashioned from two Greek verbs, *kinein* and *logus*, which mean "to move" and "to discourse." Modern phrasing has changed the meaning of the suffix *logus* to "the study of," so that *kinesiology* is literally "the study of movement." Kinesiology encompasses both the theory and practice of movement. The study of movement in physical activity has a long history in American higher education, in many institutions dating to the late nineteenth century. The field of study was primarily oriented to the practice of movement, such as physical training and the playing of sports. The beginning of the study of movement from a disciplinary perspective was a fragmented effort driven by the insight of a few individuals operating as individual scholars, practitioners of medicine, or aspiring academics in universities. Today, these various approaches to the study of movement all come under the single umbrella of kinesiology. This chapter addresses how the body moves, by way of its joints and related structures.

Articular System

The **articular system** is a series of joints that allow movement of the human body. This series of joints, combined with the neuromuscular system, enables locomotion.

When two bones come into contact, they form a **joint articulation**. Joint articulations can be freely moveable, as in the knee or hip; slightly moveable, as in the pubic symphysis, which moves slightly during childbirth; or immobile, as in the fused sutures of the skull. Many joints in the body are named by combining the names of the two bones that form the joint. An example is the sternoclavicular joint, which is the articulation between the sternum and the clavicle. The study of joints is called **arthrology**.

Classification of Joints

Joints have two main functions: they allow motion and at the same time provide stability. They are classified in three different ways:

- synarthroses, or immovable joints
- amphiarthroses, or slightly movable joints
- diarthroses, or freely movable joints

Synarthroses

Synarthroses are joints that lack a synovial cavity and are held closely together by fibrous connective tissue. Synarthroses are immovable joints. In these joints, the bones come in very close contact and are separated only by a thin layer of fibrous connective tissue. The sutures in the skull are examples of immovable (synarthric) joints. There are three structural types of synarthroses: sutures, syndesmoses, and gomphoses.

Sutures

In **sutures**, a thin layer of dense fibrous connective tissue unites the bones of the skull (Figure 3-1). They are immovable and fuse completely by adulthood. Sutures are found only in the skull.

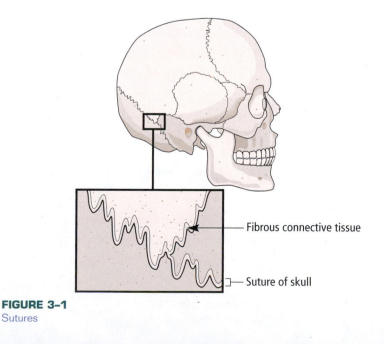

Fibrous connective tissue

Suture of skull

FIGURE 3–1
Sutures

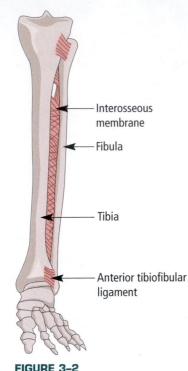

FIGURE 3–2
Syndesmosis

Syndesmoses

A **syndesmosis** is a joint in which the bones are connected by ligaments between the bones. Examples of syndesmoses are the fibula and tibia in the lower leg (Figure 3-2) and the ulna and radius of the arm. These bones move as one when we pronate (turn or rotate the hand or forearm so that the palm faces down or back) and supinate (turn or rotate the hand or forearm so that the palm faces up or forward) the forearm or rotate the lower leg. These joints do offer slight movement and thus are sometimes considered to be amphiarthroses.

Gomphosis

A **gomphosis** is a joint in which a conical process fits into a socket and is held in place by ligaments. An example is a tooth in its alveolus (socket), held in place by the periodontal ligament (Figure 3-3).

Amphiarthroses

Slightly movable joints are called **amphiarthroses**. In this type of joint, the bones are connected by hyaline cartilage or **fibrocartilage**. The connections of the ribs to the sternum are slightly movable joints connected by costal hyaline cartilage. The symphysis pubis is a slightly movable joint in which there is a fibrocartilage pad between the two bones. The joints between the vertebrae are also amphiarthroses (Figure 3-4).

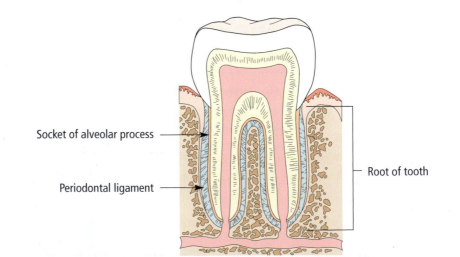

FIGURE 3–3
Gomphosis

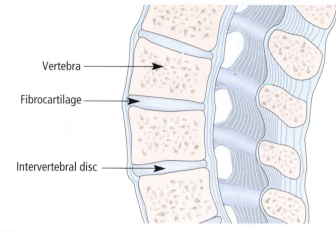

Vertebra

Fibrocartilage

Intervertebral disc

FIGURE 3–4
Amphiarthrosis

Diarthroses or Synovial Joints

Most joints in the adult body are **diarthroses**, or freely movable joints. In this type of joint, the ends of the opposing bones are covered with a type of hyaline cartilage called the **articular cartilage**, and they are separated by a space called the **joint cavity**. The components of the joints are enclosed in a dense fibrous joint capsule. The outer layer of the capsule consists of the ligaments that hold the bones together. The inner layer is the **synovial membrane** that secretes **synovial fluid** into the joint cavity for lubrication. Because all these joints have a synovial membrane, they are sometimes called **synovial joints**.

There are six different types of synovial joints. Each type of joint allows a different degree of mobility.

Pivot Joint

The **pivot joint** is a freely movable joint in which a bone moves around a central axis, creating rotational movement (Figure 3-5). An example is the joint between the radius and ulna of the lower arm.

Gliding Joint

A **gliding joint** allows bones to make a sliding motion. These movements can be back and forth or side to side. They are found in the carpals of the wrist and the tarsals of the ankle. Gliding joints are also found between the vertebrae in the spine (Figure 3-6).

Hinge Joint

The **hinge joint** allows only extension and flexion. The reason for this is that the **convex** surface of one bone fits into the **concave** surface of the

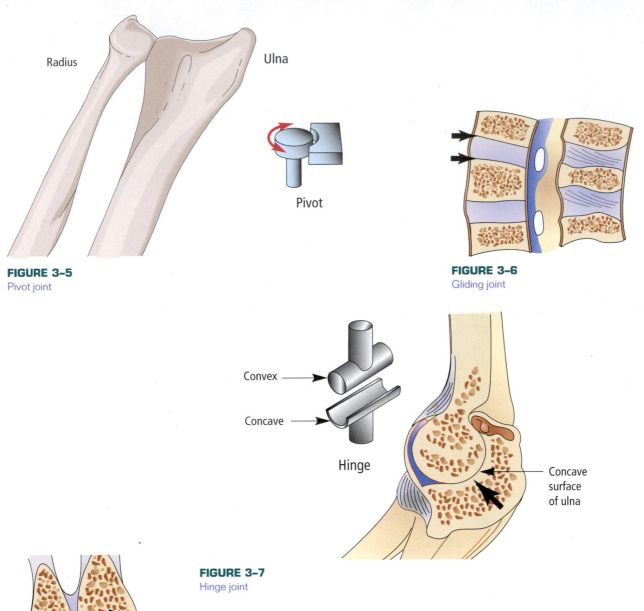

Radius

Ulna

Pivot

FIGURE 3–5
Pivot joint

FIGURE 3–6
Gliding joint

Convex

Concave

Hinge

Concave
surface
of ulna

FIGURE 3–7
Hinge joint

second bone. The knee, elbow (Figure 3-7), and phalanges of the fingers and toes are all hinge joints.

Condyloid or Ellipsoidal Joint

Condyloid or **ellipsoidal joints** are formed where bones can move about one another in many directions, but cannot rotate. This joint is named for a condyle-containing bone. A **condyle** is a curved process that fits into a fossa on another bone for its articulation. This type of joint can be found at the metacarpals (bones in the palm of the hand) and phalanges (fingers), and between the metatarsals (foot bones, excluding the heel) and phalanges (toes) (Figure 3-8).

FIGURE 3–8
Condyloid joint

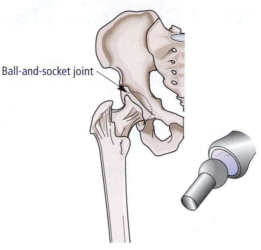

FIGURE 3–9
Ball-and-socket joint

Ball-and-Socket Joint

In a **ball-and-socket joint**, one bone has a rounded end that fits into a concave cavity on another bone. This provides the widest range of movement possible in joints; for example, the hips (Figure 3-9) and shoulders can swing in almost any direction.

Saddle Joint

The **saddle joint** occurs when two bones have both concave and convex regions, with the shapes of the two bones complementing one another. This joint also allows a wide range of movement. The only saddle joint in the body is in the thumb (Figure 3-10). This joint allows humans to turn and oppose their thumbs in cooperation with the fingers.

> **• KEY CONCEPT •**
>
> The six types of diarthroses are pivot joints, gliding joints, hinge joints, condyloid or ellipsoidal joints, ball-and-socket joints, and saddle joints. Each type of joint allows a particular type of motion.

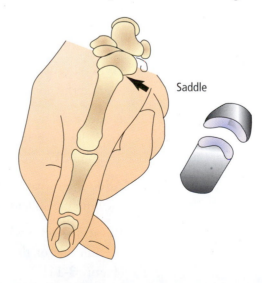

FIGURE 3–10
Saddle joint

Movements of Diarthroses (Synovial Joints)

The range of motion in movable joints varies. Some joints are only slightly movable; others are capable of a wide range of motion. The ranges of motion of the movable joints determine the positions the human body can assume, and play an important role in athletic activity.

The joints in the body that move most freely are the synovial joints. The greater the range of motion in a synovial joint, the more the joint relies on the attached muscles for stability.

The joints with the greatest amount of movement are the shoulders, with the hips a not-too-distant second. Some gymnasts have a range of motion in their hips nearly as great as in their shoulders.

The stability of a joint is determined by three factors: the shape of the bones where they come together, the ligaments that join the bones, and muscle tone. In some joints, the shapes of the bones are well matched, resulting in a very stable joint (such as the hips); in others the opposite is true. The more ligaments a joint has, the stronger it is, but joints that rely on ligaments for bracing are not very stable. For most joints, however, muscle tone is the main stabilizing factor. The shoulder and knee joints, for example, are primarily stabilized in this way. Muscle tone keeps the tendons that attach the muscles to the bones taut, reinforcing the related joints.

Synovial joints allow eighteen different types of movements:

- **Flexion** decreases the angle between two bones (Figure 3-11A).

- **Extension** increases the angle between two bones (Figure 3-11A).

- **Hyperextension** increases the angle between two bones (extends) beyond the normal range of motion (Figure 3-11B).

- **Abduction** describes movements of the limbs only; in abduction, the limb moves *away from* the midline of the body (Figure 3-11C).

- **Adduction** also describes movement of the limbs only; in adduction, the limb moves *toward* the midline of the body (Figure 3-11C).

- **Rotation** occurs when a bone turns on its axis toward or away from the midline of the body, in limbs, or between the atlas and axis (Figure 3-11D).

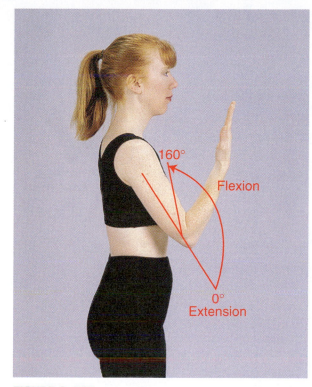

FIGURE 3–11A
Flexion and extension

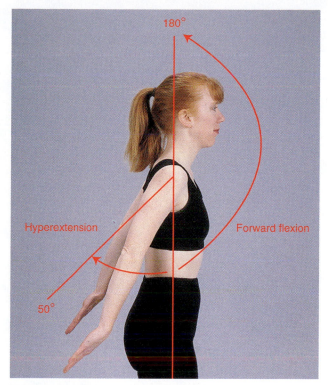

FIGURE 3–11B
Hyperextension

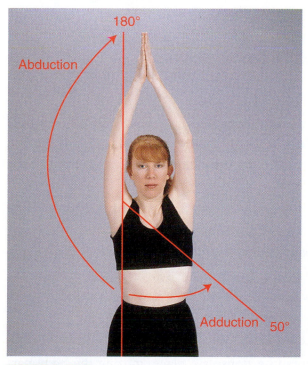

FIGURE 3–11C
Abduction and adduction

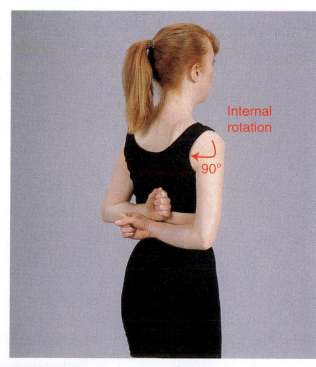

FIGURE 3–11D
Internal rotation

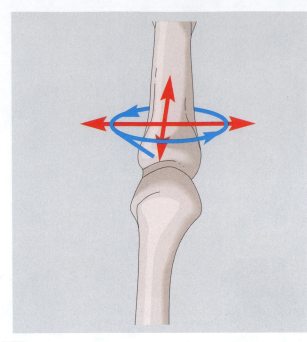

FIGURE 3–11E
Circumduction

- **Circumduction** is the ability of a limb to move in a circular path around an axis. The proximal portion of the limb remains stationary, while the distal portion moves in a circle (Figure 3-11E).

- **Supination** refers to the act of turning the palm upward, performed by lateral rotation of the forearm. When applied to the foot, it generally implies movements resulting in raising of the medial margin of the foot (Figure 3-11F).

- **Pronation** refers to the act of turning the palm downward, performed by medial rotation of the forearm. When applied to the foot, it generally implies movements resulting in lowering of the medial margin of the foot (Figure 3-11F).

- **Plantar flexion** extends the foot, with the toes pointing down (Figure 3-11G).

- **Dorsiflexion** flexes the foot, bringing the toes up toward the lower leg (Figure 3-11G).

- **Inversion** turns the sole of the foot inward (medially) (Figure 3-11H).

- **Eversion** turns the sole of the foot outward (laterally) (Figure 3-11H).

- **Protraction** occurs in a transverse plane, moving the body part forward (shoulders, mandible) (Figure 3-11I).

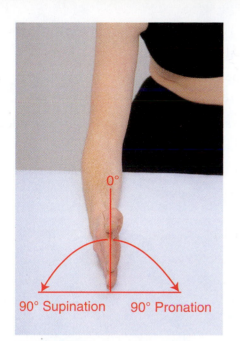

FIGURE 3–11F
Supination and pronation

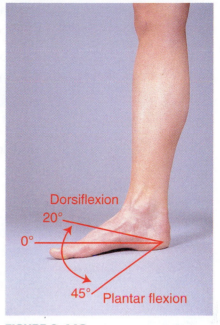

FIGURE 3–11G
Plantar flexion and dorsiflexion

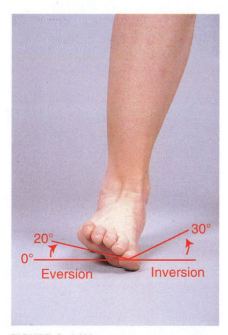

FIGURE 3–11H
Eversion and inversion

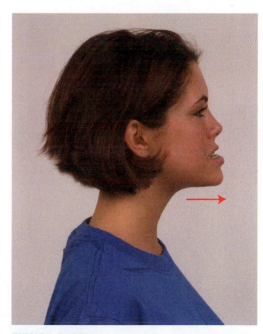

FIGURE 3–11I
Protraction

- **Retraction** also occurs in a transverse plane, moving the body part backward (Figure 3-11J).

- **Elevation** occurs in the frontal plane, lifting the body part superiorly (upward) as with the shoulders (Figure 3-11K).

- **Depression** also occurs in the frontal plane, moving the body part inferiorly (downward) (Figure 3-11L).

- **Opposition** moves the thumb to touch the tips of the other fingers (Figure 3-11M).

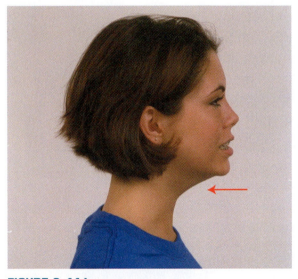

FIGURE 3–11J
Retraction

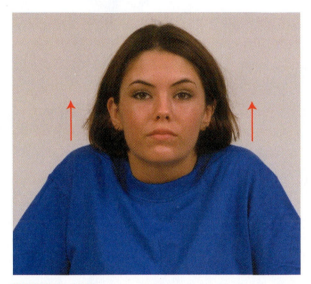

FIGURE 3–11K
Elevation

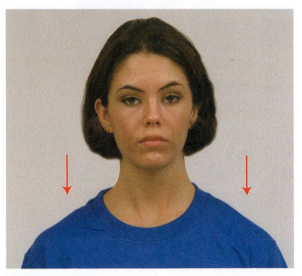

FIGURE 3–11L
Depression

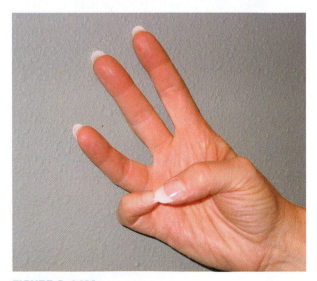

FIGURE 3–11M
Opposition

Anatomical Planes

In medicine, professionals refer to sections of the body in terms of anatomical planes (flat surfaces). These planes are imaginary lines, vertical or horizontal, which are drawn through an upright body (Figure 3-12). In the anatomical position, the human body stands erect, eyes looking forward, arms at the sides, and the palms of the hands and the toes facing forward. The following terms are used to describe the specific planes of the body.

It is important to understand how these terms and principles relate to movement about or within a specific surface or plane. Table 3-1 lists additional terms used to describe anatomical direction.

Coronal Plane (Frontal Plane)

The **coronal plane** is a vertical plane running from side to side. This divides the body or any of its parts into anterior (front) and posterior (back) portions.

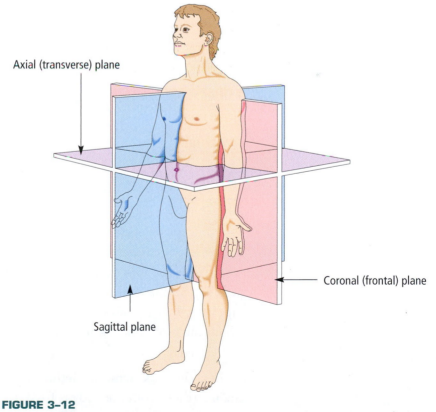

Axial (transverse) plane

Coronal (frontal) plane

Sagittal plane

FIGURE 3–12
Anatomical planes

TABLE 3-1 Anatomical Terms Relating to Direction	
Anatomical Term	**Direction**
Medial	Toward the midline of the body
Lateral	Away from the midline of the body
Proximal	Nearest to a reference point
Distal	Farthest away from a reference point
Inferior	Below
Superior	Above
Cephalad or Cranial	Toward the head
Caudal or Caudad	Toward the tailbone
Anterior	Toward the front
Posterior	Toward the back

Sagittal Plane (Lateral Plane)

The **sagittal plane** is a vertical plane running from front to back. This divides the body or any of its parts into right and left sides.

Axial Plane (Transverse Plane)

The **axial plane** is a horizontal plane dividing the body or any of its parts into upper and lower parts.

Open and Closed Kinematic Chains

The concept of open and closed chain exercise was first discussed by Dr. Arthur Steindler, in his book titled *Kinesiology of the Human Body: Under Normal and Pathological Conditions* (1955). In that book he defined *chains* as links of body parts, such as the foot, ankle, knee, and hip. Each link has an effect on each other. An example is walking, in which the foot, ankle, knee, and hip all play an important part in forward movement.

In a **closed kinematic chain** movement or exercise, the end of the chain farthest from the body is fixed; for example, in a squat the feet are fixed and the rest of the leg chain moves. Walking or performing a pull-up or push-up involve closed-chain motion.

In **open kinematic chain** movement or exercise, the end of the chain is free, such as in a seated leg extension. Waving a hand or kicking a ball are additional examples of open chain-movements.

Closed- and open-chain exercises provide different benefits. Closed-chain exercises tend to emphasize compression of joints. An example is the knee during the upright stance phase of squats (Figure 3-13). Because the distal end does not move, the knee joint is more stable.

Open-chain exercises tend to involve more shearing force parallel to the joint, and therefore, create a less stable condition for exercise. For example, during a leg extension the knee is never under compression forces (Figure 3-14).

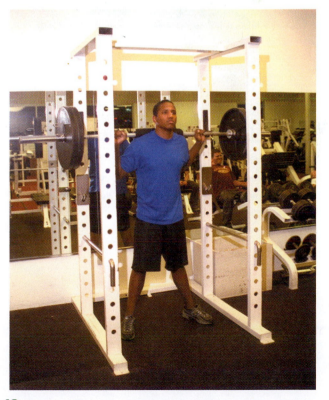

FIGURE 3–13

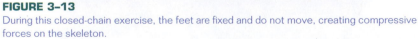
During this closed-chain exercise, the feet are fixed and do not move, creating compressive forces on the skeleton.

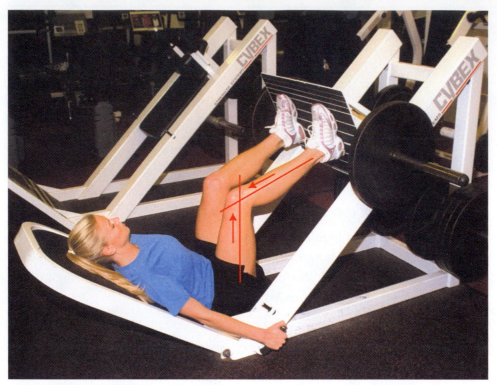

FIGURE 3–14
In this open-chain exercise, the feet move during the exercise, creating shear forces at the knee.

Closed chains tend to involve more muscles and joints than open chains, and lead to better coordination around each structure, which improves overall stability. Trunk movements are hard to categorize as open- or closed-chain because of the difficulty in assigning proximal and distal directions within the trunk.

Chapter Summary

Joints allow motion while providing stability. Joints are classified as non-movable (immobile), slightly movable, and freely movable. Besides providing stability, they allow at least eighteen different movements. This creates the dexterity needed to complete a variety of complex tasks.

Athletics involve movement in and around many different planes. The anatomical planes are used for reference as to the location and direction of movement.

Open- and closed-chain movements and exercises provide different benefits to athletes. Closed-chain exercises provide more stability for the joints and involve more muscles and joints than open chains.

Review Questions

1. What is the articular system?

2. List the three classifications of joints, including their function.

3. Give one example of where you would find a synovial joint.

4. How is the structure of the saddle joint more complex than that of the other synovial joints?

5. How are circumduction and rotation different?

6. What is the purpose of anatomical planes?

7. How are the axial and sagittal planes different?

8. Who coined the terms *open chain* and *closed chain*?

9. What is the difference between an open chain and a closed chain?

10. Give one example each of a closed- and open-chain exercise. Use examples that are not shown or described in this chapter.

Projects and Activities

1. Draw a model of a synarthrosis, an amphiarthrosis, and a diarthrosis joint.

2. Draw an example of each of the six different types of synovial joints.

3. Using stick figures, illustrate each synovial movement.

4. Draw a picture of the human body. Divide the body into its anatomical planes.

5. Research open- and closed-chain exercises for repair of the anterior cruciate ligament (ACL). In a report, explain the difference between the two chains and describe when each is used in rehabilitation.

6. Search the Web for topics on kinesiology and the various joints discussed in this chapter. Can you find additional information on programs of study or the relationship of athletics to kinesiology?

7. Are there specific joint disorders that athletes tend to suffer from?

Emergency Preparedness: Injury Game Plan

Objectives

Upon completion of this chapter, the reader should be able to:

- Define emergency preparedness.
- Discuss the importance of a written action plan for emergencies.
- List the components of the emergency plan.
- State the roles of everyone involved in an athletic emergency.
- Activate the EMS system.
- Identify the difference between defined medical emergencies and nonemergencies.
- Explain why athletic emergency cards are important.

Key Terms

Defined medical emergency

Emergency action plan (EAP)

Emergency preparedness

EMS system

Nonemergency

Emergency Preparedness

Being properly equipped and trained for any medical crisis or disaster is **emergency preparedness**. Emergency situations may arise at any time during athletic events. Expedient action must then be taken to provide appropriate care to the athletes involved in emergency or life-threatening conditions. The development and implementation of an emergency plan will help ensure the best care is provided.

Each athletic organization has a duty to develop an emergency plan that can be implemented immediately, and to provide appropriate health care (care that meets professional standards) to all sports participants. Because athletic injuries may occur at any time and during any activity, the sports medicine team must be prepared. Preparation includes formulation of an emergency plan, proper coverage of events, maintenance of appropriate emergency equipment and supplies, notification and use of appropriate emergency medical personnel, and continuing education in the area of emergency medicine. Through careful pre-participation physical screenings, adequate medical coverage, safe practice and training techniques, and other safety avenues, some potential emergencies can also be averted.

However, accidents and injuries are inherently part of sports participation, and proper preparation on the part of the sports medicine team will enable appropriate management of each emergency situation.

> **• KEY CONCEPT •**
>
> Athletic organizations have a duty to develop an emergency plan that can be implemented immediately, and to provide appropriate health care to all sports participants.

The Emergency Action Plan

Dealing with injuries without a written plan is a recipe for disaster. Programs that have well-thought-out, written action plans can deal with injuries in a systematic, logical manner that helps to avoid missteps and mistakes. The lack of a plan can lead to inadequate or inappropriate treatment of injuries (Figure 4-1).

The written **emergency action plan (EAP)** should be customized to fit the needs of the organization. The EAP should specify the needs within four basic categories: emergency personnel, emergency communication, emergency equipment, and transportation. A wealth of information is available through the Internet that can help in designing a plan for an athletic program. Visit the websites highlighted in Table 4-1, and follow the steps to view the EAPs developed by these universities and organizations.

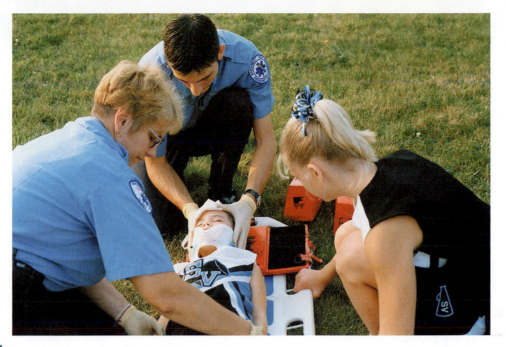

FIGURE 4–1
When an injury does occur, it is important to follow the emergency action plan.

The Sports Medicine staff at the University of Georgia, under the direction of Ron Courson, developed a template for writing a complete emergency action plan. This plan can be used in the creation of an emergency plan for any athletic program, at any level. The format of this plan is the basis of the framework for the discussion in this chapter.

Emergency Personnel

The EAP should clearly outline the roles of emergency personnel who are on the scene of a medical emergency. Generally, the first responder is a member of the athletic training staff. The athletic training staff, members of which should be available at all practices, competitions, and training events, is at a minimum trained in CPR and first aid. All members of the athletic training staff are responsible for knowing and being able to implement the emergency action plan.

Each member of the athletic training staff should be assigned specific roles to play in the event of an emergency. The most important role is providing immediate care to the injured athlete. This should be done by the most qualified member of the athletic training staff on the scene, generally the head athletic trainer or team physician. Other members of the

TABLE 4-1 Emergency Plan: Track & Field Stadium Venue

(Courtesy of Ron Courson, Director of Sports Medicine, University of Georgia)

Emergency Personnel: certified athletic trainer and student athletic trainer(s) on site for practice and competition; additional sports medicine staff accessible from Butts-Mehre athletic training facility (adjacent to track) and Stegeman Coliseum athletic training facility (across street from track)

Emergency Communication: fixed telephone line under practice shed (555-5555); additional fixed telephone lines accessible from Butts-Mehre athletic training facility adjacent to track (555-5550 and 555-5555)

Emergency Equipment: supplies maintained under practice shed; additional emergency equipment (AED, trauma kit, splint kit, spine board) accessible from Butts-Mehre athletic training facility adjacent to track

Roles of First Responders

1. Immediate care of the injured or ill student-athlete

2. Emergency equipment retrieval

3. Activation of emergency medical system (EMS)
   a. 911 call (provide name, address, telephone number; number of individuals injured; condition of injured; first aid treatment; specific directions; other information as requested)
   b. notify campus police at 555-5555

4. Direction of EMS to scene
   a. open appropriate gates
   b. designate individual to "flag down" EMS and direct to scene
   c. scene control: limit scene to first aid providers and move bystanders away from area

Venue Directions: Track and field stadium is located on Lumpkin Street (cross street Pinecrest) adjacent to Butts-Mehre Hall. Three gates provide access to track:

1. Lumpkin Street (most direct route): directly across from Catholic Student Center

2. Smith Street: opens to artificial turf practice field adjacent to track; accesses practice field drive to track

3. Rutherford Street: opens directly to practice field drive to track; gate must be activated from outside by 5-digit security code or opened by personnel from inside (either by 5-digit security code or trip switch in storage building adjacent to gate)

(Phone numbers changed from original)

TABLE 4-1 *Continued*

Venue Map

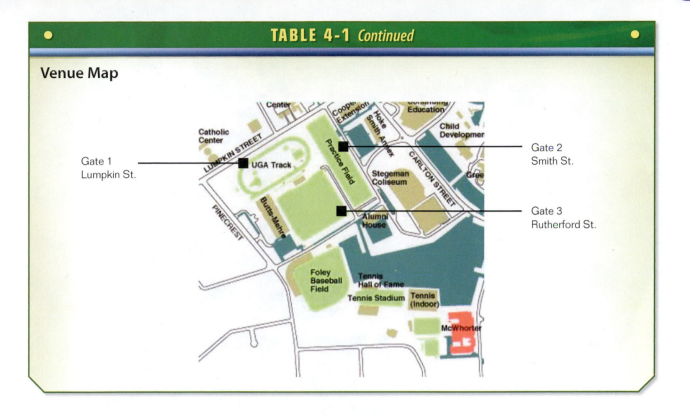

Gate 1
Lumpkin St.

Gate 2
Smith St.

Gate 3
Rutherford St.

staff should be assigned to locate and obtain any emergency equipment needed at the scene (Figure 4-2). These emergency team members must know what equipment is needed and where to get it efficiently. These duties are usually given to the coach or athletic training student aides. One member of the athletic staff on scene should be assigned to activate the **EMS system.** This is especially necessary if emergency medical services (EMS) are not already present at the sporting event. This should be done as early as possible in the emergency situation. The individual assigned to this task must be able to clearly and calmly communicate the situation over the telephone and be familiar with the venue, in order to provide the proper directions to the scene. Once EMS is summoned, someone must be available to direct EMS to the scene. This individual should be able to gain access to any locked gates or facilities.

Emergency Communication

Good working relationships between the athletic training staff and emergency medical personnel go a long way to ensuring the best care for an injured athlete. These relationships should be built long before an emergency

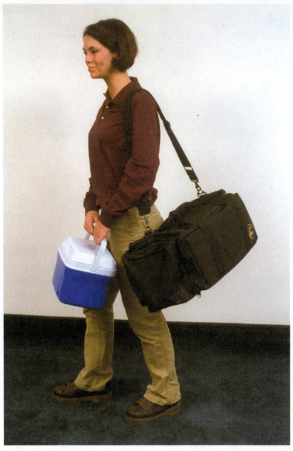

FIGURE 4–2
At least one member of the athletic training staff should be responsible for bringing the appropriate equipment to the game site or knowing where to quickly retrieve it if the need arises.

takes place. This will help establish the rapport and define the roles of the athletic training staff and the EMS providers in the event of an emergency.

Athletic training staff on the scene must have access to a working telephone or telecommunications device. Before each event, the phone system should be checked to ensure that it is in proper working order. A backup plan should be in place in case the primary communications system is inoperable.

A procedure should be in place for clearly communicating the situation to the EMS providers (Figure 4-3) after activation of the EMS system. It is important to clearly communicate to EMS the name, address, and phone number of the caller; the number of athletes injured; the condition of the injured; care and treatment being provided at the scene by the athletic training staff; specific directions to the scene; and any other information asked for by the dispatcher.

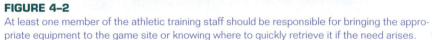

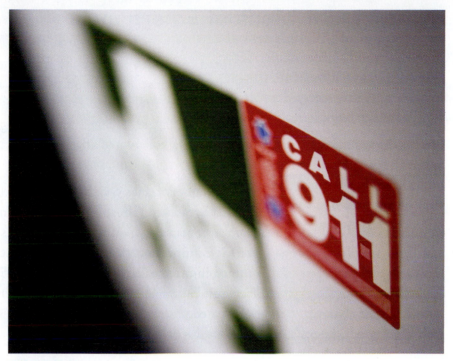

FIGURE 4–3
To activate EMS, dial 9-1-1 (if available in your area) and clearly communicate the situation in a calm and ordered tone. (Courtesy of Photo Disc)

Emergency Equipment

If the equipment needed to deal with an emergency is miles away from the site of the emergency, it will not do the athletic training staff or the injured athlete any good. All equipment that might be necessary for an emergency should be readily accessible. All equipment must also be in good working condition and should be checked before each event or competition. The individuals who will be providing care to the athlete must be knowledgeable in the use and application of the equipment that is on hand.

Transportation

EMS providers and an ambulance should be on standby at any event where there is a high risk of traumatic injury. This will lessen the response time for EMS and ensure that the injured athlete receives adequate care in a timely manner. Consideration must be given to the level of EMS providers available and the level of equipment available on the ambulance. An onsite ambulance should have clear access to the site of the event so that it can enter and exit the site without delay. Athletes with unstable injuries should never be transported in a vehicle that is not appropriately equipped to deal with the emergency. This chapter shows a completed EAP for a particular sports venue.

● **Did You Know?** ●

The "Golden Hour" is accepted as a national standard in trauma care. This name recognizes that the injury victim has 60 minutes from the time of initial injury to get the trauma center for care, in order to have the best possible outcome.

Identifying a Medical Emergency

Defined medical emergencies consist of breathing cessation, severe bleeding, no pulse, concussion with loss of consciousness, neck or spinal injury, fractures, dislocations, eye injuries, severe asthma attack, heat-related illness, or any injury causing signs of shock. Shock, which is defined as collapse of the cardiovascular system, is a precursor to death.

Nonemergencies consist of all other emergencies where life or limb is not threatened. These include abrasions, minor cuts, strains, sprains, minor concussions without loss of consciousness, contusions, and so on. It is important that athletes understand that proper treatment of minor injuries will allow continued participation. All injuries, no matter how minor, should be reported to the athletic training staff. If left untreated, minor injuries can become serious and require advanced medical care.

> **• KEY CONCEPT •**
>
> The difference between a defined medical emergency and a non-emergency is the threat of loss of limb or life. Any injury, no matter how minor, should be reported to the certified athletic trainer.

Emergency Medical Cards

Each athlete must have an up-to-date emergency information profile on record. This information is used by athletic trainers and EMS personnel to contact the athlete's guardian or nearest relative if an injury occurs. This profile also contains important medical information that could be used in case of an emergency. Hospital preference, family doctor's phone numbers, and parental permission to treat and transport are also important elements of the emergency medical card.

> **• KEY CONCEPT •**
>
> Emergency medical cards are valuable to the athletic training staff because they allow the staff to have all important contact information at their fingertips. Emergency medical cards also permit the athletic training staff to treat, and provide access to emergency care for, an injured minor athlete in the event the parents or guardians are unavailable.

Chapter Summary

Emergency preparedness is the central element of a good sports medicine program. Emergencies become manageable when everyone involved understands his or her role and works as a team. The emergency preparedness team consists of everyone involved in athletics. These include certified athletic trainers, athletic training student aides, support medical staff, EMS, coaches, athletes, and (if needed) bystanders.

The emergency plan must be written down and agreed upon by all parties, including the local emergency medical services personnel. Practice makes perfect. An emergency plan that has never been set into action will encounter challenges. It is important to have practice sessions at least once a year to familiarize everyone involved with the process.

The importance of being properly prepared when athletic emergencies arise cannot be stressed enough. An athlete's survival may hinge on how well-trained and prepared athletic health care providers are. It is prudent to encourage athletic department "ownership" of the emergency plan by involving the athletic administration and sport coaches, as well as sports medicine personnel, in its development. The emergency plan should be reviewed at least once a year with all athletic personnel, along with CPR and first aid refresher training.

As important as the emergency plan is, it is also important to understand the difference between defined medical emergencies and nonemergencies.

Emergency medical cards should be on the sideline of every practice and game. No athlete should be involved in athletics without an emergency card on hand.

Review Questions

1. Define the four basic components of the emergency plan discussed in this chapter.

2. What are the four roles within the emergency team?

3. How is the EMS system activated in your school or facility?

4. List the defined medical emergencies described in this chapter.

5. What are nonemergencies?

Projects and Activities

1. Review the emergency action plan for your school. What are its primary components? When was the plan written and last revised? Is there a separate written plan for athletic emergencies?

2. Create a detailed map of each sport venue located on school grounds. This map should easily direct EMS personnel to the site. Include in your map any access doors/gates, as well as any special instructions that might be needed.

3. See Table 4-1 for a list of colleges and programs that have EAPs.

4. Visit www.nata.org and read the NATA position statement on planning for emergencies at athletic events.

5. Visit the website of your local EMS agency, and see if they have any information available on responses to athletic events.

Prehabilitation and Preseason Conditioning

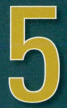

Objectives

Upon completion of this chapter, the reader should be able to:

- Discuss how prehabilitation can decrease the chance of injury.
- Explain how preseason conditioning will help the body adapt to the demands placed upon it.
- Describe isometric, dynamic, and isokinetic exercise and how they are used in a conditioning program.
- Compare and contrast manual resistance training, circuit training, and special individualized programs.
- Describe the science behind progressive resistance exercise.
- Explain how stretching and flexibility are important components of an overall fitness program.
- Explain the benefits of cardiorespiratory training.

Key Terms

Adaptation
Atrophy
Ballistic stretching
Cardiorespiratory
   conditioning
Circuit training
Dynamic exercise
Fast-twitch fiber

Flexibility
Hypertrophy
Isokinetic exercise
Isometric exercise
Isotonic exercise
Manual resistance
   training
Motor unit

Overload
Prehabilitation
Preseason
   conditioning
Progressive
   resistance
   exercise
Proprioceptive

neuromuscular
   facilitation (PNF)
Rehabilitation
Reversibility
Slow-twitch fiber
Specificity
Static stretching
Stretching

Prehabilitation

Most people have heard the term **rehabilitation**, meaning a programmed exercise program designed to return an athlete to fitness and competition. This is accomplished after an injury occurs. **Prehabilitation** is trying to prevent injuries before they occur, through a preventative management program. This program addresses concerns or deficits recognized by the athlete's family physician or other sports medicine specialists prior to sports participation. Addressing these concerns early will enable the athlete to participate with a greater chance of success and lower incidence of injury.

In the United States, more than 50 percent of boys and 25 percent of girls in the 8- to 16-year-old age range are engaged in some type of competitive, scholastic, organized sport during the school year. Children and adolescents are becoming more involved in sports at earlier ages and with higher levels of intensity. According to research done at Children's Hospital in Boston, foot and ankle problems are the second most common musculoskeletal problem facing primary care physicians in children under ten years of age, next to acute injury (Omey & Micheli, 1999). Additional research reported in *Clinical Sports Medicine* suggests that 30 percent to 40 percent of all sports injuries result from overuse (Herring & Nilson, 1987).

These statistics make it clear that a personalized prehabilitation program designed to address the total body, as well as sport-specific needs, should be an integral component of the total athletic fitness program.

> **• KEY CONCEPT •**
>
> Prehabilitation decreases the chance of injury by addressing areas of concern or deficit identified before participation in a sporting event. A program can be implemented to strengthen and develop these areas, thus reducing the chance of injury during participation.

Preseason Conditioning

Whenever athletes start a fitness program, or after they take an extended period of time off, their bodies need time to adjust to the new stresses and demands. The terms **preseason conditioning** and *prehabilitation* are similar, yet each has a slightly different focus. Preseason conditioning works on developing the athlete in the off-season. Athletes can work on overall conditioning as well as concentrating on specific weaknesses.

Athletes often must train harder and longer to excel in sports. A preseason conditioning program, beginning six to eight weeks prior to sports participation, allows the body to gradually adapt to the demands to be placed on it. Doing too much, too soon, at too high an intensity, will not allow the body to adapt effectively and therefore, increases the risk of injury.

Sports medicine physicians, certified athletic trainers, and qualified youth coaches should prescribe a preseason conditioning program and provide athletes with information on the type, frequency, intensity, and duration of training. Sharing this information with parents can be helpful so that they can reinforce the importance of preseason conditioning at home.

There are many different approaches to conditioning. After the athlete has set the goals that he or she would like to achieve in the conditioning program, the types of exercises can be selected and tailored to fit those needs.

Strength Training

Strength training is a highly adaptive process whereby the body changes in response to increased training loads. **Adaptation** is the whole purpose of strength training. Adaptation requires a systematic application of exercise stress. The stress should be sufficient to stimulate muscle fatigue, but not so severe that breakdown and injury occur.

Skeletal muscle is highly adaptable. If a muscle is worked beyond its normal limits, it adapts and becomes larger, or **hypertrophies**. In doing so, the muscle improves its strength, allowing it to accommodate an increased workload. The reverse is also true. If a muscle is worked less than normal, it **atrophies**, or becomes smaller, and therefore cannot accommodate the workload it once did.

The purpose of **progressive resistance exercise** is to allow the body to adapt to the increased demand placed upon it by training. The nature of the muscles adapting must always be considered when designing the training program. Factors that determine the rate and type of strength gains include overload, specificity, reversibility, and individual differences.

Overload

Muscles increase in strength and size when they are forced to contract at tensions close to maximum. Muscles must be **overloaded** to improve strength. If consistent gains in strength are to occur, muscles must be overloaded at a progressively increased rate.

Muscular tension must be attained at an adequate intensity and duration for optimal development of strength. Studies have found that the ideal number of repetitions is between four and eight. These repetitions should be done in multiple *sets* of three or more. Strength gains are less when either fewer or greater numbers of repetitions are used. It is important to include proper rest intervals between sets. This allows the muscles to recover from exertion and prepare for the next work interval. The optimal period of rest between sets has not been scientifically determined.

Specificity

Muscles adapt specifically to the nature of the work performed. This is known as **specificity**. If the leg muscles are exercised, they hypertrophy, whereas the muscles of the shoulders remain the same. If a football player wants to increase leg strength, he will have to work the muscles in his legs.

When muscles contract, they recruit different types of **motor units** to carry out the contraction. There are two different muscle fiber types (motor units). Each has different characteristics while contracting. **Slow-twitch fibers** are relatively fatigue-resistant; **fast-twitch fibers** can contract more rapidly and forcefully, but also fatigue rapidly.

The low-threshold, slow-twitch fibers are recruited for low-intensity activities such as jogging (and for that matter, most tasks of human motion). However, for high-speed or high-intensity activities, such as sprinting or weight lifting, the fast-twitch motor units are engaged.

The amount of training that occurs in a muscle fiber is determined by the extent to which it is recruited. High-repetition, low-intensity exercise, such as distance running, uses mainly slow-twitch fibers. Low-repetition, high-intensity activity, such as weight training, causes hypertrophy of fast-twitch fibers, though there will also be some changes to the lower threshold slow-twitch fibers. The training program should be structured to produce the desired training effect.

Increases in strength are very specific to the type of exercise, even when the same muscle groups are used. Specific motor units are recruited for specific tasks. If a person uses weight training to improve strength for another activity, the exercises should mimic the desired movements of that activity as closely as possible. Likewise, when one is attempting to increase strength after an injury or surgery, rehabilitation should include muscle movements that are as close as possible to those made in normal activities.

Muscle fiber type appears to play an important role in determining success in some sports. Successful distance runners have a high proportion of slow-twitch muscles (the percentage of slow-twitch fibers is closely related to maximum oxygen consumption). Sprinters have a predominance of fast-twitch muscles. Several studies have shown that large numbers of fast-twitch fibers are a prerequisite for success in progressive resistance training.

Not all sports have preferred fiber characteristics. For example, world-class shot-putters show surprisingly diverse muscle fiber composition. In those athletes, larger muscle fibers, rather than percent fiber type, accounts for excellent performance. There are differences in the relative percentage of fast-twitch fibers in explosive-strength athletes. Having a high percentage of fast-twitch fibers is not necessarily critical for success. Many strength athletes have a higher fast-to-slow twitch fiber ratio than sedentary persons or endurance athletes. Individual differences in training intensity and technique can make up for deficiencies in the relative percentage of fast-twitch fibers in these athletes.

Training programs that are designed to stimulate both strength and endurance have been found to interfere with gains in strength. Strength athletes may inhibit their ability to gain strength by participating in vigorous endurance activities. Muscles may be unable to adapt optimally to both forms of exercise.

Reversibility

Muscles will atrophy with disuse, immobilization, and starvation. Disuse leads to a decrease in strength and muscle mass. This process is called **reversibility.**

Fast-twitch and slow-twitch fibers do not atrophy at the same rate. If a joint is immobilized as a result of an injury, the slow-twitch fibers will atrophy faster. After immobilization, it will be important to undertake a program of strength and endurance exercises. This will allow the atrophied muscle fibers to regain the strength they had prior to the disuse.

Progressive resistance training allows the body to adapt to the demand placed on it through training. The rate and type of strength gain are determined by four factors:

1. Overload: the overwork of muscles at tensions close to their maximum.

2. Specificity: the targeting of a particular muscle group to improve and gain strength in that muscle group alone.

3. Reversibility: the characteristic of muscles that causes decreases in strength and mass with disuse.

4. Individual differences, which also account for an individual's ability to strengthen certain muscles at a particular rate. Genetics have a strong influence on strength gain.

Individual Differences

As with other forms of exercise, people vary in the rate at which they gain strength. Some of these differences can be attributed to the relative predominance of fast- and slow-twitch motor units in muscles. Usually, endurance athletes will have more slow-twitch fibers in their active muscles. Strength athletes will have more fast-twitch fibers (Figure 5-1). Intense, progressive resistance training mainly enlarges fast-twitch fibers. People who have more fast-twitch fibers will tend to gain strength faster than those who do not. Fast-twitch fibers tend to be stronger than other fiber types, so people who have more of them will tend to be stronger and have greater potential for strength gains.

Several studies reported by the Internet Society of Sports Medicine have shown that fiber composition is genetically determined (Fahey, 1998). Genetics is not the sole determinant of individual differences in strength, though genetics exert a strong influence on the ability to gain strength. A good training program can make up for genetic deficiencies.

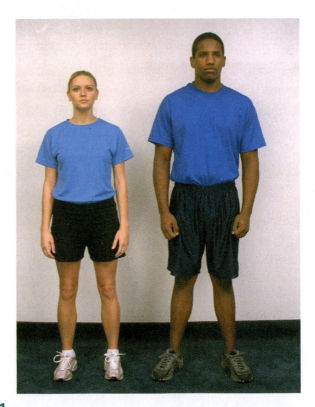

FIGURE 5–1
Endurance athletes will have more slow-twitch fibers in their active muscles. Strength athletes will have more fast-twitch fibers.

Strength Training Exercises

A variety of exercises and techniques can be used to build up strength based on the principles of progressive resistance training. The athlete should work with the certified athletic trainer or a personal trainer to determine the goals of the strength training program and the exercises and techniques that will best meet those goals.

Isometric Exercise

During **isometric exercises**, muscles contract, but there is no motion in the affected joints. The muscle fibers maintain a constant length throughout the entire contraction. Isometric exercises are usually performed against an immovable surface or object, such as pressing the hand against the wall. The muscles of the arm are contracting, but the wall is not reacting or moving as a result of the physical effort.

Isometric exercise is often used for rehabilitation because the exact area of muscle weakness can be isolated and strengthening can be administered at the proper joint angle. This kind of training provides a relatively quick and convenient method for overloading and strengthening muscles, without the need for any special equipment and with little chance of injury. Static exercise improves strength but also increases blood pressure quickly. People with circulation problems and high blood pressure should avoid strenuous isometric exercises.

Dynamic Exercise

Dynamic or **isotonic exercise** differs from isometric exercise in that there is movement of the joint during the muscle contraction. A classic example of an isotonic exercise is weight training with dumbbells and barbells. As the weight is lifted throughout the range of motion, the muscle shortens and lengthens (Figure 5-2). Calisthenics are also isotonic exercises. These include chin-ups, push-ups, and sit-ups, all of which use body weight as the resistance force. Blood circulation, strength, and endurance are improved by these continuous movements.

Manual Resistance Training

Manual resistance training is a form of dynamic exercise that is accomplished with a training partner. The training partner assists by adding

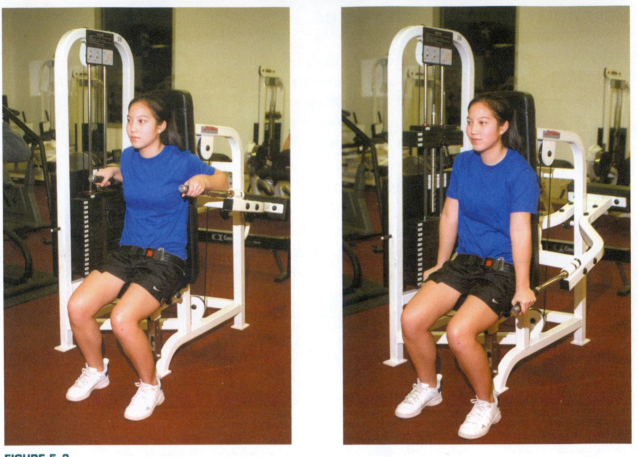

FIGURE 5–2
Dynamic exercise works muscle groups through the range of motion.

resistance to the lift as the lifter works the muscles through the full range of motion (Figure 5-3). The training partner, or spotter, adds enough resistance to allow the lifter to fatigue the muscles, and then releases enough resistance so that the lift can be completed.

Advantages of manual resistance training are:

- It requires minimal equipment.
- The spotter can help control technique.
- Workouts can be completed in less than thirty minutes.
- Training can be done anywhere.

The disadvantages are that a spotter is required, and both the lifter and spotter must be trained so that the exercise will be safe and effective.

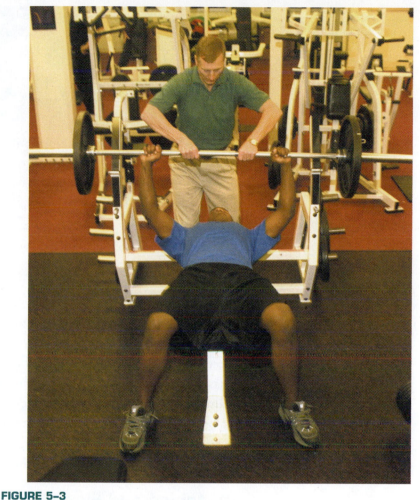

FIGURE 5–3
The training partner, or spotter, adds enough resistance to allow the lifter to fatigue the muscles, and then releases enough resistance so that the lift can be completed.

Isokinetic Exercise

Isokinetic exercise uses machines that control the speed of contraction within the range of motion. Isokinetic exercise attempts to combine the best features of both isometrics and weight training. It provides muscular overload at a constant, preset speed while the muscle mobilizes its force through the full range of motion. For example, when an isokinetic stationary bicycle is set at 90 revolutions per minute, no matter how hard and fast the exerciser works, the isokinetic properties of the bicycle will allow the exerciser to complete only 90 revolutions per minute. Machines such as the Cybex and Biodex provide isokinetic results; they are generally used by physical therapists and are not readily available to the general population.

- In isometric exercise, the muscles maintain a constant length throughout the contraction. This is a good type of exercise to target an exact area of weakness due to an injury.
- In isotonic or dynamic exercise, there is movement of the joint during muscle contraction. This type of exercise helps improve blood circulation, strength, and endurance.
- Isokinetic exercises use machines to control the speed of the contraction within a range of motion. These exercises provide muscle overload at a constant, preset speed and full range of motion.

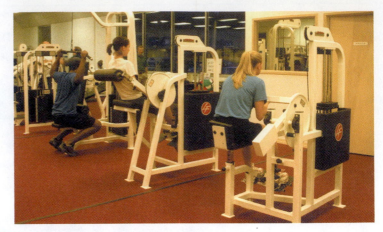

FIGURE 5–4
Circuit training utilizes six to ten strength exercises that are completed as a circuit, one exercise after another.

Circuit Training

Circuit training is an excellent way to improve strength and stamina. Circuit training utilizes six to ten strength exercises that are completed as a circuit, one exercise after another (Figure 5-4). Each exercise on the circuit is performed for a specified number of repetitions or a specific period of time before moving on to the next exercise. Each exercise is separated by a brief, timed rest interval. If more than one circuit is to be completed, the circuits will be separated by a longer rest period. The total number of circuits performed may vary depending on the athlete's training level.

Stretching and Flexibility

Stretching means moving the joints beyond the normal range of motion (Figure 5-5). **Flexibility** is the ability of a joint to move freely through its full range of motion (Figure 5-6).

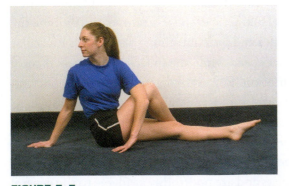

FIGURE 5–5
The athlete is able to increase the length of muscles as a result of stretching.

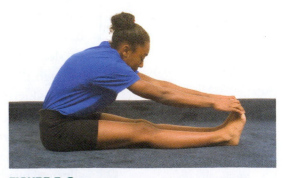

FIGURE 5–6
Greater flexibility allows the joint to move further before an injury occurs.

Stretching is useful for both injury prevention and injury treatment. One of the benefits of stretching is that the athlete increases the length of the muscles. This leads to an increased range of movement, which means the limbs and joints can move further before an injury occurs.

Before doing stretching exercises the athlete should warm up. Warming up is an essential component of stretching. Warming up increases the heart rate, blood pressure, and respiratory rate, which in turn increase the delivery of oxygen and nutrients to the muscles. This allows the muscles to prepare for strenuous activity. For most activities, the warm-up period should be nonstrenuous but allow the athlete to begin to perspire. It is known that:

- An active person tends to be more flexible than an inactive person.
- Females tend to be more flexible than males.
- Older people tend to be less flexible than younger people.
- Flexibility is as important as muscular strength and endurance.
- To achieve flexibility in a joint, the surrounding muscles must be stretched.

There are three basic types of stretching: static, ballistic, and proprioceptive neuromuscular facilitation (PNF).

Static Stretching

Static stretching is a gradual stretching of a muscle through the muscle's entire range of motion. This is done slowly until a pulling sensation occurs. This position should be held for 20 to 30 seconds. Stretching should not be painful; if it is, injury may occur.

Ballistic Stretching

Ballistic stretching was popular a couple of decades ago. This method of stretching involves a rhythmical, bouncing action. Ballistic stretches were done ten to fifteen times, stretching the muscles a little further each time. This method has fallen out of favor as a result of the increased incidence of injury. It was found that the bouncing action actually activates the stretch reflex, resulting in small muscle tears, soreness, and sometimes injury.

Proprioceptive Neuromuscular Facilitation

Proprioceptive neuromuscular facilitation (PNF) involves a combination of contraction and relaxation of the muscles. *Proprioceptive* refers to stimuli originating in muscles, tendons, and other internal tissues. *Neuromuscular* pertains to muscles and nerves. *Facilitation* is the

TABLE 5-1 Advantages and Disadvantages of Flexibility Training

Type	Advantages	Disadvantages
Static	safest form of stretching	takes longer to complete
Ballistic	good for dynamic flexibility	increased chance of injury
		increased chance of soreness
		reduces static range of motion
PNF	allows for greater reflex inhibition, greater stretch	need for a trained assistant
	increased neuromuscular response by stimulating neural proprioceptors	relying on assistant could increase chance of injury

hastening or enhancement of any natural process. This method requires an initial isometric contraction against maximum resistance at the end of the range of motion. This position is typically held for six seconds, followed by relaxation and a passive stretch. This is repeated several times. PNF is designed to be done with a qualified assistant.

Table 5-1 illustrates the advantages and disadvantages of flexibility training.

Cardiorespiratory Conditioning

Cardiorespiratory conditioning, also known as *aerobic* or *endurance training*, refers to activities that put an increased demand on the lungs, heart, and other body systems. Aerobic training can improve performance in all types of sports and activities.

Cardiorespiratory conditioning uses large muscle groups in activities such as walking, jogging, swimming, cross-country skiing, and cycling. Certain team sports, such as soccer and water polo, are excellent for aerobic conditioning. The goal of aerobic conditioning is to train the heart and other muscles to use oxygen more efficiently. The better efficiency of the cardiovascular system allows the person to perform exercise for longer periods of time, therefore improving the overall fitness level.

Muscular endurance is the ability of muscles to sustain high-intensity, aerobic exercise. An example of this is a weight lifter who has trained to

● **KEY CONCEPT** ●

Cardiorespiratory training conditions the heart and other muscles to use oxygen more efficiently. This allows the athlete to perform for longer periods of time.

complete twenty bench presses at 150 pounds in 60 seconds. Cardiorespiratory endurance relates to the whole body's ability to sustain prolonged, rhythmical exercise; an example is a cross-country runner completing a 5-mile run.

The body adapts to prolonged cardiovascular exercise in many different ways. The heart increases in size, thereby increasing pumping volume. Because the size of the heart increases (as does any muscle with increased exercise), the resting heart rate decreases. This also contributes to a decrease in blood pressure.

The lungs adapt to aerobic conditioning as well. A well-conditioned athlete will be able to increase the amount of air exchanged, providing more efficient oxygen transfer to the blood. This allows the athlete to work, condition, and compete at a higher level. Cardiorespiratory conditioning has also been proven to increase resting metabolism.

The design of an aerobic conditioning program should take into account several factors, to account for individual differences. These factors include beginning fitness level, age, sex, and physical limitations. The training program should be carefully matched to the athlete's individual needs to maximize the physiological benefit.

Additional benefits of cardiovascular conditioning include:

- Reduced fatigue
- Improved self-confidence
- Improved muscle strength and tone
- Increased endurance
- Reduced stress levels
- Reduced body fat
- Improved overall physical and mental health

An aerobic conditioning program starts with a check up by the family doctor. A physician can check overall health to be sure that there are no physical limitations on beginning a conditioning program.

Individualized Programs

Athletes who wish to have personalized assistance with their training program can contact a variety of individuals or organizations for help. The cost of a personal trainer depends on the type of program desired and the amount of time for personalized instruction. Personal trainers can assist in strength training, cardiovascular fitness, speed, and endurance work, as well as helping with body composition. Personal trainers should have the proven knowledge and expertise to set up a personal training program, or be certified by one of the following associations:

- The National Federation of Professional Trainers (NFPT)
- The International Sport Sciences Association (ISSA)
- The American College of Sports Medicine (ACSM)

Personal trainers can set up programs to meet the athlete's objectives and do so in a safe and controlled manner (Figure 5-7). Referrals are very important. Just because a person has a certification does not mean that he or she is the best choice for a given athlete. The athlete should ask around to find a personal trainer to fit his or her needs.

Certified athletic trainers are allied health professionals who have a considerable knowledge of anatomy and physiology. These professionals are involved in setting up personalized programs for athletes and are an excellent resource for training needs. Certified athletic trainers can be found at many high schools and most colleges and universities.

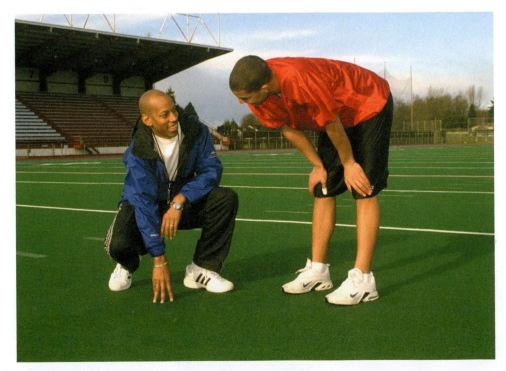

FIGURE 5–7
Personal trainers tailor workouts to the specific needs of the athlete.

Chapter Summary

Trying to prevent injuries before they occur is known as prehabilitation. Personalized programs designed to address the total body, as well as sport-specific needs, should be an integral component of the total athletic fitness program.

There are many different ways to achieve fitness. The use of isometric, dynamic, and isokinetic exercises will help the athlete develop a program tailored to fit his or her needs.

Stretching and flexibility are important components of fitness. A well-thought-out stretching and flexibility program will help with injury prevention and treatment.

Review Questions

1. Using all of the key terms listed at the beginning of the chapter, create a "matching" puzzle. Your key words and answers should be scrambled. At the bottom of your puzzle, show the answer key.

2. Describe the elements of a well-rounded preseason conditioning program.

3. Give three examples each of isometric, isotonic, and isokinetic exercise.

4. How can a personal trainer help you achieve your conditioning goals?

5. In a one-page paper, explain the science of progressive resistance exercise.

6. Stretching and flexibility exercises are the first to be neglected by athletes. Why is this a bad idea?

7. Explain the differences between static, ballistic, and PNF stretching.

8. Describe the benefits of cardiorespiratory training.

Projects and Activities

1. Interview three athletes from different sports in your school. How do their preseason conditioning programs differ?

2. Call, e-mail, or write to a college or professional athlete that you admire. Ask your athlete how he or she prepares in the off-season (prehabilitation) for the sport. Share this information with your class.

3. Visit the weight training facility at your school. Ask your strength coach to give you information on circuit training. Compile your information and set up an individualized program for yourself. Submit your plan to your teacher.

4. Pick one key term, from the list at the beginning of the chapter, that interests you the most. Research this term, and write a one-page paper describing the term and why it interests you.

5. Visit the websites of the National Federation of Professional Trainers (www.nfpt.com), the International Sport Sciences Association (www.issaonline.com), and the American College of Sports Medicine (www.acsm.org). How do the requirements for certification to be a personal trainer differ among these organizations? How are they similar?

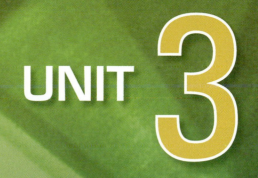

UNIT 3

Adaptive Physical Education

Adaptive Physical Education

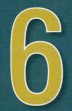

Objectives

Upon completion of this chapter, the reader should be able to:

- Define and describe what is meant by adaptive physical education.
- Discuss the qualifying standards utilized in determining eligibility for adaptive physical education.
- Explain how assessments are used in addressing the individualized needs of those with disabilities.
- Describe several adaptations that could be used to modify activities.

Key Terms

Adapted Physical Education National Standards

Adaptive physical education

Individualized Education Program

Individuals with Disabilities Act

Least restricted environment

Adaptive Physical Education

Adaptive physical education (APE) is physical education which may be adapted or modified to address the individualized needs of children and youth who have gross motor developmental delays.

Adaptive physical education comprises a program of individualized programs and developmental activities. These activities include exercises, games, rhythms, and sport designed to meet the unique needs of individuals with disabilities who may not safely or successfully engage in unrestricted participation in the vigorous activities of the general physical education program or a modified program in a regular class (Figure 6-1).

Adaptive physical education may take place in regular physical education classes where students are mainstreamed, or in self-contained classrooms. Although an adaptive physical education program is individualized, it can

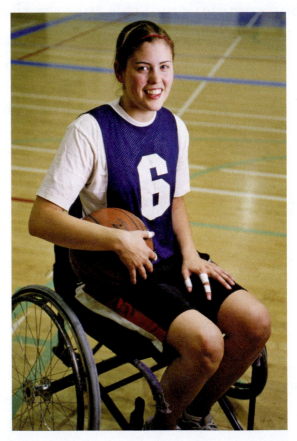

FIGURE 6–1
Adaptive physical education should be safe, relevant, and enjoyable. (Courtesy of Getty Images)

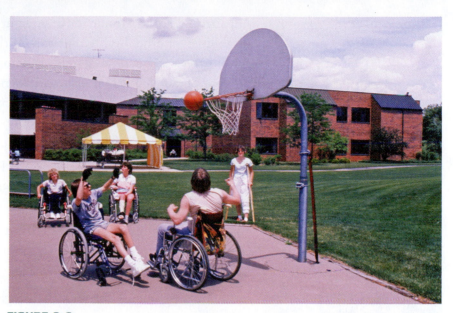

FIGURE 6–2
Team games should be modified to allow maximum participation. (Courtesy of Getty Images)

be implemented in a group setting (Figure 6-2). It should be geared to each student's needs, limitations, and abilities. Students receiving an adaptive physical education program should be included in regular physical education settings whenever appropriate.

Adaptive physical education is an active program of physical activity rather than a sedentary alternative program. It supports the attainment of the benefits of physical activity by meeting the needs of students who might otherwise be relegated to passive experiences associated with physical education. In establishing adaptive physical education programs, educators work with parents, students, teachers, administrators, and professionals in various disciplines. Adaptive physical education may employ developmental, community-based, or other orientations and may use a variety of teaching styles. It takes place in schools and other settings responsible for educating individuals.

Qualifying Standards

Students who qualify for adaptive physical education include people with disabilities specified in the **Individuals with Disabilities Education Act** (IDEA). This includes children who have mental retardation, deafness or other hearing impairment, speech or language impairment, blindness or other vision impairment, serious emotional disturbance, orthopedic impairment, autism, traumatic brain injury, a learning disability, multiple disabilities, or other health impairments that require special education or related services. Infants and toddlers who need early intervention services because of developmental delays in cognitive, physical, communication, social, emotional, or adaptive development can also qualify for adaptive physical education. The state can choose to include infants and toddlers younger than three years who are at risk of experiencing a developmental delay if early intervention services are not provided.

Students who qualify under Section 504 of the Rehabilitation Act of 1973 can also receive adaptive physical education. In Section 504, a person with a disability is anyone who has a physical or mental impairment that limits one or more major life activities, has a record of impairment, or is regarded as having an impairment.

A fourth group of students that might qualify for adaptive physical education is students who are recuperating from injuries or accidents, are recovering from noncommunicable diseases, are overweight, have low skill levels, or have low levels of physical fitness. This group is not covered by legislation, but a school district can decide to develop a plan to meet these students' physical education needs. Adaptive physical education only serves people from the ages of 0 to 21.

> **● KEY CONCEPT ●**
>
> Adaptive physical education only serves people from the ages of 0 to 21.

Determining Educational Needs Through Assessment

Adaptive physical education programs should include the following:

- Assessment and instruction by qualified personnel. These professionals are specially trained and prepared to gather assessment data and provide physical education instruction for children and youth with disabilities and developmental delays.

- Accurate assessment, including diagnostic and curriculum-based data

- **Individualized Education Program** (IEP) goals and objectives that are measurable with objective statements written by the physical education instructor. These goals and objectives should reflect the physical education instructional content and be monitored and evaluated according to district policy. This will ensure that goals and objectives are being met in a timely manner.

- Instruction in a **least restricted environment** (LRE), which refers to adapting or modifying the physical education curriculum and/or instruction to address the individual abilities of each child. Adaptations are made to ensure that each student will experience success in a safe environment. Placement is outlined in the IEP and may include one or more of the following options:

  - general physical education setting
  - general physical education setting with a teaching assistant or peers (Figure 6-3)
  - separate class setting with peers
  - separate class setting with assistants
  - one-to-one setting including a student and an instructor

Adaptive physical education assessment focuses on identifying activity needs of the individual and interpretating measurements obtained through testing. Assessment is also used to make decisions

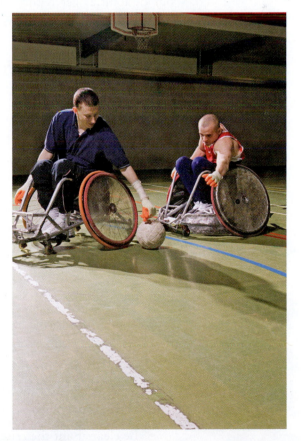

FIGURE 6–3
Adaptive Physical Education in the gymnasium (Courtesy of PunchStock)

about placement and program planning. It forms the foundation for the instruction given to an individual with disabilities so he or she can safely and successfully participate in physical education class. The Individuals with Disabilities Education Act (IDEA) Amendments of 1997 stated that parents need to be involved in the assessment of their child and the development of their child's IEP. Consequently, parental input and observations are vital to the assessment process.

Another aspect of assessment is determining the physical education grade a student receives on his or her report card. IDEA 97 added the requirement that children with disabilities be included in all assessments. This means that if the regular curriculum calls for physical fitness, motor, or content knowledge assessments, the instructor must give that assessment to students with disabilities or be prepared to provide alternative assessments. The 1997 amendment also requires that students with disabilities be given grades and progress reports on the same schedule as regular education students. This means that if parents of children without disabilities get report cards every nine weeks, parents of students with disabilities must also receive a report card every nine weeks.

> **• KEY CONCEPT •**
>
> If parents of children without disabilities get report cards every nine weeks, parents of students with disabilities must also receive a report card every nine weeks.

Assessment Tips for Physical Education Instructors

The following tips may be helpful to physical education teachers who are using assessment techniques in their classrooms.

- Be very clear about what is being assessed. (Is it worth learning and demonstrating?)

- Know why you are assessing. (What will you do with the information? Is the feedback for students, parents, the instructor, or the program?)

- Assessment is more than grading. Assessments should demonstrate what students know or are able to do. Assessments can "show off" learning in your program.

- Share the information with students, administrators, other teachers, and parents as appropriate. (This will lend credibility to your program.)

- Start small. (Begin with your most cooperative group or start with one group, one class, one grade level, or even just a few students).

- Be clear about the criteria (rubric standard, exemplary model, etc) for making judgments.

- Let students in on the process. (Using your criteria they can evaluate self, partner, or others. Allow students some choices in the manner in which they want to be assessed and include the criteria for each assessment.)

- Performance assessments involve students doing a task; they can be based on products, performances, or processes.

- The authenticity of an assessment can be either real or perceived. The more real-life, the more authentic.

- There are many types of assessments (peer, group, project-based, oral response, observation, debate, video, paper/pencil).

- If you are too busy to have students complete paper and pencil assessments, consider asking classroom teachers to help administer assessments in their classrooms.

Adapted Physical Education National Standards

In 1995 the National Consortium for Physical Education and Recreation for Individuals with Disabilities published the results of their **Adapted Physical Education National Standards** (APENS) Project. The purpose of the project was to develop national standards for adaptive physical educators and develop a national certification examination to measure knowledge of the standards. The published standards are an initial attempt to describe the roles, responsibilities, and perceived needs of practicing adapted physical educators. The national APENS exam is an evaluation of how well practicing teachers know and understand the standards.

The goal of APENS is to ensure that all students who qualify for specially designed physical education services receive them from a qualified teacher. Only a few states have adapted physical education certifications or endorsements. This lack of standards has impeded the hiring of qualified adaptive physical educators to provide services to students that need and deserve adaptive physical education.

The APENS exam is for all teachers who consider themselves qualified, competent adaptive physical educators. The minimum qualifications to take the exam are a bachelor's degree in physical education, 200 hours of experience providing adaptive physical education services, one three-credit survey course in adaptive physical education, and a valid teaching certificate.

Special Adaptations of Physical Activities

Quality adaptive physical education involves modifying a physical activity so it is as appropriate for the person with a disability. There are numerous ways that some sports and activities can be modified. The goal is to have an activity where all students can be successful. Listed below are some strategies for modifying various activities. (Source: PE Central: Adaptive Physical Education: Adaptations for Physical Activities.)

Environment–General

Decrease distance
Use well-defined boundaries
Simplify patterns
Adapt playing area (make it smaller, remove obstacles)

Actions–General

Change locomotor patterns
Modify grasps
Modify body positions
Reduce number of actions
Use different body parts

Time

Vary the tempo
Slow the activity pace
Lengthen the time
Shorten the time
Provide frequent rest periods

Bowling

Simplify/reduce the number of steps
Use two hands instead of one
Remain in stationary position
Use a ramp
Use a partner
Give continuous verbal cues

Basketball

Use various balls (vary size, weight, texture, color)
Allow traveling
Allow two-handed dribble
Disregard three-second lane violation
Use larger/lower goal
Slow the pace, especially when students are first learning the sport
If student uses wheelchair (Figure 6-4), allow him or her to hold ball on lap while pushing wheelchair
Use beeper ball, radio under basket for individual with visual impairment

Golf

Use a club with a larger head
Use shorter/lighter clubs
Use colored/larger balls
Practice without a ball
Use tee for all shots
Shorten distance to hole

Soccer

Use walking instead of running
Have well-defined boundaries
Reduce playing area
Play six-a-side soccer
If students use wheelchairs, allow them to hold ball on their laps while pushing the wheelchair

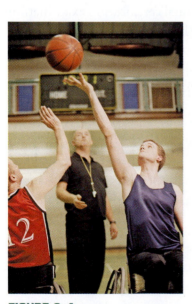

FIGURE 6–4
Athletes using specially designed wheelchairs to compete (Courtesy of PunchStock)

Use a deflated ball, Nerf™ ball, beeper ball, or brightly colored ball

Use a target that makes noise when hit

Softball

Use Velcro™ balls and mitts

Use larger or smaller bats

Use a batting tee

Reduce the base distances

Use Incrediballs™

Shorten the pitching distance

If individuals are in wheelchairs, allow them to push ball off ramp, off lap, or from tee

Use beeper balls

Provide a peer to assist

Have players without disabilities play regular-depth defense

Require students without disabilities to count to ten before tagging out person with disability

Volleyball

Use larger, lighter, softer, brightly-colored balls

Allow players to catch ball instead of volleying

Allow student to self-toss and set ball

Lower the net

Reduce the playing court area

Stand closer to net on serve

Allow ball to bounce first

Hold ball and have student hit it

Tennis

Use larger, lighter balls

Use shorter, lighter racquets

Use larger-headed racquets

Slow down the ball

Lower the net or do not use a net

Use brightly colored balls

Hit ball off tee

Allow a drop serve

Stand closer to net on serve

Do not use service court

Use a peer for assistance

> **• KEY CONCEPT •**
>
> Quality adaptive physical education involves modifying, a physical activity so it is as appropriate for the person with a disability.

CASE STUDY

The following is a disability awareness unit developed to help students, faculty, and staff discover and explore the world of a disabled individual. This creates an awareness of what the world is like from the perspective of a disabled person, and promotes understanding of what it takes to include persons with disabilities in our physically active lives. This unit was developed by Don Knitt at Jewett Middle Academy School in Winter Haven, Florida. (Reprinted with permission of Don Knitt.)

Name of Unit: Disability Awareness in Physical Activity

Rationale/Purpose of Event: This unit was designed for our students, faculty, and staff to discover and explore together the world of a disabled individual.

Suggested Grade Level: all

Materials Needed: Wheelchairs, walkers, crutches, blindfolds, variety of balls, bowling pins, jump ropes, batting tee, plastic bat and ball (larger than normal), paddles with fluff tennis balls, playground balls, medicine balls, scooters.

Disability Awareness in Physical Activity

This program incorporated a progression of activities from learning basic maneuvering and manipulating skills with adaptive equipment to developing the skills to participate in small adaptive games and other physical tasks. After each day students wrote reflective paragraphs in their "Sportfolios" regarding their feelings and experiences.

Day 1: Introduction of the week's activities. Students learned the proper use of a wheelchair, crutches, and walkers. All students had multiple opportunities to practice, and if they wanted to leave the physical education field for a water break they had to choose one of the types of equipment to travel to and from the fountains. The terrain was not too smooth! At the end of the class session we had a cool-down session and discussed each student's feelings toward the types of equipment they tried. They also talked about family and friends that have disabilities and how it affects them.

Day 2: Students were shown a video produced by the National Sports Center for the Disabled, which showed athletes participating in winter sports in Winter Park, Colorado. Special attention was given to the blind snow skiers. Students chose a buddy to escort them from the locker room to the physical education area (about 100 yards). One person kept their eyes closed the entire way; the other used verbal and tactile cues to have them walk safely. During our daily warm-up routines all students stretched with eyes closed, focusing on feeling their bodies and muscles. Then we sat in total silence and darkness to listen for sounds we normally ignore. This inspired some very insightful comments in the students' daily journals.

Activity Awareness

Station 1: Wheelchair weave through cones (100 yards)

Station 2: Travel with walker around cones (about 50 yards)

Station 3: Blind run—Run 50 yards blindfolded, holding a baton that is attached to and slides on a rope, with students on each end giving verbal cues

Station 4: Kicking a soccer ball while walking with crutches

Station 5: Water break—Travel 25 yards from playground over sand, grass, and uneven pavement, using either a chair, walker, or crutches

Closure: Discussion about the difficulty of performing the tasks. Students also reflected on the accessibility of our school facilities for a truly disabled person.

Day 3: We have cross curricular reading at our school, so today we read an article from the United States Olympic Committee regarding a wheelchair rugby player. Students answered some questions based on the article about this athlete's motivation and determination. Additional stations were created.

Station 1: The wheelchair station was changed to an 880-yard oval

Station 6: Scooter volleyball

Station 7: Paddle ball played sitting on the ground

Station 8: Wheelchair bowling

Closure: Each day more stations were added or adapted. Students discussed the new challenges, and also the concept of adapting games for different types of disabilities. In their daily journals, students were asked to reflect on how their muscles felt after doing activities that they were not used to.

Day 4: On our final day we added a few more stations. A rubric was created in the form of a checklist. Students were asked to try every station and rate the activity according to difficulty.

Station 9: Wheelchair basketball on adapted lower rims

Station 10: Blind jump rope

Station 11: Wheelchair baseball using a batting tee

Station 12: Passing and catching balls between two wheelchairs. (Equipment varied from a playground ball to a 2-lb. medicine ball.)

Closure: Students were reminded to complete their journal reflections. We discussed our progress from start to finish. Students offered comments and suggestions on how to improve the unit next year. (One suggestion was that selected students would spend an entire day in a wheelchair in order to really experience the challenges.) We closed by watching a video from Special Olympics produced in Florida. It featured some local athletes that our students know.

Integration: Our art teacher showed students a video on blind and disabled artists. Students experimented with writing their name or drawing with a pencil in their mouth and in their toes. Language arts classes read short stories about people with disabilities. We arranged for guest speakers from various civic organizations to tell how they help people with disabilities and how they can get students involved. The school's TV crew videotaped the week's activities and used still photos in a multimedia presentation. Students were interviewed about people they know and how they relate to their disability.

Culminating Event: We are scheduling a school-wide assembly with a wheelchair basketball game between a team of students and faculty; and a local team of wheelchair athletes.

Chapter Summary

Adaptive physical education is a subdiscipline of physical education. It is an individualized program created for students who require a specially designed program. The program involves physical fitness, motor fitness, fundamental motor skills and patterns, aquatics skills, dance skills, and individual and group games and sports.

For people with disabilities, adaptive physical education provides safe, personally satisfying, and successful experiences related to physical activity, rather than a sedentary alternative program.

There are numerous standards and assessment programs that are utilized in adaptive physical education. Assessments are used to find the proper level and program for each student.

Chapter Review Questions

1. What type of activities does an adaptive physical education program generally consist of?

2. Why is it important for the adaptive physical education program to be active?

3. What type of disabilities are specified in the Individuals with Disabilities Act?

4. What is the age range that adaptive physical education can serve?

5. What type of placement options may be utilized through assessment?

6. Are students with an IEP graded differently than the general population? Why?

7. List three of your favorite assessment tips for physical education instructors. Why are these three your favorites?

8. Will national standards for adaptive physical education result in higher quality and greater opportunities for those with disabilities?

9. Pick an activity not listed in this chapter and create adaptations that will allow students with disabilities to participate.

10. What was your impression of the case study presented at the end of the chapter?

Projects and Activities

1. Volunteer at a local secondary school's adaptive physical education program. Record your findings in a journal.

2. Research federal legislation enacted to protect students with disabilities in physical education. Write a paper describing what you have found.

3. Expand on the assessment tips for physical education instructors listed in this chapter. Create an additional list of creative ideas of your own.

4. Shadow a special needs student throughout his or her school day. Describe what hardships and barriers he or she must endure during the day.

Website Resources

Adaptive Physical Education

A wealth of resources on adaptive physical education can be found at the following site:

http://www.csupomona.edu/~pvetter/ape/web_links.html

Developing and Administering the Individualized Education Program

Objectives

Upon completion of this chapter, the reader should be able to:

- Explain the different laws that ensure the rights of students with disabilities.
- Describe the purpose and use of the individualized education program.
- List the ten steps in the development of an IEP for a student with disabilities.

Key Terms

Individualized Education Program (IEP)

Section 504 of the Rehabilitation Act of 1973

Education for All Handicapped Children Act (Public Law 94-142)

The Individuals with Disabilities Education Act (IDEA)

The Americans with Disabilities Education Act

No Child Left Behind Act of 2001 (NCLB)

Developing and Administering the Individualized Education Program

Developing and administering individualized education programs for special needs children require an understanding of the legal parameters associated with development of these programs. The ultimate, attainable goal is enhancing the quality of life for all learners, including those with disabilities. Educators not only need to understand legal issues, but also have the knowledge of techniques for modifying instructional methods, curricular materials, technology, and the learning environment (Figure 7-1).

Legislation and Adaptive Physical Education

Section 504 of the Rehabilitation Act of 1973

Section 504 of the Rehabilitation Act of 1973 declared that individuals with disabilities cannot be excluded, based solely on the disability, from any program or activity receiving federal funds. In physical education, intramurals, extracurricular or interscholastic athletics, a reasonable accommodation must be made to include a student with disabilities who wishes to participate.

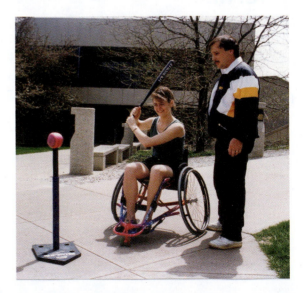

FIGURE 7–1
Administering an Individual Education Program includes students with disabilities. (Courtesy of Kim A. Duchane, Manchester Sport Sciences College)

The Individuals with Disabilities Education Act (IDEA)

Congress enacted the **Education for All Handicapped Children Act (Public Law 94-142)** on November 29, 1975. The law was intended to support states and localities in protecting the rights and individual needs of children and youths with disabilities, as well as their families.

Prior to the enactment of Public Law 94-142, many children were denied access to education and opportunities to learn. For example, in 1970, U.S. schools educated only one in five children with disabilities, and many states had laws excluding certain students, including children who were deaf, blind, emotionally disturbed, or mentally retarded, from their schools.

The Individuals with Disabilities Education Act (IDEA), which evolved from Public Law 94-142, is designed to ensure the following rights for students with disabilities:

- Right to a free, appropriate education
- Right to nondiscriminatory testing, evaluation, and placement procedures

The Individuals with Disabilities Education Act is the primary federal legislation that has a direct impact on adaptive physical education.

Americans with Disabilities Act

The Americans with Disabilities Education Act prohibits discrimination in employment, public accommodations, transportation, state and local government services, and telecommunication relay services. ADA broadened the scope of Section 504 and mandated nondiscrimination in the private sector as well.

The primary impact of this legislation on adaptive physical education was that it mandated access to leisure and travel services and recreation and sport facilities such as bowling alleys, golf courses, curling centers, downhill and cross-country skiing centers, and boat and canoe rentals.

Legislative Outcome

Today, early intervention programs and services are provided to more than 200,000 eligible infants and toddlers and their families, while about 6.5 million children and youths receive special education and related services to meet their individual needs. More students with disabilities are

> • **Did You Know?** •
>
> In 1970, U.S. schools educated only one in five children with disabilities.

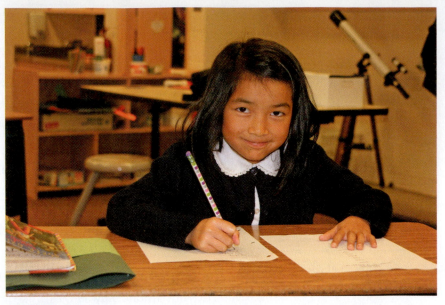

FIGURE 7–2
Students that have extra time to finish assignments benefit from the learning experience.

attending schools in their own neighborhoods that may not have been open to them previously. Fewer students with disabilities are in separate buildings or separate classrooms on school campuses, and are instead learning in classes with their peers (Figure 7-2).

When President George W. Bush and Congress set out to reauthorize the IDEA legislation in 2004, they made sure it called for states to establish goals for the performance of children with disabilities that are aligned with each state's definition of "adequate yearly progress" under the **No Child Left Behind Act of 2001 (NCLB)**. Together, NCLB and IDEA hold schools accountable for making sure students with disabilities achieve high standards.

IDEA is now aligned with the important principles of NCLB in promoting accountability for results, enhancing the role of parents, and improving student achievement through instructional approaches that are based on scientific research. While IDEA focuses on the needs of individual students and NCLB focuses on school accountability, both laws share the goal of improving academic achievement through setting high expectations and requiring quality education programs. These efforts go beyond physical access to the education system. They aim to provide full access to high-quality curricula and instruction and improve education outcomes for children and youth with disabilities.

> **• KEY CONCEPT •**
>
> The Individuals with Disabilities Education Act (IDEA) is the primary federal legislation that has a direct impact on adaptive physical education.

Evidence that this approach is working can be found in the increase in the number of students with disabilities who graduate from high school instead of dropping out. The National Longitudinal Transition Study-2 (NLTS2), which documents the experiences of a national sample of students with disabilities over several years as they move from secondary school into adult roles, shows that the incidence of students with disabilities completing high school rather than dropping out increased by 17 percent between 1987 and 2003. During the same period, their postsecondary education participation more than doubled to 32 percent. In 2003, 70 percent of students with disabilities who had been out of school for up to two years had paying jobs, compared to only 55 percent in 1987.

The Individualized Education Program (IEP)

> **• KEY CONCEPT •**
>
> The IEP guides the delivery of special education support and services for the student with a disability and is the cornerstone of a quality education.

Each public school child who receives special education and related services must have an **Individualized Education Program (IEP)**. Each IEP must be designed for one student and must be a truly individualized document. The IEP creates an opportunity for teachers, parents, school administrators, related services personnel, and students (when appropriate) to work together to improve educational results for children with disabilities. These individuals pool knowledge, experience, and commitment to design an educational program that will help the student be involved in, and progress in, the general curriculum. The IEP guides the delivery of special education support and services for the student with a disability and is the cornerstone of a quality education.

Federal guidelines require certain information to be included in each child's IEP. States and local school systems often include additional information in IEPs in order to document that they have met certain aspects of federal or state law. The flexibility that states and school systems have to design their own IEP forms is one reason why these forms may look different from school system to school system or state to state.

The writing of each student's IEP takes place within the larger picture of the special education process under (IDEA). There are ten steps by which a student is identified as having a disability, needing special education and related services, and, thus, needing an IEP.

Step 1. Child is identified as possibly needing special education and related services. The state must identify, locate, and evaluate all children with disabilities in the state who need special education and related services. To do so, states conduct "Child Find" activities. Child Find is a component of (IDEA) that requires states to identify, locate, and evaluate all children with disabilities, aged birth to twenty one, who are in need of early intervention or special education services. A child may be identified by "Child Find," and parents may be asked if the "Child Find" system can evaluate their child. Parents can also call the "Child Find" system and ask that their child be evaluated. A school professional may ask that a child be evaluated to see if he or she has a disability. Parents may also contact the child's teacher or other school professional to ask that their child be evaluated. This request may be oral or in writing. Parental consent is needed before the child may be evaluated. Evaluation needs to be completed within a reasonable time after the parent gives consent.

Step 2. Child is evaluated. The evaluation must assess the child in all areas related to the child's suspected disability. The evaluation results will be used to decide the child's eligibility for special education and related services and to make decisions about an appropriate educational program for the child. If the parents disagree with the evaluation, they have the right to take their child for an independent educational evaluation (IEE). They can ask that the school system pay for this IEE.

Step 3. Eligibility is decided. A group of qualified professionals and the parents look at the child's evaluation results. Together, they decide if the child is a child with a disability, as defined by IDEA. Parents may ask for a hearing to challenge the eligibility decision.

Step 4. Child is found eligible for services. If the child is found to be a child with a disability, as defined by IDEA, he or she is eligible for special education and related services. Within thirty calendar days after a child is determined eligible, the IEP team must meet to write an IEP for the child.

Step 5. IEP meeting is scheduled. The school system schedules and conducts the IEP meeting. School staff must:

- contact the participants, including the parents
- notify parents early enough to make sure they have an opportunity to attend
- schedule the meeting at a time and place agreeable to parents and the school

- tell the parents the purpose, time, and location of the meeting
- tell the parents who will be attending
- tell the parents that they may invite people to the meeting who have knowledge or special expertise about the child.

Step 6. IEP meeting is held and IEP is written. The IEP team gathers to talk about the child's needs and write the student's IEP. Parents and the student (when appropriate) are part of the team (Figure 7-3). If the child's placement is decided by a different group, the parents must be part of that group as well. Before the school system may provide special education and related services to the child for the first time, the

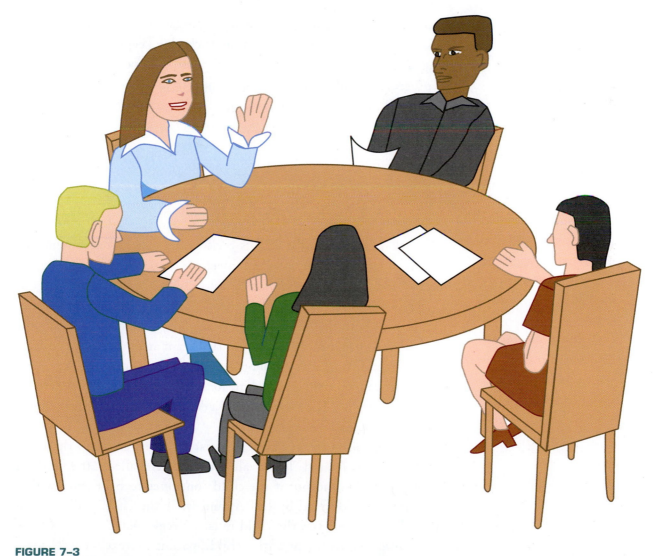

FIGURE 7–3
The IEP team is composed of professionals, the parent, and occasionally the student.

parents must give consent. The child begins to receive services as soon as possible after the meeting.

If the parents do not agree with the IEP and placement, they may discuss their concerns with other members of the IEP team and try to work out an agreement. If they still disagree, parents can ask for mediation, or the school may offer mediation. Parents may file a complaint with the state education agency and may request a due process hearing, at which time mediation must be available.

Step 7. Services are provided. The school makes sure that the child's IEP is being carried out as it was written. Parents are given a copy of the IEP. Each of the child's teachers and service providers has access to the IEP and knows his or her specific responsibilities for carrying out the IEP. This includes the accommodations, modifications, and supports that must be provided to the child in keeping with the IEP.

Step 8. Progress is measured and reported to parents. The child's progress toward the annual goals is measured, by the criteria stated in the IEP. His or her parents are regularly informed of the child's progress and whether that progress is enough for the child to achieve the goals by the end of the year. These progress reports must be given to parents at least as often as parents are informed of their nondisabled children's progress.

Step 9. IEP is reviewed. The child's IEP is reviewed by the IEP team at least once a year, or more often if the parents or school ask for a review. If necessary, the IEP is revised. Parents, as team members, must be invited to attend these meetings. Parents can make suggestions for changes, can agree or disagree with the IEP goals, and can agree or disagree with the placement. As stated before, if parents do not agree with the IEP and placement, they may discuss their concerns with other members of the IEP team and try to work out an agreement. There are several options, including additional testing, an independent evaluation, or asking for mediation (if available) or a due process hearing. They may also file a complaint with the state education agency.

Step 10. Child is reevaluated. At least every three years the child must be reevaluated. This evaluation is often called a *triennial*. Its purpose is to find out if the child continues to be a child with a disability, as defined by IDEA, and what the child's educational needs are. However, the child must be reevaluated more often if conditions warrant or if the child's parent or teacher asks for a new evaluation.

Modifications involved in an adaptive physical education IEP

Current Level of Performance—This states how your child is currently performing in physical education. This statement is a reflection of abilities seen at home and school. Parents will need to contribute to this list of abilities and needs. The current level of performance will be used to determine goals, short-term objectives, and any services needed.

 CASE STUDY

John, a student with cerebral palsy, is very attentive during physical education class. He works best in small groups. He works cooperatively with his peers during skill practice. When throwing something at a target, John demonstrates side orientation and eyes on target. Because of his cerebral palsy, he has a difficult time with weight transfer and balance when attempting to step in opposition. John can kick a stationary ball, but he does not use any knee action in his kick or much range of motion in his hips. Balance is a real problem when kicking. During game-like situations, John is very aware of his abilities. He enjoys having peers assigned to be his helper. He understands rules and strategies for most activities. Most of his skills are limited by his lack of balance and strength on his affected side.

Annual Goal or Long Term Goals: A statement describing what the child can reasonably accomplish within a twelve-month period. There should be a connection between this and the present level of performance.

Example
John will demonstrate the skills necessary to participate in a game of baseball with assistance as needed with his friends.

Short-term Objectives: Measurable, intermediate steps taken to reach the long-term goal

Example
John will demonstrate the following components of a functional throw so that the ball travels a minimum of 15–20 feet within 2 feet of a peer in three out of five trials, four days in a row.

Throwing components:

• Rotates body to side

• Extends throwing arm behind body while at the same time pointing non-throwing arm toward target.

- Forcefully rotates body forward while lagging throwing arm behind body as long as possible.

- Forcefully brings arm forward and releases the ball.

- Follows through by leaning body forward and bringing throwing arm down.

Example

John will demonstrate the following components of a functional catch from a stationary position so that he successfully catches a softball-sized foam ball four out of six times four days in a row.

Catching components:

- Shows ready position by looking at ball and having hands outstretched at chest height.

- Opens hands as ball is tossed and leans into ball with chest to intercept ball (using affected hand as much as possible).

- Traps ball against body if necessary or catches ball with two hands and brings it in toward chest to secure it.

Example

John will independently hit a regulation softball that is placed on a tee using a two-handed striking pattern (if possible) including body rotation so that the ball travels 10–15 feet in the air and rolls another 5–10 feet in four out of six trials.

Chapter Summary

The individualized education program requires an understanding of the legislation governing special needs students and its implementation. (Figure 7-4) Laws were passed to protect students with disabilities and ensure their rights. The development of the IEP requires a team approach of all stakeholders in the decision. This includes the parents and sometimes the student. An effective IEP will ensure that the student will receive a meaningful education in the least restrictive environment possible.

Chapter Review Questions

1. What does it mean to develop an IEP?

2. Write a brief paragraph outlining the federal laws that govern adaptive physical education.

3. Research how many students are eligible to receive special education services in your state.

4. What is IDEA and what are its goals?

5. What did The National Longitudinal Transition Study-2 conclude?

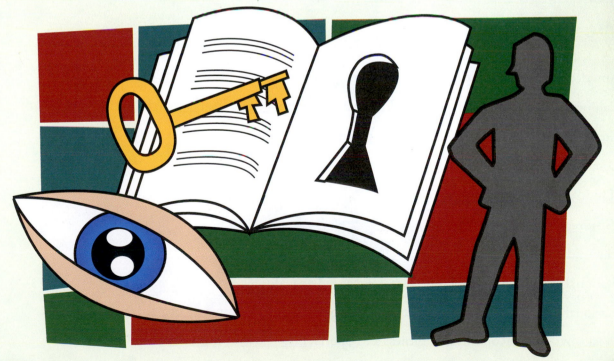

FIGURE 7–4

6. List the ten steps in the development of an IEP for a student with disabilities.

7. What can happen if a school district doesn't comply with legislation governing adaptive physical education?

8. What is "Child Find"?

9. Who are the stakeholders involved in a student's IEP?

10. If the parents do not agree with the IEP and placement, what can they do?

Projects and Activities

1. Set up a meeting with the special education director of a local school district. Ask the director several questions pertaining to adaptive physical education and the school district's compliance. Record or take notes of your conversation. Write a summary of what was said.

2. Using Appendix 4 at the end of the book, write a sample IEP for the student used in the case study.

3. Meet with a parent of a student with an IEP. Ask a series of questions about adaptive physical education. Write a summary of your conversation.

Website Resources

American Alliance for Health, Physical Activity, Recreation and Dance: http://www.aahperd.org

California State Council on Adapted Physical Education: http://sc-ape.org

Coalition for Active Living (Canada): http://www.activeliving.ca/

Disability Resources.org: http://www.disabilityresources.org

IDEA97 regulations: http://www.ed.gov/

ISBE regulations: http://www.isbe.net/

Law and Exceptional Students: http://www.unc.edu/

National Center on Accessibility: http://www.indiana.edu/

National Center on Physical Activity and Disability: http://www.ncpad.org

President's Council on Physical Fitness and Sports: http://www.fitness.gov

World Association of Persons with Disabilities: http://www.wapd.org

Coaching: The Challenges and the Benefits

Coaching: The Challenges and the Benefits

Objectives

Upon completion of this chapter, the reader should be able to:

- Explain the challenges associated with coaching.
- Describe the qualities of successful coaches.
- Describe why the coaching code of ethics is important.
- Explain the importance of a sound coaching philosophy.

Key Terms

Coaching code of ethics
Coaching philosophy

Coaching: The Challenges and the Benefits

Coaching sports is a challenge. As children we loved to play sports; whether on the playing field, in the backyard, at a friend's house, or in an organized arena. As adults, the enjoyment and personal satisfaction of sports is no less than it was in our youth. The transition from playing sports to coaching sports is a natural progression. To be a successful coach there are many things that you must understand (Figure 8-1).

Statistically, many of the young athletes that you coach will not even play varsity sports in school; most of them will not play in college, and almost none will ever play professional sports. So, what does this mean for coaches? Coaches need to emphasize all the other aspects of sports and the life lessons that make young athletes love playing the game. For the most part, coaches need to make the experience of sport fun.

Sports allow young athletes to learn success and failure, winning and losing, sportsmanship and teamwork, and how to respond to different situations while under pressure. None of these are easy lessons. Winning with grace is just as hard to teach as losing with dignity. How can coaches accomplish this and make sure that everybody has a great season? That's the trick.

> ● **KEY CONCEPT** ●
>
> Statistically, many of the young athletes that you coach will not even play varsity sports in school; most of them will not play in college, and almost none will ever play professional sports.

> ● **KEY CONCEPT** ●
>
> Sports allow young athletes to learn success and failure, winning and losing, sportsmanship and teamwork, and how to respond to different situations while under pressure.

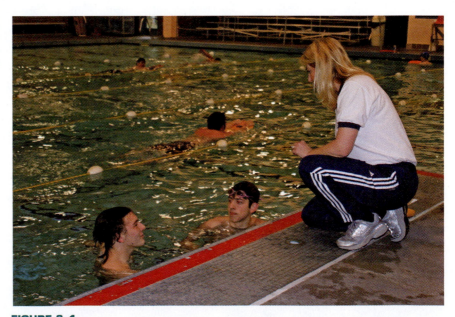

FIGURE 8–1
Head coach Carla Boone works with her men's swim team.

Every team you will ever coach, especially teams of younger kids, will be split between kids that are talented and kids that are not. The goal that you have as a coach is to make sure that every one of those kids has a great experience and wants to play again next season. The way to do this is to emphasize things other than on-field performance.

Qualities of Successful Coaches

Sports coaches help athletes develop their full potential. They are responsible for training athletes in a particular sport by analyzing their performance, instructing them in relevant skills, and providing encouragement. Therefore, the roles of the coach will be many and varied. The coach will be an instructor, assessor, friend, mentor, facilitator, chauffeur, adviser, supporter, motivator, counselor, organizer, planner, and the fountain of all knowledge (Figure 8-2).

In relation to sports, the role of the coach is to create the right conditions for learning and to find ways of motivating the athletes. Most athletes are highly motivated and therefore the task is to maintain that motivation and to generate excitement and enthusiasm. The coach will need to be able to help athletes build new skills by providing prepared training programs

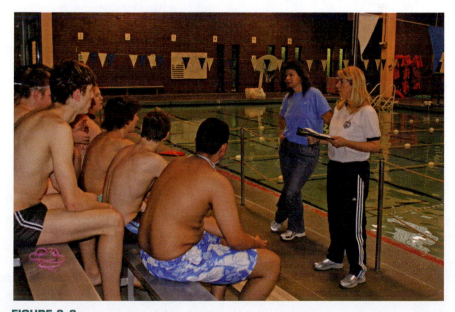

FIGURE 8–2
Coaches Carla Boone and Tammy Taylor prepare their team for morning practice.

that predict and monitor training progress and performance. A successful coach must always communicate effectively with his or her athletes.

Traits of Successful Coaches

- A goodwill ambassador for youth sports
- Able to inspire, encourage, and motivate
- An advisor to athletes on nutrition and safety
- Approachable
- Someone who cares about people
- Someone who demonstrates personal integrity
- An effective communicator
- Someone who enjoys working with people
- Enthusiastic
- Able to evaluate the athlete's and coaching performance
- A hard worker
- Honest and fair
- A careful listener

- A monitor of training progress
- Able to set reasonable goals
- Someone who has a solid understanding of the techniques of the sport
- Unbiased
- Understands the causes and recognizes the symptoms of over-training
- Understands and appreciates the rules of the sport
- Understands his or her own strengths and weaknesses
- Understands the capabilities of growing children
- Understands the learning process and training principles
- Understands various coaching styles
- Works well with parents and the community

> **• KEY CONCEPT •**
>
> The coach will need to be able to help athletes build new skills by providing prepared training programs that predict and monitor training progress and performance.

Coaching Code of Ethics

The function of a coach is to educate students through participation in interscholastic competition. An interscholastic program should be designed to enhance academic achievement and should never interfere with opportunities for academic success. Each student-athlete should be treated as though he or she was the coach's own child, and his or her welfare should be the highest priority at all times. Accordingly, the following guidelines for coaches have been adopted by the Board of Directors of the National Federation of High Schools (NFHS).

- The coach shall be aware that he or she has a tremendous influence, for either good or ill, on the education of the student-athlete and, thus, shall never place the value of winning above the value of instilling the highest ideals of character.

- The coach shall uphold the honor and dignity of the profession. In all personal contact with student-athletes, officials, athletic directors, school administrators, the state high school athletic association, the media, and the public, the coach shall strive to set an example of the highest ethical and moral conduct.

- The coach shall take an active role in the prevention of drug, alcohol, and tobacco abuse.

- The coach shall avoid the use of alcohol and tobacco products when in contact with players.

- The coach shall promote the entire interscholastic program of the school and direct his or her program in harmony with the total school program.

- The coach shall master the contest rules and shall teach them to his or her team members. The coach shall not seek an advantage by circumvention of the spirit or letter of the rules.

- The coach shall exert his or her influence to enhance sportsmanship by spectators, both directly and by working closely with cheerleaders, pep club sponsors, booster clubs, and administrators.

- The coach shall respect and support contest officials. The coach shall not indulge in conduct which would incite players or spectators against the officials. Public criticism of officials or players is unethical.

- Before and after contests, coaches for the competing teams should meet and exchange cordial greetings to set the correct tone for the event.

- A coach shall not exert pressure on faculty members to give student-athletes special consideration. A coach shall not scout opponents by any means other than those adopted by the league and/or state high school athletic association.

Coaching Philosophy

As new coaches begin their coaching careers, it is important that they spend time and effort on developing their coaching philosophy. Everyone knows the great coaches of the past and present, but what is it about them

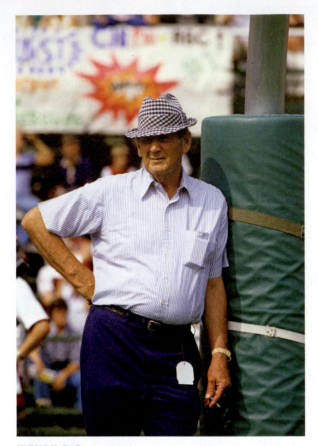

FIGURE 8–3
Paul "Bear" Bryant. (Photo © Rich Clarkson/Rich Clarkson and Associates)

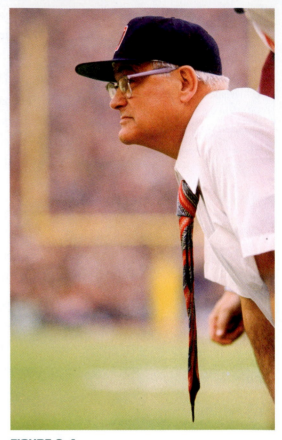

FIGURE 8–4
Woody Hayes. (Photo © Rich Clarkson/Rich Clarkson and Associates)

• Did You Know? •

Under the guidance of John Wooden, the Bruins set all-time records with four perfect 30–0 seasons, eighty-eight consecutive victories, thirty-eight straight NCAA tournament victories, twenty PAC 10 championships, and ten national championships, including seven in a row.

that made the difference in the eyes of their players? Was it the signature hat worn by the late, great Paul "Bear" Bryant of Alabama (Figure 8-3)?

Was it the fierce intensity shown by Ohio State's late, great Woody Hayes (Figure 8-4)?

Was it the result of one of the finest teachers the game of basketball had ever seen, the great John Wooden of UCLA (Figure 8-5)?

Is it the fiery emotion shown by basketball's great Bobby Knight of Texas Tech (Figure 8-6)?

Or the one-liners and positive team approach to football shown by the recently retired great Frosty Westering of Pacific Lutheran University (Figure 8-7)?

What is it that makes these coaches, and others just like them, stand out? Is it winning percentage? All of the coaches mentioned above were

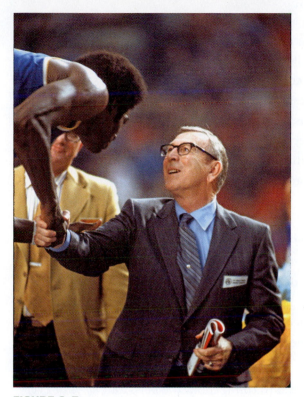

FIGURE 8–5
John Wooden (Photo © Rich Clarkson/Rich Clarkson and Associates)

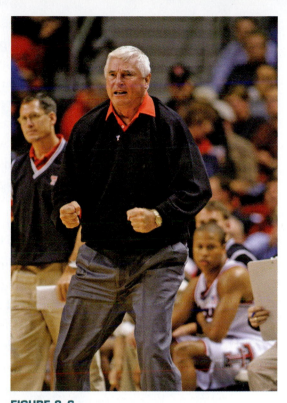

FIGURE 8–6
Bobby Knight (Photo © Rich Clarkson/Rich Clarkson and Associates)

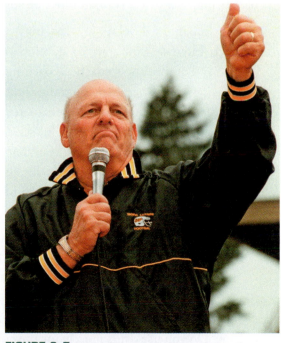

FIGURE 8–7
Frosty Westering (Courtesy of Pacific Lutheran University)

highly successful, national championship–winning coaches. But all of them would probably agree that winning is only a by-product of what you do as an athlete and how you prepare. Making the team goal be winning every game, or the conference championship, or the state title, is a road to failure, not success. Only one team or individual will ever win a league or state championship each year. What happens to individual and team goals if winning everything is the primary goal? As stated at the beginning of this chapter, athletics should be fun, enjoyed by everyone, and secondary to getting a good education.

Developing a Coaching Philosophy

Coaches beginning their careers will often spend the majority of their time planning drills and deciding practice schedules. The excitement of coaching will often cause beginning coaches to put coaching philosophy off to the side. To be successful, new coaches need to spend almost as much time developing their coaching philosophy as they do coming up with their practice plan.

Specifically, coaches need to think about the *hows* and *whys* of everything they will do as a coach. What basis or reasons do you have for your approach? This is a critical step for all new coaches. Even experienced coaches may want to reevaluate their philosophy.

The thought of developing a coaching philosophy is a fairly daunting prospect. How do you start to develop your philosophy of coaching? That's easy. For most new coaches, coaching philosophy begins with their own playing experience. Providing they had a positive experience, most of their basic philosophy probably emanates from their high school and college coaches. This is a very natural start, because this is the approach with which beginners are most familiar and comfortable. To grow individually as a coach, think about the following ten questions. These questions may help you in your effort to formulate or analyze your own philosophy of coaching.

1. **Is your approach educationally sound?** Several things should be considered as you analyze your coaching techniques and methods. Ask yourself the following questions:
   - Do your drills serve a purpose? For example, do they teach a part of your offense, defense, or appropriate skills that are needed?
   - Do you use drills merely for the enjoyment or entertainment of the athletes and coaching staff?

- Are your drills structured to provide the necessary repetition for each athlete?
- Are your drills and the skills they teach relative to your athletes' ability level?

Coaching involves teaching, and athletics should have sound educational value. Your answers to the questions posed above will be extremely important in developing your personal coaching philosophy.

2. **Is your approach appropriate for your players?** For example, many soccer coaches imitate the system employed by the last World Cup champion. But do their players have the ball control and skills to implement it? Probably not. It may be an excellent system, but not suited to their high school players.

As another example, a basketball coach attended a clinic and came away with what seemed to be a great new offense. When practice began for the season, the coach immediately implemented it. However, the players struggled with the offense and it took the coach almost half a season to realize that the talent differential from the college squad to his was the real difference. While the offense was good for the college team, it was not the answer for the high school team.

The ultimate answer is to use an approach which is developmentally appropriate for your players.

3. **Is your philosophy ethical?** In basketball, for example, many coaches who are losing in the waning minutes of a close game instruct their players to foul in order to stop the clock. While this tactic may be annoying to some fans, it is certainly within the limits of the rules. Can the same be said for faking an injury in order to stop the clock? No, that is unethical.

Consider what you do in all aspects of your coaching. Is it ethical? It should be and, if not, your philosophy should change. Because there is great educational value involved in athletics, coaching from an ethical standpoint is an extremely important way to provide a model for the athletes.

4. **Will your approach last over the years or is it based on a one- or two-year fad?** Successful programs and the systems that they employ are usually perpetual, continuing efforts, whereas, fads will disappear after a few brief years. Analyze your approach.

• **KEY CONCEPT** •

Because there is great educational value in athletics, coaching from an ethical standpoint is an extremely important way to provide a model for the athletes.

- How many other programs use the offense or defense that you use?
- How long have other programs used their approach?
- How successful (and success has to first be defined) have they been while using their system?

Remember, that imitation is a real indicator of success. If no one else is using your offense, defense, or other elements of your approach, this should give you a real hint. Using a system year after year is another very good indicator of its success and soundness.

5. **Do you stick with your philosophy and insert your players into it, or do your adapt to the players that are available?** Unlike colleges, most high schools, cannot recruit players. A college coach can, therefore, find players to insert into his system and philosophy.

Most high school coaches have to develop the talent on hand. Realistically, there may be some years in which the athletes may not possess the ability or skills to fit into your philosophy. You cannot change the players, but you can alter your approach.

6. **Is there a better way of doing what you are doing?** Apply this question to all aspects of your coaching philosophy: offense, defense, motivation of your athletes, conditioning, etc. Keep an open mind.

For example, if an opponent successfully attacks your defense, can you adapt their offense for your own use? Or does the success of your opponent's offense prove that your defense simply isn't effective?

It is extremely important to constantly analyze everything you do. Learning should be a life-long pursuit and so should developing your coaching philosophy.

7. **Can you explain why you use or do something?** In order to instruct and to motivate your athletes, you have to be able to justify what you do. Can you? It is no longer good enough to simply say, "Well, this is the way we are going to do it," and stop at that. You also have to be able to explain why. There is no way that you can justify anything associated with your program to athletes and parents without being able to explain it.

8. **Is what you do in practice sessions and games safe?** There is considerable information available concerning proper techniques and

skills. Staying abreast and aware of risk management aspects is vital. After all, unsafe approaches can lead to injuries and potential lawsuits. Some of the areas that need particular attention by coaches are:

- weather-related conditions such as lightning and heat/temperature
- injuries and their treatment
- equipment
- methods of training or conditioning
- teaching proper skill techniques

Anything unsafe needs to be immediately eliminated from your coaching philosophy. The safety of the athletes must be paramount.

9. **Is your coaching philosophy compatible with your personality?** For example, are you normally
- cautious or a risk taker?
- controlling or laid back?
- patient or impatient?
- an analytical planner or impulsive?
- deliberate or aggressive?

You will probably be more successful in coaching if your philosophy and personality are compatible. Is your approach with coaching in line with your personality or does your philosophy go against your basic nature?

10. **Is there anything unsportsmanlike about your philosophy?** Certain situations arise in some games that could be considered unsportsmanlike by your opponent, officials, or fans. One needs to consider how everything is perceived, such as:
- running up the score
- playing starters long after the outcome has been determined
- allowing taunting

While these are just a few examples, they need to be seriously considered. If any of these exist within your approach to coaching, you will have to make some changes, because these practices do not exhibit good sportsmanship.

After analyzing all the factors involved in coaching and developing your own philosophy, another very good exercise is to put it into written form. As mentioned previously, it is extremely important to be able to express and to explain your approach to athletes, parents, and supervisors.

• KEY CONCEPT •

Only you, with time and honest effort, can develop your own coaching philosophy.

A written document can also give you something concrete to re-examine and evaluate annually. In this way, you can easily update and improve your coaching philosophy.

The ten questions listed above are intended to promote thought, introspection, and, hopefully, some revelation. They are obviously not intended to provide the complete or definitive answer to developing your coaching philosophy. Only you, with time and honest effort, can develop your own coaching philosophy.

CASE STUDY: ADULTS HURTING YOUTH SPORTS

(The following case study is used with permission of the *San Jose mercury New* © 2007. All rights reserved.)

A national report card released Wednesday probably only confirmed what many parents who enroll their children in athletic programs already suspected. There are serious problems in the world of youth sports. And the finger of blame is being pointed squarely at adults for spoiling the fun.

The first Youth Sports National Report Card, prepared by a group called Citizenship Through Sports Alliance, issued low grades for parents' behavior and a win-at-all-cost mentality fostered by the grown-ups who oversee kids' sports. "We really hope that this will be a wake-up call," said Jim Thompson, executive director of Stanford's Positive Coaching Alliance. "This is such an important part of kids' lives. And if there's something wrong with youth sports, then we ought to start thinking about the ways we can change it."

A panel of experts based its results on evaluations of youth sports programs for children 6 to 14. But the report is a sharp rebuke of adults. The worst grades—Ds—were issued in the categories of parental behavior and "child-centered" philosophy. And a C-minus was given for coaching. The report card indicates that adults are micro-managing their kids' sports careers, placing too much emphasis on winning and setting bad examples with their own poor sportsmanship.

This assessment of kids' sports doesn't come as a surprise. Reports of violence at events, usually perpetrated by angry parents, have become more common. And even if those incidents remain the exception and not the rule, any parent of a sports-playing child probably has witnessed uncomfortable scenes in which adults took the game too seriously.

"Nearly all the problems in youth sports are caused by people over the age of 18," said panel member Doug Abrams, a University of Missouri School of Law professor. "I coach hockey and I know some parents can learn from the behavior of their 7-year-olds. The kids are the role models."

The panelists indicated there are some bright spots: They gave a B-minus for officiating and a C-plus for health and safety. But overall, the assessment was negative.

"There is a real silent majority of parents who don't like what's going on and are uncomfortable with the direction youth sports has taken," said Thompson, a member of the panel. "Yet even though they have this anxiety, they also don't know what to do."

Dan Gould, director of Michigan State's Institute for the Study of Youth Sports, said part of the problem is what he calls the "professional-ization" of children's athletics. Adults are applying a professional model of training at ever-younger ages. Even parents who are interested solely in a healthy experience for their kids can find themselves navigating a system where the philosophy is shifting away from making sure all kids get to play and toward developing only the most talented youngsters.

That's evident in the growing phenomenon of traveling teams and club sports, for which parents shell out thousands of dollars so their kids can compete year-round and receive the best training. "Youth sports has become an arms race," Abrams said. "If some team has nicer uniforms than ours, then we've got to get better ones next year. If they play 20 games, then we've got to play 25. Next thing you know, you have year-round specialization with 75 games a season and all the problems that come with it."

John Murphy, chairman of the Pleasanton-based California Youth Soccer Association, had mixed feelings about the report card. He agreed with the criticism directed at the "elite" programs that stress winning. But he noted that the vast majority of the 217,000 kids and 25,000 or so adults in CYSA are involved at the recreation level. "We're a volunteer organization and most of our adults are in this for the right reasons," said Murphy, whose three grown children all played soccer. "We're not trying to put anyone on the U.S. World Cup team."

One concern that all youth sports experts share is research that shows 70 percent of kids drop out of sports by 13—and the primary reason is pressure exerted by adults. That age is about when kids begin to face the influences of drugs and alcohol. "This is exactly the time we should be encouraging kids to participate in sports," Abrams said. Both Thompson and Abrams said there is more good than bad in youth sports. But they also defended the report card's negative tone. "There are coaches and parents all across the country who are doing great things in youth sports," Thompson said. "But that's not the trend."

Clark Kellogg, CBS Sports basketball studio analyst, offered a unique perspective on CTSA's efforts. "Because sports participation can have such a positive impact on young people, it's extremely important that parents and coaches keep the games in perspective and the interests of the participants at the very top of the priority list," Kellogg said. "Unfortunately, there are a growing number of examples where that is not the case. As one who has enjoyed the benefits of athletic participation, and as the father of three young athletes, that is terribly disheartening to me. And it needs to change. I welcome the opportunity to be part of the process to help parents and coaches be the role models they can be and should be for youth in sports."

The Citizenship Through Sports Alliance is committed to promoting positive behavior in youth sports by harnessing the collective resources of major U.S. sports organizations to provide practical and proven tools for parents and coaches in youth sports.

The members of the CTSA are: National Collegiate Athletic Association (NCAA); Major League Baseball (MLB); National Basketball Association (NBA) and Women's National Basketball Association (WNBA); National Hockey League (NHL); National Federation of State High School Associations (NFHS); National Association of Intercollegiate Athletics (NAIA); National Association for Sport and Physical Education (NASPE); National Junior College Athletic Association (NJCAA); and National Association of Collegiate Directors of Athletics (NACDA).

Contributed by Mark Emmons, Mercury News

Chapter Summary

Effective coaching and effective coaches both rely on a strong code of ethics and coaching philosophy that they employ at every practice and competition. Understanding that kids play sports for fun is the most important aspect of coaching. Few, if any, of your players will play college or professional sports. Therefore, the goal of organized sports should be to develop the athlete, both personally and educationally. Your effectiveness as a coach will have more to do with preparating and motivating athletes than winning percentage. Athletics should be fun, enjoyed by everyone, and secondary to getting a good education (Figure 8-8).

Chapter Review Questions

1. Statistics indicate that a coach will probably never have one of his or her athletes play professional sports. Why is this a factor in developing a coaching philosophy?

2. What important items should coaches emphasize to their athletes?

3. How can a coach ensure that every kid will want to turn out for their team next year?

4. After rereading the coaching code of ethics, explain what you would consider your top three codes of ethics.

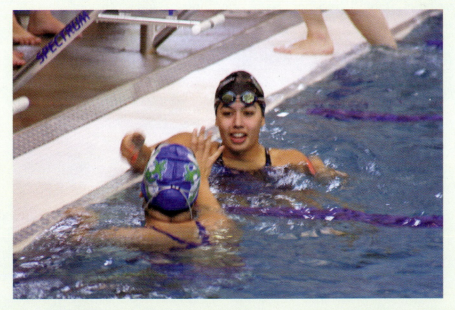

FIGURE 8–8
Fun, sportsmanship, and competition make all the hard work pay off. (Courtesy of Federal Way Community Center)

5. Give a detailed summary of a coaching philosophy.

6. How does a new coach develop a coaching philosophy?

7. What does it mean to coach ethically?

8. How can you create a coaching philosophy that is compatible with your personality?

Projects and Activities

1. Create your own coaching code of ethics. This should be a detailed working document that can be used at a later date.

2. Develop your own personal coaching philosophy. This should be a detailed working document that can be used at a later date.

3. Think back on all of the coaches you had in sports. Which coach was your favorite? Why? What was this coach's code of ethics and philosophy?

Website Resources

SportsKids: http://www.SportsKids.com

National Federation of State High School Associations: http://www.nfhs.org

Gatorade Sports Science Institute: http://www.gssiweb.com/

National Collegiate Athletic Association (NCAA): http://www.ncaa.org

International Association of Athletics Federations: http://www.iaaf.org

The Roles of the Assistant and Head Coach

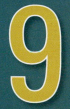

Objectives

Upon completion of this chapter, the reader should be able to:

- Describe the roles of the assistant and head coach.
- Explain how defining goals and measuring results are important in coaching.
- Discuss the important attributes that make a successful coach.
- Explain the importance of state and national coaching standards.

Key Terms

Coaches

Coaching evaluations

Coaching standards

Communication skills

Conflict resolution

Decisiveness

Delegation

Goals

Influence

Initiative

Motivation

Sportsmanship

Teamwork

The Assistant and Head Coaches

Coaches provide a range of critical leadership capabilities. First and foremost, coaches provide leadership in the guidance and motivation of student-athletes. Win, lose, or draw, the athletic experience should be a constructive life lesson in working hard to accomplish goals, supporting teammates during stressful times, and celebrating the effort. Student-athletes deserve the opportunity to compete in a context that values hard work, achievement, and respect for all concerned (Figure 9-1).

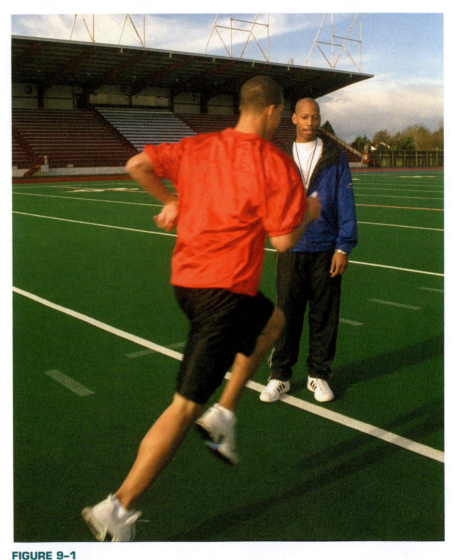

FIGURE 9–1
Personal trainers work one-on-one with athletes to pinpoint training needs and build strength and endurance.

Coaches further provide leadership through their faculty colleagues. Principals, school staff, athletic directors, and assistant coaches all want their student-athletes to exemplify behaviors of strong teamwork, competitive spirit, and good sportsmanship. A smooth, collaborative effort is required to produce optimum results. Coaches orchestrate this team effort and, in turn, take responsibility for the outcome.

Coaches confront the challenge of sustaining a well-coordinated support system with the parents of their athletes. Parents have a strong and often emotionally-vested interest in seeing their child succeed. They have been known to express their enthusiasm in a manner which is not always in accord with the coach's plans or values. Responsibility for educating parents, and transforming them into allies who advocate appropriate values, rests squarely with the coach (Figure 9-2).

Most great coaches have simple goals: improve the performance of their student athletes and, by doing so, enable them to experience a sense

> ● **KEY CONCEPT** ●
>
> Responsibility for educating parents, and transforming them into allies who advocate appropriate values, rests squarely with the coach.

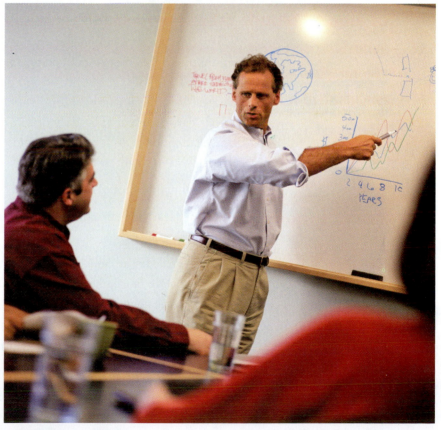

FIGURE 9–2
Coaches leadership skills are often called upon to help engage or motivate staff. (Courtesy of Photodisc)

of pride that accompanies achievement. Coaches further seek to field teams that demonstrate respect for each other, their teammates, and the sport. All too easily, coaches can get seduced into focusing more energy on improving their win/loss ratio than on the experience of the student athletes. Success in coaching has much more to do with character development than it does with counting trophies.

The Coaching Challenge

Individuals approach new challenges with a range of different attitudes. Some relish a new test of their skills and embrace the opportunity to find solutions to novel problems. Others tend toward a more conservative approach, preferring to accumulate confidence by mastering one new task at a time.

Coaching presents a consistent diet of new challenges. Your attitude about dealing with new challenges will influence your success and, most likely, the future path of your career.

Defining Goals and Measuring Results

Well-defined **goals** focus energy and attention. Research has consistently demonstrated that clearly-defined goals provide coherent direction to behavior and actually create incentives for achievement. Coaches need to define skill-achievement goals and time frames for athletes, so that they have a clear picture of what they need to strive for. When coaches articulate well-defined goals for a team, athletes have a clear, common vision of what they need to accomplish (Figure 9-3).

> **● KEY CONCEPT ●**
>
> Well-defined goals focus energy and attention.

The following should be considered when clarifying goals:

- Is it clear how an athlete's goals are designed to complement the teams' goals?

- Are goals for athletes sufficiently challenging? Appreciate that there are a wide range of individual variations with regard to what represents a challenging goal. You should be able to describe how different athletes vary with regard to their readiness for different challenges.

- Are the goals realistic and attainable? Individual athletes and teams should have an excellent chance of achieving goals they set.

- Do individual athletes have a solid plan for how to achieve their goals?

- Does the team have goals that change over time? For example, do you engineer the team's performance to peak at the end of the season.

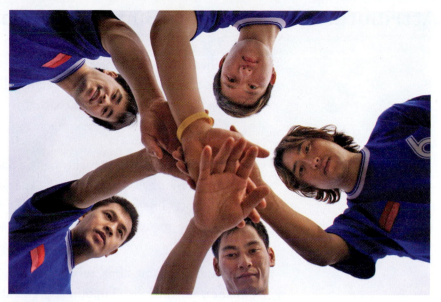

FIGURE 9–3
Goals and teamwork help focus energy to provide for a positive outcome. (Courtesy of PunchStock)

Gauging Results

Gauging results in the coaching profession can be a highly controversial topic. Is success measured in terms of your win/loss record? It's difficult to argue that winning doesn't matter. However, success when coaching student-athletes really boils down to creating conditions under which athletes experience a sense of pride and accomplishment from achieving personal goals and experiencing team success.

Results may come in the form of increased self-confidence. Results may come in the form of inspired teamwork, even if it does not produce a consistent winning record. Teaching young athletes to respect themselves, respect others, pursue competitive success with a passion, and have fun doing it represents success.

Building a solid relationship with each athlete sets the stage for a positive sports experience. Setting appropriate goals gives athletes the opportunity to experience success. Further, athletes need consistent and structured feedback to understand what they do well and what they need to do differently in order to improve.

Coaches inspire and motivate athletes in a variety of ways. Some are consistently positive; others are more strenuous and outspoken. Whatever your style, make sure that you preserve the dignity of the athlete and instill the belief that he or she is capable of better things. Help them experience the sense of pride that comes with consistent improvement of their performance.

Attributes That Make a Successful Coach

Coaches accomplish their goals with a variety of techniques. Different people get results with different styles. The following attributes can help define the assistant and head coach.

Decisiveness

Obviously, coaches must make many decisions on the spot. The quality of those decisions is a function of experience, intuition, and knowledge. People have different ways of preparing for the moment when decisions have to be made. Some spend hours analyzing relevant information. Others rely mostly on their gut instinct.

Studying game films, reviewing data about athletes and team performance, and analysis of opponents, can all help make informed decisions. Are you more analytical and reflective, or are you likely to use your intuitive expertise to guide your decisions?

Communications

• KEY CONCEPT •

Perhaps no other skill is as important to success in coaching as is communication.

Perhaps no other skill is as important to success in coaching as is communication. Developing strong connections to your athletes, working collegially with the coaching and athletic staff, and relating to school administration and staff all require highly developed **communication skills**. It's essential to assess the effectiveness of your communication tactics. Getting direct feedback is the best way to accomplish that.

Interpersonal Skills: Influence and Initiative

Coaches provide leadership in many ways:

- By modeling behavior that includes an optimistic attitude and good **sportsmanship**.
- By utilizing ongoing analysis of strategies, players, and opponents.
- By setting appropriate goals for achievement.
- By motivating individual athletes and inspiring the team to higher levels of performance.
- By modeling positive stress-management behaviors.
- By showing respect for teammates and opponents.
- By responding to losses with renewed determination and perseverance.

To inspire others requires strong **motivation** to function in a position of authority and influence, the skillful use of influence tactics, and the constant readiness to initiate action. This motivational characteristic can be the starting point for notable success.

Coaches often bring a personal sense of mission to their role and start with a strong commitment to help student-athletes achieve new levels of performance. The best coaches tailor their tactics to the specific needs of different individuals and situations. There is no way to understand those specific needs unless you are skilled at listening to the way that your athletes think about different situations.

Influence

Being able to **influence** others represents another critical competency for successful coaching leadership. Coaches often find themselves in a situation where they need to persuade or motivate athletes to accomplish specific tasks; this ability is essential when teaching, motivating and supporting athletes. Coaches with the ability to influence others are often successful because they can get athletes to focus on priority goals and to collaborate in order to achieve those goals.

Initiative

Initiative is an essential leadership behavior for coaches. Planning and goal setting represent critical blueprints for action, but initiative makes a vital contribution to translating those plans into goal-directed behavior. Taking initiative incites action on the part of others. Coaches model positive problem-solving techniques by taking the initiative to improve processes that need to work more effectively.

Teamwork, Delegation, and Conflict Resolution

Successful leaders are gifted at mobilizing people's energy to work toward the achievement of a common goal. Coaches have to build teams constantly. The athletic team needs to believe in the importance of the common interest above individual glory. Similarly, coaches and parents form an alliance for the benefit of the student-athlete. School officials, including the principal, teachers, athletic director, and coaches, act in concert to create a supportive educational experience for students and to promote a positive image of the school. Coaches play a central, and often pivotal, role in the formation and sustenance of all these teams.

To make this happen, coaches need to delegate responsibility, either implicitly or explicitly, to athletes, parents, and colleagues. As with all teams with a great deal at stake, conflicts arise out of differences in perspective. How those conflicts are managed has a substantive impact on the quality of **teamwork**. Developing sophisticated skill in each of these areas can help coaches and student-athletes achieve goals born of mutual interest and commitment.

Teamwork

Teams need leaders to take initiative and emphasize the mutual benefits of supporting a collaborative effort. Coaches are perceived as models for team play and will be expected to show and model teamwork with parents and colleagues, working toward a common goal. As Andrew Carnegie once said, "Teamwork is the ability to work together toward a common vision. The ability to direct individual accomplishments toward organizational objectives. It is the fuel that allows common people to attain uncommon results."

Delegation

As the head coach, it is important to hand off responsibility for component pieces of the coaching process. This allows the head coach, in essence, to be in more than one place at a time. No coach can do everything him- or herself; the coach who fails to delegate is destined to fail. As a head coach, you will need to develop effective systems for enabling others to achieve the same results that you would produce if you did it yourself. This doesn't mean that you assign a new coach critical duties, such as play-calling or defensive strategy. Assistant coaches need to grow with your program. Delegate simple tasks at first; Later, when you feel the assistant coach is ready for more important tasks, allow them to take on more important duties. With **delegation** comes the commitment to perform at a high level and to take responsibility when things go wrong.

The head coach must act as teacher and mentor to all of the coaches and people involved with his or her program. Anyone can make a mistake or make the wrong call. Part of the success of the program as a whole is how the head coach handles these situations. Assistant coaches are adults that have a great deal of pride in what they are trying to accomplish. If the head coach comes down hard on an assistant for making a mistake, he will probably lose the respect of that coach—and possibly the other coaches as well.

Delegation also brings with it ownership in the program as a whole. It is critical that your assistant coaches feel that they are important to the success of the overall program. You will notice that the most successful programs are those with coaching staffs that have been together for many years. It is important that the people to whom you delegate have the resources they need to succeed.

Conflict Resolution

Coaches will be called on to resolve conflicts several times during a season. Most will be minor disagreements among players, but others may be significant. It is important that coaches respect the emotional realities of the situation and work toward a mutual resolution. To respect those emotional realities, you will have to spend time listening to different perspectives. Understanding the following points will help increase the chance that your **conflict resolution** tactics will be successful.

Consider the following in creating structure for resolving conflict:

- Do not suggest that serious conflicts be hashed out without a structured process to resolve differences. Find a skilled facilitator to help.

- Make sure that all parties really want to achieve a solution. If one party lacks the motivation to resolve the conflict, chances are good that progress will be slow and painstaking.

- Emphasize common interests. In most cases, both parties have a stake in producing common outcomes.

- Discourage blaming behavior and scapegoating. Encourage both parties to consider what behavior of theirs has contributed to the conflict.

- Encourage parties to be candid and diplomatic. Brutal verbal assaults do not help the process of resolving conflicts.

- Encourage both parties to move beyond global negative characterizations and describe specific behaviors that are problematic.

- Encourage both parties to articulate how they interpreted the other person's behavior. Frequently, someone's interpretation does not match up with the other party's intentions.

- Attempt to stay in the present. Dredging up ancient history rarely helps in making progress.

- Explore several different options as part of a resolution. Avoid having to choose one party's solution or the other.

- Try to incorporate suggestions from both sides in recommending a path forward. Give everyone something they want.

- Get each party to make an explicit verbal statement that they will positively contribute to a solution.

- Provide for followup. Commit to revisiting the issue to check on progress.

Job Descriptions for Assistant and Head Coaches

Table 9-1 and Table 9-2 give sample job descriptions that may be encountered when applying for a coaching position.

TABLE 9-1 Sample Head Coach Job Description

Title: Head Athletic Coach

Qualifications:

1. Has the ability to organize and supervise a total sports program.

2. Has previous successful coaching experience in the assigned sport.

3. Must have substantial knowledge of the technical aspects of the sport and, at the same time, must continue to examine new theories and procedures pertinent to the field.

Reports to: The athletic director, who provides overall objectives and final evaluation in conjunction with the high school principals.

Supervises: A staff of high school assistant coaches and middle school coaches (in conjunction with the athletic director and respective principal).

Job Goals:

To instruct athletes in the fundamental skills, strategy, and physical training necessary for them to realize individual and team success. To assist athletes in the formulation of moral values, pride of accomplishment, acceptable social behavior, self-discipline, and self-confidence. To upgrade his or her knowledge and skills through coaching clinics, observations, consultation.

General:

1. The success of athletic programs has a strong influence on the community's image of the entire system. The public exposure is a considerable responsibility and community/parent pressure for winning performance is taxing, but must not override the objectives of good sportsmanship and good mental health.

2. The position includes other unusual aspects such as extended time, risk injury factor, and due process predicaments.

3. It is the express intent of this job description to give sufficient guidance to function. In cases not specifically covered, it shall be assumed that a coach shall exercise common sense and good judgment.

TABLE 9-1 *Continued*

Duties and responsibilities:

1. Has a thorough knowledge of all the athletic policies approved by the Board of Education and is responsible for their implementation by the entire staff of the sports program.

2. Has knowledge of existing system, state, and league regulations; implements same consistently and interprets them for staff.

3. Understands the proper administrative line of command and refers all requests or grievances through proper channels. Is aware of all public, staff, and departmental meetings that require attendance.

Staff responsibilities:

1. Establishes the fundamental philosophy, skills, and techniques to be taught by staff. Designs conferences, clinics, and staff meetings to ensure staff awareness of overall program.

2. Trains and informs staff, encourages professional growth by encouraging clinic attendance according to local clinic policy.

3. Delegates specific duties, supervises implementation, and, at season's end, analyzes staff effectiveness and evaluates all assistants.

4. Maintains discipline, adjusts grievances, and works to increase morale and cooperation.

5. Performs other duties as assigned by the athletic director or principal.

Administrative duties:

1. Assists the athletic director in scheduling, providing transportation, and developing requirements for tournaments and special sport events.

2. Assists in the necessary preparations for scheduled sport events or practices; adheres to scheduled facility times. Coordinates program with maintenance and school employees.

3. Provides documentation to fulfill state and system requirements concerning physical examinations, parental consent, and eligibility.

4. Provides proper safeguards for maintenance and protection of assigned equipment sites.

5. Advises the athletic director and recommends policy, method, or procedural changes.

Student responsibilities:

1. Provides training rules, and any other unique regulations of the sport, to each athlete who is considered a participant.

2. Gives constant attention to a student athlete's grades and conduct.

3. By his or her presence at all practices, games, and while traveling, provides assistance, guidance, and safeguards for each participant.

Continued

TABLE 9-1 *Continued*

4. Initiates programs and policies concerning injuries, medical attention, and emergencies.

5. Completes paperwork on all disabling athletic injuries on proper forms and submits to athletic office within 24 hours.

6. Directs student managers, assistants, and statisticians.

7. Determines discipline, delineates procedures concerning due process when the enforcement of discipline is necessary, and contacts parents when a student is dropped or becomes ineligible.

8. Assists athletes in their college or advanced educational selection.

Finance and equipment:

1. Participates in the budgeting process with the athletic director by establishing requirements for the next season. Recommends equipment guidelines as to type, style, color, or technical specifications. Is responsible for operating within budget appropriations.

2. Is accountable for all equipment and collects the cost of any equipment lost or not returned. Arranges for issuing, storing, and reconditioning of equipment, and submits annual inventory and current records concerning same.

3. Properly marks and identifies all equipment before issuing or storing.

4. Monitors equipment rooms and coaches' offices; authorizes who may enter, issue, or requisition equipment.

5. Permits athletes to be in authorized areas of the building only at appropriate times.

6. Examines locker rooms before and after practices and games, checking on general cleanliness of the facility. Responsible for cleanliness and maintenance of specific sport equipment.

7. Secures all doors, lights, windows, and locks before leaving building (if custodians are not on duty).

8. Instills in each player a respect for equipment and school property, its care and proper use.

Public relations:

1. Organizes preseason meetings for parents, coaches, players, and guests.

2. Promotes the sport within the school through recruiting athletes who are not in another sports program. Promotes the sport outside the school through news media, Little League programs, or in any other feasible manner.

3. Responsible for the quality, effectiveness, and validity of any oral or written release to local media.

4. Responsible for maintaining good public relations with news media, booster club, parents, officials, volunteers, and fans.

5. Presents information to news media concerning schedules, tournaments, and results.

TABLE 9-2 Sample Assistant Coach Job Description

Title: Assistant and/or Junior High Coach

Responsible to: Head coach, athletic director, and principal

Function: To cooperate with the head coach in the assigned interscholastic sport in maintaining a quality program within the policy framework of the school district.

Duties:

1. cooperate with the head coach, athletic director, and the principal in performing the following duties related to the school athletic program.

2. Assure that players under his or her jurisdiction understand the training rule policy. The signed parental permission form shall be in the hands of the coach or athletic office prior to an athlete beginning practice. All parental forms are to be returned to the athletic director.

3. Support the head coach in conducting the athletic program of that particular sport and the overall athletic program of the school district.

4. Remain loyal to the head coach and to the team. May have to give up some personal opinions or ideas (for example regarding team strategy), in order to fit into the overall pattern as set forth by the head coach.

5. Attend all practices for the entire season, as well as all staff meetings and scouting assignments.

6. Assume the responsibility for maintenance of facilities and personnel in the absence of the head coach.

7. Report all injuries, misconduct, or other unusual situations to the head coach, athletic director, or principal.

8. Assist the head coach in checking in and inventorying all equipment at the end of the season.

9. Assume all duties as assigned by the head coach.

10. Complete and return a Coach's Annual Report form to the athletic director within two weeks after the last contest.

11. Complete and return a supplemental pay voucher to the athletic director after all responsibilities have been fulfilled.

12. Perform other duties as assigned by the head coach or athletic director.

13. Complete all requirements mandated by the State and National organizations.

Defining the term "coaching" is complicated by the fact that those persons affected by the ability and influence of a coach perceive the coach differently. The school administrator views the coach as the teacher who directs the competitive play and behavior of all athletes who represent the school. The team sees the coach as a highly skilled teacher who builds game skills, teaches competitive play, and fosters an appreciation for both virtue in cooperation and excellence in competition.

Coaching is highly skilled teaching of a limited number of individuals. Coaching develops skills beyond the fundamentals and combines the abilities of individuals into a team effort with the focus on enthusiastic competition in the spirit of fair play, good sportsmanship, and friendship. The experience and demands of competitive play are complex; all persons concerned undergo a degree of intensity of effort and psychological stress.

The following is a list of topics designed to assist the coach in preparing for the competitive season.

- Coaching is in-depth teaching of the advanced skills and strategies of the sport.
- Coaching requires expert knowledge of the sport.
- The coach must be willing to be a specialist.
- The coach must be willing to devote a large amount of time to a relatively small group of students.
- A coach must be sensitive, firm, insightful, adaptable, and flexible.
- A coach must be consistent.

Personal Knowledge

Every coach needs to refresh and review before beginning the season. This may consist of concentrated reading, attending workshops or clinics, or visiting other coaches and teams to observe and ask questions. Many theories of play and techniques of skills and strategy change over time. It is the coach's responsibility to be aware of changes.

Coaching Standards

The coaching profession is bolstered by local, state, and national standards that require coaches to meet qualifying standards prior to working with athletes. Table 9-3 shows the national standards for athletic coaches as the result of a consensus project facilitated by the National Association for Sport and Physical Education (NASPE).

The Washington Interscholastic Activities Association (WIAA) has set specific **coaching standards** that must be met by all individuals who wish to coach in the state of Washington. These standards are an example of what is being expected of coaches throughout the nation. Table 9-4 lists these standards.

TABLE 9-3 NASPE National Coaching Standards

The National Standards for Athletic Coaches are the result of a consensus project facilitated by the National Association for Sport and Physical Education (NASPE), an association of the American Alliance for Health, Physical Education, Recreation and Dance (AAHPERD).

These standards and competencies are viewed as part of a dynamic compilation of the knowledge, skills, and values that are associated with the effective and appropriate coaching of athletes. New information will demand that this document be reviewed and updated on a regular basis. The overriding premise in the development of this document is that its contents be used to ensure the enjoyment, safety, and positive skill development of America's athletes.

It is not intended that the National Standards for Athletic Coaches be a certification program or be the basis of a single national assessment for all coaches. The Standards are put forth to help organizations and agencies who currently certify coaches, provide coach education/training, evaluate select coaches, or design programs to meet the needs of prospective and practicing coaches. Also, the standards are not sport-specific. Therefore, it will continue to be the role and responsibility of all sport-sponsoring organizations to develop appropriate sport-and situation-specific programs using the National Standards for Athletic Coaches as a basis or framework for program design.

Description of Coaching Levels:

The 37 standards are grouped in eight domains and appropriate competencies are identified to further define and delineate the meaning of each standard. The eight domains are as follows:

- Injuries: prevention, care, and management
- Risk management
- Growth, development, and learning
- Training, conditioning, and nutrition
- Social/psychological aspects of coaching
- Skills, tactics, and strategies

Continued

TABLE 9-3 Continued

- Teaching and administration
- Professional Preparation and Development

Domain: Injuries: Prevention, Care, and Management
Standard 1
Prevent injuries by recognizing and insisting on safe playing conditions.

Standard 2
Ensure that protective equipment is in good condition, fits properly, and is worn as prescribed by the manufacturer; ensure that equipment and facilities meet required standards [American Society for Testing Materials, (ASTM) and U.S. Consumer Product Safety Commission, (USCPSC)].

Standard 3
Recognize that proper conditioning and good health are vital to the prevention of athletic injuries.

Standard 4
When planning and scheduling practices and contests and implementing programs for physical conditioning, minimize the risk of injuries by considering the effects of environmental conditions on the circulatory and respiratory systems.

Standard 5
Be able to plan, coordinate, and implement procedures for appropriate emergency care.

Standard 6
Demonstrate skill in the prevention, recognition, and evaluation of injuries and the ability to assist athletes with the recovery and rehabilitation from injuries that are generally associated with participation in athletics in accordance with guidelines provided by qualified medical personnel.

Standard 7
Facilitate a unified medical program of prevention, care, and management of injuries by coordinating the roles and actions of the coach and a National Athletic Trainers Association (NATA) certified athletic trainer with those of the physician.

Standard 8
Educate coaching assistants, athletes and parents/guardians about injury prevention, injury reporting, and sources of medical care.

Domain: Risk Management
Standard 9
Understand the scope of legal responsibilities that accompanies a coaching position, i.e. proper supervision, planning and instruction, matching participants, safety, first aid, and risk management.

TABLE 9-3 *Continued*

Standard 10

Properly inform coaching assistants, athletes, and parents/guardians of the inherent risks associated with sports so that decisions about participation can be made with informed consent.

Standard 11

Know and convey the need for, and availability of, appropriate medical insurance.

Standard 12

Participate in continuing education regarding rules changes, improvements in equipment, philosophical changes, improved techniques, and other information in order to enhance the safety and success of the athlete.

Domain: Growth, Development and Learning

Standard 13

Recognize the developmental and physical changes that occur as athletes move from youth through adulthood; know how these changes influence the sequential learning and performance of motor skills in a specific sport.

Standard 14

Understand the social and emotional development of the athletes being coached, know how to recognize problems related to this development, and know where to refer them for appropriate assistance when necessary.

Standard 15

Analyze human performance in terms of developmental information and individual body structure.

Standard 16

Provide instruction to develop sport-specific motor skills and refer the athletes to appropriate counsel as needed.

Standard 17

Provide learning experiences appropriate to the growth and development of the age group being coached.

Domain: Training, Conditioning, and Nutrition

Standard 18

Demonstrate a basic knowledge of physiological systems and their responses to training and conditioning.

Standard 19

Design programs of training and conditioning that properly incorporate the mechanics of movement and sound physiological principles, taking into account each individual's ability and medical history,

Continued

TABLE 9-3 *Continued*

avoiding contra-indicated exercises and activities, and guarding against the possibility of overtraining; be able to modify programs as needed.

Standard 20
Demonstrate knowledge of proper nutrition; educate athletes about the effects of nutrition upon health and physical performance.

Standard 21
Demonstrate knowledge of the use and abuse of drugs, and promote sound chemical health.

Domain: Social/Psychological Aspects of Coaching
Standard 22
Subscribe to a philosophy that acknowledges the role of athletics in developing the complete person.

Standard 23
Identify and interpret the values that are to be developed from participation in sports programs to coaches, athletes, concerned others, and the general public.

Standard 24
Identify and apply ethical conduct in sports by maintaining emotional control and demonstrating respect for athletes, officials, and other coaches.

Standard 25
Demonstrate effective motivational skills and provide positive, appropriate feedback.

Standard 26
Conduct practices and competitions to enhance the physical, social, and emotional growth of athletes.

Standard 27
Be sufficiently familiar with the basic principles of goal-setting to motivate athletes toward immediate and long-range goals.

Standard 28
Treat each athlete as an individual while recognizing the dynamic relationship of personality and sociocultural variables such as gender, race, and socioeconomic differences.

Standard 29
Identify desirable behaviors (self discipline, support of teammates, following directions, etc.) and structure experiences to develop such behaviors in each athlete.

Domain: Skills, Tactics, and Strategies
Standard 30
Identify and apply specific competitive tactics and strategies appropriate for the age and skill levels involved.

TABLE 9-3 *Continued*

Standard 31
Organize and implement materials for scouting, planning practices, and analysis of games.

Standard 32
Understand and enforce the rules and regulations of appropriate bodies that govern sports and education.

Standard 33
Organize, conduct, and evaluate practice sessions with regard to established program goals that are appropriate for different stages of the season.

Domain: Teaching and Administration
Standard 34
Know the key elements of sport principles and technical skills as well as the various teaching methods that can be used to introduce and refine them.

Standard 35
Demonstrate objective and effective procedures for the evaluation and selection of personnel involved in the athletic program and for periodic program reviews.

Domain: Professional Preparation and Development
Standard 36
Demonstrate organizational and administrative efficiency in implementing sports programs, such as event management, budgetary procedures, facility maintenance, and participation in public relations activities.

Standard 37
Acquire sufficient practical field experience and supervision in the essential coaching areas to ensure an adequate level of coaching competence for the level of athlete coached. This would include a variety of knowledge, skills, and experiences.

TABLE 9-4 Washington State Coaching Standards

Purpose: The purpose of the Washington Interscholastic Activities Association (WIAA) Coaching Standards program is to enhance the training of student-athletes by assuring that their coaches maintain a certain level of professional development throughout their careers.

Requirements: A coach is required, prior to the beginning of his or her third year of coaching, to 1) complete the NFHS Coaching Principles Course OR 2) participate in at least thirty (30) hours of activities, courses or programs that provide some level of professional development for the coach. After achieving this, paid high school coaches are require to maintain a minimum of fifteen (15) hours of professional development activities each three year period following the initial two year cycle. Individuals who graduate

Continued

TABLE 9-4 *Continued*

from an accredited college or university with a P.E. or coaching major or minor (or hold a P.E. endorsement on his or her teaching certificate) are exempt from the initial 30 hour requirement.

In addition to meeting the above requirements, each coach must also maintain a current CPR/First Aid card (and Red Cross Safety Training for Swim Coaches), a Washington State Patrol criminal background check, an OSPI Character/Fitness Supplement, be 21 years of age if head coach, (19 years if assistant coach), and attend a WIAA/WOA Rules Clinic (if a high school varsity head coach).

Qualifying activities: WIAA maintains standards only in terms of the number of hours required; beyond that, it is up to the administration of the member schools to determine which activities qualify toward the 30/15 hour marks (aside from the aforementioned Coaching Principles Course, which automatically qualifies for the middle level mark and counts toward initial or continuing high school standards). The types of activities that are typically qualified toward the coaching hours requirements include, but are not limited to, the following:

- WIAA rules clinics
- League coaches meetings
- Chemical awareness training
- Sports psychology courses

- CPR/first aid training
- In-school coaching staffing
- WIAA/school policy review
- Injury prevention/rehab course

- Sport-specific clinics
- Liability training
- Coaching roundtables
- Motivation training

Documentation: Each year, every WIAA member school is required to file with the WIAA office an overview of compliance for each coach, paid and volunteer, that coaches for that school. Each coach is required to maintain his or her own records of activities taken to meet the hour requirements and to provide a copy of such documentation to the school for compliance records.

School standards: Each school must have at least 80% of its coaching staff in compliance with the above-stated requirements in order for that school to meet WIAA compliance. Each school must also provide a plan to attain 100% compliance. For schools not in compliance, a progressive penalty is incurred.

Coaching Evaluations

There are two primary types of evaluations: head coaches evaluating their assistants and head coaches being evaluated by the athletic director. Both types of evaluations are important indicators of the coach's success during the season. Evaluations serve two purposes. The first is to inform the coach about how he or she performed in a number of different categories, and the second is to help the athletic director decide whether or not to retain the coach for the next season.

Assistant Coach Evaluations

In most school districts, head coaches evaluate their assistants. The primary reason for this is obvious: the head coach has worked closely with his or her assistants all season long. In some districts, the athletic director evaluates all assistant coaches with direct input from the head coach. Both methods are effective and both require careful thought and detailed analysis.

The evaluation process must not be rushed. Coaches need to take as much time evaluating the strengths and weaknesses of their assistants as they do planning for their next opponent. This takes time, but the benefits of a well-thought-out evaluation will reap rewards down the line. The assistant coaching evaluation should specify very specific strengths and weaknesses the coach possesses. The specifics should include everything from preseason work through the final season meeting. This type of detail will assist the coach in preparing for the next season. Coaches that avoid listing weaknesses risk problems or litigation if there is ever reason to fire or (in the example given next) hire the coach.

For example, a head coach had a volunteer coach that worked for him for two years. The volunteer came to practice as much as he could, but didn't make it to team meetings or special events. The head coach went along with this because it allowed another adult with the background in the sport to help out with drills and coaching. A paid assistant position became available the next year. The volunteer applied for the position, but wasn't hired. The volunteer filed a grievance and fought hard to have the decision reversed, claiming that he didn't have any problem areas (except missing an occasional practice and meetings) listed on his evaluation. Since the volunteer coach wasn't being paid, the head coach had not been critical in his evaluation. If the head coach had given the volunteer an honest, detailed evaluation, this situation might not have happened.

A written evaluation is only the first step in evaluating coaches. The head coach must set up a private meeting with all of his or her assistants after the evaluations have been written. Evaluations should give the head coach and assistants an opportunity to end up on the same page when the evaluation meeting is over. This meeting should be constructive and allow both sides to explain how they perceived the season went. If the evaluation needs to be revised after the meeting is held, this is fine. Often a clearer picture arises once both sides have time to talk out specific items. Once the evaluation is complete, both the head and assistant coach will sign, date, and deliver it to the athletic director for his or her signature. Figure 9-4 is a sample of a coaching evaluation form.

COACHING EVALUATION FORM

Personal Information:

Coach_____Sport_____Position_____

Total years experience as Head Coach_____Assistant_____Salary Placement_____

CPR expires_____First Aid expires_____Date of Pathogen training_____

Sports Rules Clinic_____ Approved coaching hours past year_____

Other courses or clinics_____ Student Survey Completed_____

Collaborative Assessment:

	Needs Improvement	Meets Expectations	Exceeds Expectations
Coaching Skills (instruction, strategy, game management, etc.)	☐	☐	☐
Organizational Skills (equipment, budget, supervision, etc.)	☐	☐	☐
Professional Relations (faculty, peers, media, etc.)	☐	☐	☐
Student/Parent Relations	☐	☐	☐
Personal Characteristics (poise, enthusiasm, commitment, etc.)	☐	☐	☐

Comments _____
_____
_____

Coaching Goals_____
_____
_____

Overall Performance Assessment:

Satisfactory ☐   Needs Improvement ☐   Unsatisfactory ☐

_____   _____   _____
Signature of Athletic Director   Signature of Coach   Date

_____   _____
Signature of Principal   Date

Recommendation to Rehire: *(Does not apply to positions added based on numbers.)

Yes ☐   Yes ☐

FIGURE 9–4
Sample coaching evaluation that would be used to assess a coach's performance during the past season

Head Coach Evaluation

Most head coaches are evaluated by their athletic director. The athletic director has the responsibility to maintain a focused and educationally sound athletic program. This includes all aspects of every sport in the school. Head coaches will be evaluated on their performance in numerous areas involving their sport. These areas include, but are not limited to supervision of athletes and coaches, implementing local, state, and national rules and regulations, school and public relations, discipline, practice and game schedules, training rules, medical protocols, budgets, equipment, facility management, relationship with the press, and knowledge of their sport.

CASE STUDY: SPORTSMANSHIP, A SECOND PERSPECTIVE

"Targeting Sportsmanship"

Reprinted with permission from the June 2006 issue of *The School Administrator.*

Superintendent David Prescott heard about the verbal pressure, the parents calling coaches to complain about the player who wasn't any good, the play they couldn't comprehend, and the playing time their kids didn't get. He witnessed the bad behavior of raucous spectators at sporting events heckling and ranting vitriol under the watchful eye of impressionable youngsters.

He grew concerned as good coaches resigned and others threatened to, and he noticed that able coaching prospects often were reluctant to step up to the plate because it was not worth their time and sanity to withstand the berating and taunting of out-of-bounds spectators. "We have actually asked people to leave sporting events, but it doesn't necessarily mean it's going to be better the next time," says Prescott, superintendent of the 3,700-student Albert Lea Area Schools in south-central Minnesota. "Most people will cool it when you talk to them. But the others, you can pick them out because they're usually sitting alone because nobody wants to sit with them. And what they yell certainly doesn't set the right tone for our students."

Behavioral Rules

Spurred on by incidents of bad sportsmanship, the Albert Lea district, working through a committee of stakeholders, published a set of standards that spell out for players, coaches, students, parents, and community members the school district's expectations for good sportsmanship at interscholastic athletic events. Taking effect this year with the winter season, players and their coaches and families were asked to sign, before play commenced, a compact to uphold the principles of appropriate behavior relative to each group. A parent, for example, signs a promise not to berate or taunt officials, coaches or opposing teams; a coach signs a promise not to force athletes to specialize too soon in one sport at the expense of all others.

The document, titled "Athletics the Right Way," was influenced by last year's "Sports Done Right" report produced at the University of Maine. It takes a broad look at a myriad of issues involving many groups—with a notable focus on spectators at interscholastic sports events in Albert Lea.

Indeed, many school districts have begun to use the comprehensive "Sports Done Right" report, which emphasizes seven core principles and supporting core practices for creating an environment conducive to "discipline, respect, responsibility, fairness, trustworthiness and good citizenship." The report identifies "out-of-bounds" issues—troubling trends in behavior on and off the field that should be remedied.

"The biggest problem we have at interscholastic events is with parents; because how do we discipline parents?" Prescott says. "We don't have much control over them. What we're trying to do with this document is encourage peer pressure from other parents. Parents know appropriate behavior, and when they see inappropriate behavior, we hope they will intercede."

When push comes to shove, however, Dudley says a school district's best defense lies with its coaching staff. Having capable basketball coaches, she says, is what prevented the fan fracas in February from becoming something worse and that allowed her student athletes an opportunity to demonstrate their poise under pressure, which she reinforced with praise at the school board meeting.

"The coach is one of the more important parts of your team," Dudley says. "They set the standards. They set the expectations, they model those expectations and they work with the kids every day. Our job is much more than coaching a team and winning a ball game. We're raising children. It's a big responsibility and we have a hand in how those children turn out and what kind of adults they become. We need to take that obligation seriously."

Chapter Summary

The role of the assistant and head coach is varied; good coaches are crucial to the success of the overall sports program. Coaches wear many hats, and are responsible for creating an environment in which the athlete can grow and mature as a player.

Coaches work closely with School administration, with staff, and with parents. Strong communication skills are necessary in order to gain everyone's "buy-in" to the coach's goals and to "their" team. The greater the coach's communication skills, the greater the success the program will have.

Creating an atmosphere of teamwork with the entire coaching staff will help everyone feel closely connected to the overall outcome of the program. Head coaches need to develop trust in their assistants by delegating responsibilities of the program. As trust is earned, more important responsibilities can be delegated to assistants.

Assistant coaches need to be loyal to the head coach and project an image of respect and professionalism. Assistants can often mitigate conflicts that players and parents have with the head coach. This is done through supporting the head coach and helping parents and players understand why certain decisions are made.

Overall, coaching young athletes is an exciting and highly meaningful endeavor. It's well worth the time and the hard work to see athletes progress and accomplish their goals. Some of the greatest memories athletes have in their lives are of coaches who cared, motivated them, and were willing to listen.

Chapter Review Questions

1. Write a detailed job description of an assistant and head coach.

2. In your opinion, what are the top five characteristics of a head coach?

3. How does an assistant coach support the head coach and the athletic program?

4. What are some of the challenges that coaches experience today?

5. What types of goals are most effective in individual and team sports?

6. How do coaches clarify goals to their athletes?

7. Once the goals have been set, how do you gauge results?

8. Why is decisiveness an important attribute of a coach?

9. If a coach is having trouble communicating with his or her team, what would you tell the coach?

10. What types of interpersonal skills are important in coaching?

11. What does teamwork mean to you?

12. Explain how delegation works and why it is important in coaching.

13. What is conflict resolution? Why is it important in coaching?

14. How can coaching standards elevate the status of coaches?

15. How does the assistant and head coach get evaluated? What's similar and what's different?

Projects and Activities

1. In Chapter 10, a few notable head coaches were mentioned by name. Select one of these coaches to write a report on. Your report should concentrate on motivation and goal setting.

2. Pick the coach you admire most from your playing past. Interview him or her about the challenges of coaching (past and present).

3. Select a book of your choice on coaching (past and present). Write a report on what you read and what you thought was important.

4. Search the Internet for information on state coaching standards. What did you find? Do the standards go far enough, or too far?

Website Resources

American Sport Education Program: http://www.asep.com

Institute for International Sport: http://www.internationalsport.com/

Josephson Institute: http://www.josephsoninstitute.org

National Alliance for Youth Sports: http://www.nays.org

National High School Coaches Association: http://nhsca.com

Positive Coaching Alliance: http://www.positivecoach.org/

Pursuing Victory with Honor program: http://www.aiaonline.org/

Working with Parents and Booster Clubs

CHAPTER 10

Objectives

Upon completion of this chapter, the reader should be able to:

- Understand the dynamics of working with parents.
- Describe the areas in which parents may have disagreements with the coach.
- Describe ways to minimize conflicts with parents.
- Explain how to run a coach-parent meeting to resolve a conflict.
- Discuss the function of an athletic booster club.
- Understand the challenges of working with booster clubs.

Key Terms

Athletic booster clubs

Title IX

Working with Parents and Booster Clubs

Of all the duties that head and assistant coaches have, the most important may be working with parents and booster clubs. Parents and booster clubs have an immediate link to the athletic program and can either help or hinder the goals of the coaching staff (Figure 10-1).

Working with Parents

Coaching can be fun and rewarding. It can be a great experience to work with young players, help them improve their skills, and watch their development over a period of time. All coaches wish all of their players could become stars. All coaches wish they could substitute people at any position without missing a beat. All coaches try their best to benefit and help their team and the individual players.

However, as hard as coaches may try, there will be mistakes. A wrong substitution, a wrong play called, or a perceived wrong call or play—whatever you can think of—it will happen at some point. Despite the best intentions, a coach will eventually draw the ire of a parent. Many

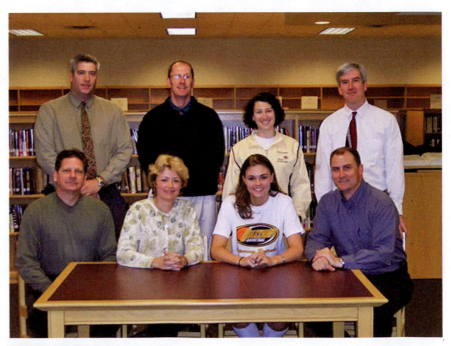

FIGURE 10–1
Student athlete receives a scholarship to continue playing sports in college.

coaches are also parents, and so understand that no parents like to see their child hurting. For example, if players play as much as they think they should, they can become upset. Many parents handle these situations very well and can get their child to understand the coach's reasoning. However, some parents immediately put the blame on the coach. Seeing their child hurting leaves them frustrated. They need to vent at someone, and since they think the coach is the one at fault, that is who is going to bear the brunt of their frustration.

The coach-parent relationship has become a very important subject, partly because of the recent increase in physical violence in coach-parent conflicts. Most coaches and parents are level-headed people. Even so, emotions can run high in many situations, especially ones involving children and athletics.

Coaches need to be careful to anticipate situations that might present problems. For an individual and a team to succeed, parents and coaches must work together. Keeping the lines of communication open will help everyone understand what is transpiring with the team.

No matter how good a coach you think you are, not all parents will agree with you 100 percent of the time. If you have a team with ten players on it, everyone will agree on some issues, but you might have ten different opinions on other issues. There are four main areas that parents have disagreements with: playing time, skills being taught, style of coaching, and competitive level of play.

> ● **KEY CONCEPT** ●
>
> Despite the best intentions, a coach will eventually draw the ire of a parent.

> ● **KEY CONCEPT** ●
>
> Playing time is the number-one topic of parent complaints.

Playing Time

Playing time is the number-one topic of parent complaints. Parents all to see their child play as much as possible. At the younger grades, this is usually not a problem. Coaches should allow all their athletes considerable play time; that's the only way they are going to learn. But in a competitive environment, some players will play more than others, especially in high school. This can lead to frustration on the part of the athlete and, in turn, the parents (Figure 10-2).

Skill Development

The skills being taught can also be a source of conflict. Parents sometimes believe that they have an advanced knowledge of the game beyond what the coach may have. Even though most, if not all, coaches stress the fundamentals, such as passing, dribbling, defense, and shooting, this will still not

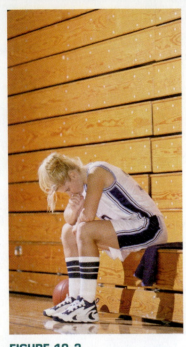

FIGURE 10-2
Balancing playing time and the needs of the team is a struggle all coaches face every season. (Courtesy of Photodisc)

satisfy everyone. Coaches need to communicate with the parents. Parents who continue to needle the coach, either face-to-face or through others, will need to be talked with rather than allowing this behavior to go further. The longer a coach puts off talking with difficult parents, the more difficult the situation will become. It may eventually become a cancer on the entire team, draining resources and energy from the coaching staff. Sometimes difficult parents just want to be involved. Allowing them to volunteer with the team in some capacity may turn an adversary into an ally.

Coaching Style

A coach's style and method of coaching can also pose a problem for some parents. Some coaches are laid back, while others are very intense. Some have strict rules to follow, while others let players come and go as they please. Some say nothing on the sidelines, while others are always yelling instructions.

Parenting styles aren't much different. Parents whose style is in conflict with the coach's may become irritated. This is normally because they don't have control over how the team is handled. This is a good topic to cover in the preseason parent meeting.

Competitive Level of Play

The competitive level of play is another potential source of conflict. As athletes progress through the competitive levels of play, from T-ball through high school, winning games becomes more important. Beginning levels of play are designed to include all players are in every game. Having fun is the number-one priority. Even so, some parents, even at the earliest levels, want to play to win every game. Some parents feel that everyone should play in every game, while others feel that playing time should be equal at all levels. This is just another possible problem area that coaches face.

How to Minimize Conflicts

What can be done to help minimize these possible conflicts? The most successful approach is to meet with the parents on your team right at the beginning of the season. Many parents want to be supportive but don't understand every sport. You must educate the parents as well as the players. Start by opening the lines of communication. Explain to parents the level of play, how much playing time their child can expect (if it's equal, or if they get a certain amount of time, or if there is no guaranteed playing time), what your goals for the season are, and what you expect of both players and parents. Fully explain any rules that you have and the level of commitment that you are expecting. Explain to parents that any concerns that they may have during a game will not be dealt with until the next day at the earliest. This will give angry parents time to cool off and rethink their concerns. Explain to parents in the preseason meeting that immediately after a game you have the players to worry about, and that you can't give the players your full attention if you are involved in another issue. However, this won't stop every parent. Even so, by telling parents up front what you expect, the number of complaints goes way down. There still will be some, but at least this way, parents can't say they weren't informed.

Consider this scenario:

Your team has just played a great game, and you walk off the court feeling proud of their effort. Just as you are exiting, a parent comes up to you, obviously upset, and says, "We need to talk right now!" What do you do? Your first reaction, being human, is to get defensive. But you can't do that in this situation; you must remain calm. If you give a loud response, or one that the parent doesn't like, the situation could escalate very quickly. A shouting match could ensue, and things could get ugly.

The best solution is to acknowledge parents and, explain that you need to be with your team. Assure parents that you are interested in their concern and you will be available to talk with them the next day. This does two things: it stops a scene from developing in front of the players and fans, and it gives both parents and coach time to collect their thoughts. If it is a simple question that you can answer right there, go ahead and do it. But if it is an involved issue or if emotions are running high, tell parents that you will gladly sit down with them at a different time and discuss it, but that you cannot discuss it at this time. As stated above, it is very important, if at all possible, not to meet with angry parents immediately following the game. If parents insist, ask the athletic director, an administrator, or an assistant coach to intervene in setting up a meeting the next day.

Parent Meeting

As explained earlier, nothing good comes of a situation in which one or both parties are not acting like adults. That is why both parents and the coach need a cooling-off period. As the coach, you now know the problem, so you can prepare an answer. The parents have now had time to cool down and be more reasonable. In the heat of the moment, hurtful things are sometimes said. By letting a day or two pass, the coach and parents can both put the situation into perspective. Cooler heads will prevail, and both sides can calmly discuss the issues at hand. This also makes it more likely that parents will listen to what the coach is saying. They may or may not agree, but at least they are listening and trying to understand the coach's point of view.

Try to meet in person, not by telephone. Phone conversations have a tendency to turn into one-sided arguments, with the other side unable to get a word in. Meet at your school in a private setting. A large office or other private setting is important to ensure that what is discussed remains private.

When meeting with a parent, it is highly recommended that you have an assistant coach, athletic director, or another adult with you in the meeting. If you are meeting with a parent of a different gender, it is also advisable to have someone of the opposite sex attend. There are two main reasons for having an additional person attend:

- First, you want someone else to hear the conversation. You don't want to be misquoted and misunderstood in a situation like this. Their main purpose is to just listen to the conversation, and get the two parties back on track if the conversation turns personal or away from the original issues being discussed. If anything else should develop, or the problem goes to the next level, that person can explain to your athletic director what took place.

- Second, you want someone else there in case there is trouble. You never know what an upset person might do, so for your own safety, make sure you have another adult there with you. It's better to be overly cautious in this situation. It is highly unlikely that anything will happen, but don't take any chances.

After you have introduced everyone, invite parents to describe their concerns to you again. Sometimes parents just need to vent to someone; let them talk as long as they need to, while you sit listening attentively. If a parent thinks you are taking their concerns seriously, that is half the battle. If you act uninterested, you are only going to make the situation worse. Don't interrupt parents while they are talking. Even if you completely disagree with their story, just listen. Don't make any facial gestures either, and don't shake your head "NO" the whole time. This will only add fuel to the fire. The only time you should interrupt is if parents are not acting in a civil manner. Personal attacks against you or the use of profanity are grounds to end the meeting. Remind parents that all of you are here to help their child, that all want to find a resolution, and that uncivil behavior is not going to help. When parents are finished talking, then you can give your response. Speak calmly and answer their questions point by point. Stick to the issues that were raised and avoid going off on a tangent. If a valid point has been raised, agree with the parents and admit you need to work on the situation. However, don't compromise your principles. If you are doing what is in the best interest of all the players, don't change everything to please one parent. Allowing one player to get away with something, or allowing a player to follow his or her own rules, will cause dissention between the other parents and the other players as well.

If parents interrupt you, remind them that you listened to their concern, and that, now they need to listen to your whole response. Also remind them that you are meeting with them with the goal of resolving any problems. You as a coach want their children to be successful just as their parents do; you are both working toward the same goal.

After you're finished talking, often parents will see that you are really trying to be helpful and will be satisfied with your answers. Many times, just the process of talking about the situation helps parents to feel better. Either way, the primary goal of the meeting is to walk away with both sides feeling satisfied.

Unfortunately, not all conferences will go that well. If you and parents can't reach an agreement, then you need to give them other options. Whether there is a conflict-management plan to refer them to, or an athletic director or school official, tell parents what their options are and how they go about pursuing them.

Working with Booster Clubs

Athletic booster clubs are an important function of today's athletic programs. As schools scramble to fund more with less, outside help is generally appreciated. The athletic booster club is a nonprofit organization made up of parents, teachers, and community members. Well-organized booster clubs can help fill the gap for a struggling athletic budget.

The role of an approved booster club is to assist and support, but not to direct, interfere with, nor supplant the staff, existing facilities, or athletics programs of the school district. It must be clearly understood by all booster club members that all school district sponsored activities are under the control, direction, and supervision of the board of school directors through its building principals and their designee, the district, and/or building athletic director. The athletic director should serve as the immediate liaison to the booster organizations.

Booster organization activities may strive to achieve the following objectives:

- To promote fan support, spirit, and sportsmanship.
- To assist the school district by providing supplemental benefits and services to student-athletes.
- To increase the opportunity for communication between parents and coaches in areas of common interest.

Before approving any booster club related to the athletic program, the athletic director, with approval from the building principal, should require a copy of the booster club's constitution and bylaws giving specifics of the purpose, functions, control, membership, and leadership selection procedures of the club. The document submitted must include the provision that the club's activities will be limited to financial and other activities in support of the school group.

The athletic director and principal who approve the organization of the booster club have the responsibility of verifying that the booster club meets the following stipulations:

- Activities of the booster club must conform to school and district regulations and must be supportive of the school program involved.
- The club must have a written statement of purpose and organizational control and procedures; these must be approved by the athletic director and principal.
- Booster clubs must have a school employee as an advisory member.
- Fund-raising activities should have the approval of the athletic director and principal. Lotteries, and other activities construed as gambling, are prohibited.
- Assets acquired through booster club fundraising must be properly accounted for, and must be deposited promptly in the name of the booster club in a local bank or savings institution, unless the activity has been approved by the Associated Student Body (ASB) cabinet for deposit in an ASB trust fund, which also requires prompt

• KEY CONCEPT •

The role of an approved booster club is to assist and support, but not to direct, interfere with, nor supplant the staff, existing facilities, or athletics programs of the school district.

deposit. School districts are not liable for the assets or obligations of any booster club.

- Booster clubs and booster club officers may not obligate the ASB or the school in any financial way. Booster club officers and members may obligate the club only in the specific manner authorized in the club's written rules.

- Promoting, advertising, selling, or giving information about booster club activities on the school premises, or through school bulletins, must have approval of the building principal.

- Individual students or staff may assist a booster club in its activities.

The difference between helping and hindering of booster clubs will be the constitution and bylaws, giving specifics of the organization's purpose, and careful oversight by the athletic director.

Booster Club Challenges

One of the challenges faced by high school athletic directors is working with parent-run booster clubs to ensure that male and female participants are being treated equitably. Booster clubs often generate considerable amounts of money; these funds are used to support athletic teams, sometimes with the oversight of the athletic director. Some booster clubs strongly resist being told how to spend "their" money. This can lead to problems when their generosity positively impacts one gender more than the other.

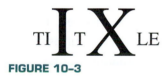

FIGURE 10-3

Title IX (chapter 15) does not require that budgets for sports be equal for each gender. In fact, the law allows schools to take into account the very real differences in outfitting athletes in equipment that is of comparable quality. Outfitting football players, for example, is more costly than outfitting field hockey players. The criteria for equality of equipment and supplies, then, are to assess the quality, quantity, suitability, maintenance, and availability of equipment for the athletic programs on the whole. Further, schools are allowed to privilege one sport over another, provided that a gender bias does not exist and that the overall quality of opportunities is equal for boys and girls. For example, a school district can choose to provide better facilities for baseball than softball teams, as long as this gap is balanced elsewhere in the programs (say, by providing outstanding facilities for field hockey) (Figure 10-3).

Often, it is money generated and earmarked for a specific sport that leads to an overall imbalance between boys' and girls' sports. When inequity results from gifts given along gender lines, it is the responsibility of the district to correct the inequity by allocation of its own resources. When powerful booster clubs garner strong community support, this task can be difficult.

District officials must assess whether booster gifts are creating disparate athletic opportunities and experiences along gender lines. Then, if inequity exists, they must remedy the problem. The district can allocate greater funds to the gender that does not receive booster support, it can seek to control the booster budget and to allocate it to create equality of experience for both genders, or in extreme cases, it can reject the donations outright. Whatever a district chooses, it has the sole responsibility for complying with Title IX and cannot shift the responsibility to the booster club. It is not uncommon for this requirement to force the district to incur unforeseen expenses when balancing booster gifts.

> **• KEY CONCEPT •**
>
> When inequity results from gifts given along gender lines, it is the responsibility of the district to correct the inequity by allocation of its own resources.

CS FLORIDA CASE STUDY

A Florida case underscores the difficulty of treating athletes equitably when booster money is flowing to a specific sport. The case involved a disparity in baseball and softball facilities. Booster money had been used to outfit the baseball field with new bleachers, an announcer's booth, an electronic scoreboard, a batting cage, bathrooms, and lights for night games. The softball field featured none of these things. Further, there was no other girls' team receiving favorable treatment sufficient to offset the inequity between baseball and softball. The court ordered the district to equalize the situation. Claiming it did not have the funds to improve the softball facility, the district began to dismantle the baseball facility. The court ordered the district to cease the dismantling and gave it a timeline to rectify the situation through improvements to the softball field. The most important outcome, for this district, was that the School Board directed the building principals to oversee expenditures to ensure gender equity, regardless of funding source (whether it be school funds, district funds, or booster donations).

Athletic directors can face any number of difficult situations as they work with booster clubs. The job of raising and allocating funds while ensuring gender equity is not an easy one. Through the challenges of handling earmarked gifts, managing splintered booster clubs, and transferring money from boosters to teams, athletic directors have a clear legal responsibility to provide equitable treatment to those under their charge.

Chapter Summary

Working with parents can be both rewarding and challenging. Supportive parents can be worth his or her weight in gold, while a difficult one can cause many sleepless nights. Communication is the greatest tool coaches have at their disposal. The better the communication, the fewer problems the coach and administration will have to deal with during (and sometimes after) the season.

Parent-run booster clubs are separate from the school system and team, yet very much entwined. Their support to the athletic department is very helpful, both financially and on a volunteer basis.

As a separate organization, a booster club has a great deal of autonomy; however, booster clubs must understand the ramifications of their actions in regard to gender-specific support of individual programs. Title IX does not permit discrimination in athletic programs. Booster clubs will need guidance and support in adhering to the rules and regulations of Title IX and the school district.

Chapter Review Questions

1. What are the four main areas in which parents have disagreements with coaches?

2. If a coach has an angry parent demanding satisfaction, what should the coach do?

3. Why is it unwise to meet with an angry parent right after a game?

4. What procedures should be taken in setting up a parent meeting?

5. If a parent is not satisfied with the outcome of the parent meeting, what is the next step?

6. What is an athletic booster club?

7. What role(s) can a successful booster club play in the athletic department?

8. What objectives should a booster club organization strive to achieve?

9. What stipulations should the athletic director and principal insist upon prior to approving a booster club?

10. Describe some of the challenges faced by high school athletic directors in working with parent-run booster clubs.

Projects and Activities

1. Go to the website www.dsr.nsw.gov.au/. Locate and write a detailed summary of its Sport Rage information guides. This program is sponsored by the New South Wales (Australia) Department of the Arts, Sport and Recreation.

2. Find two news stories on the Internet concerning coaches and angry parents. Report on what you find.

3. Meet with the president of a local booster club. Ask specific questions dealing with the relationship they have with the school and coaches. How is their booster club organized? Does it meet Title IX regulations?

Website Resources

Sport rage: http://www.dsr.nsw.gov

The North American Booster Club Association, Inc.: http://www.boosterclubs.org

Sports Psychology

Objectives

Upon completion of this chapter, the reader should be able to:

- Discuss the importance of sports psychology to athletic performance.
- Describe goal setting and its effect on motivation.
- Draw up a personal goal-setting program.
- Explain the difference between imagery and simulation.
- Explain the benefits and dangers of stress.
- Discuss the dangers of burnout.
- Describe career opportunities in the field of sports psychology.

Key Terms

Burnout

Goal setting

Imagery

Motivation

Simulation

Sports psychology

Stress

Sports Psychology

Sports psychology is the study of sport and exercise, and the mental (psychological) factors influencing performance. Sport psychologists apply psychological principles and a number of different techniques to the field of sport and exercise, all aimed at improved performance and positive self-image. The connection of mind, body, and athletic performance is a powerful one. Athletes do so much physical preparation to get an edge on the competition that they often forget about the mental aspects of their sport. It is often said that performance in a sport is 95 percent mental; however, most of the athlete's time is spent in physical preparation for competition.

Until a couple of decades ago, the general perception was that sport psychologists and consultants dealt only with athletes who had a problem of one kind or another—definitely not with athletes who were healthy and successful. Today, sports psychology has become a booming field, in which practitioners guide athletes at all levels to find increased success and happiness (Figure 11-1). Sport psychologists can help athletes develop

- goals
- self-confidence

> ● **KEY CONCEPT** ●
>
> Sports psychology is a rapidly growing field in which practitioners guide athletes at all levels to find increased success and happiness. Sport psychologists can help athletes set goals, boost self-confidence, stay motivated, enhance self-image, and cope with stress and disappointment.

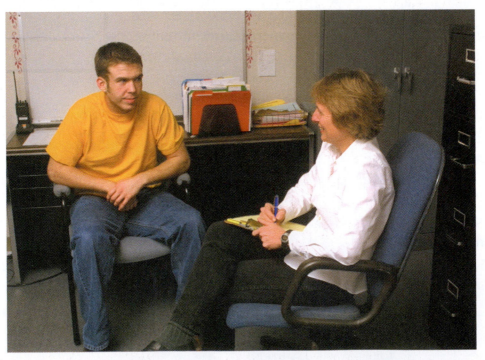

FIGURE 11–1
Sport psychologists can help athletes improve performance through motivation, goal setting, and development of a positive self-image.

- motivation
- positive self-image
- strategies to cope with stress and disappointment.

Motivation

In 1981, Kleinginna and Kleinginna defined **motivation** as an internal state or condition (sometimes described as a need, desire, or want) that serves to activate or energize behavior and give it direction.

There are two types of motivation: extrinsic and intrinsic. *Extrinsic* means from the outside. One who is extrinsically motivated is motivated by some type of external reward, such as money or praise. Extrinsic motivation is based on the goals, interests, and values of others. *Intrinsic motivation* comes from within. It is behavior for its own sake, rather than for the rewards or outcomes the behavior might reap. Intrinsically motivated behaviors, such as personal achievement, enjoyment, self-confidence, or feeling positive emotions, require no external support or reinforcement.

Goal Setting

Goal setting is one of the most powerful techniques for human motivation. Goal setting gives long-term vision and short-term motivation. By setting clearly defined, specific goals, an athlete can measure progress and take pride in the achievement of those goals. With goals in mind, an individual can

- achieve more
- improve performance
- improve the quality of training
- increase motivation to achieve at a higher level
- increase pride and satisfaction in performance
- improve self-confidence.

Research has shown that people who use goal setting effectively

- suffer less from stress and anxiety
- concentrate better

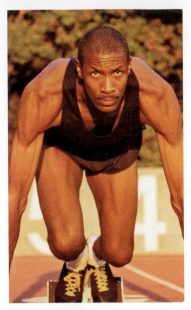

FIGURE 11–2
An athlete must have confidence and believe that he will be able to reach higher and more difficult goals. (Courtesy of Photodisc)

- show more self-confidence
- perform better
- are happier with their performances.

By setting goals and measuring their achievement, athletes can see what they have accomplished and think about how much more they are capable of achieving. This gives them the confidence and belief that they will be able to reach higher and more difficult goals (Figure 11-2).

The way in which goals are set determines their effectiveness. Before just setting goals, an athlete should understand the level he or she wishes to reach and know the skills needed to achieve these goals. The following broad guidelines apply to setting effective goals.

Express Goals Positively

It is very difficult to achieve a goal when an athlete secretly believes it cannot be done. Negative phrasing only highlights difficulty and focuses attention on *not* doing, rather than positive performance. An athlete should express goals in ways that allow him or her to envision success. For example, "By X date, I will improve Y by 20 percent" or "I will be able to do A by B date." Taking small steps and celebrating each accomplishment keeps motivation high and the desire to continue strong. Positive reinforcement from friends and colleagues will help when motivation is low. Posters and positive visual reminders assist in keeping the goal in sight.

Set Priorities

If an individual is striving to attain several goals, each goal should be given a priority. Setting priorities helps one avoid feeling overwhelmed by too many goals and directs attention to the most important goal.

Write Goals Down

Writing goals down helps to avoid confusion and gives the goals more power. Specific, written goals make an individual focus his or her energy in a specific direction and keep from straying off course. Written goals should be visible and read each day. Writing goals down and putting them in a drawer just means the goals will be forgotten or ignored. A visible, written list of goals acts as a constant reminder of what is to be accomplished.

Keep Operational Goals Small

Operational goals are the mini-goals that help accomplish larger goals—a little at a time. An example is an athlete whose goal is to run a mile in eight minutes. If the starting point is ten minutes, a weekly operational goal of shaving off fifteen seconds will allow an athlete to work progressively toward the ultimate goal. If a goal is too large, it can appear that progress is not being made. Keeping goals small and incremental gives more opportunities for reward. Today's operational goals should be derived from larger goals.

Set Performance Goals, Not Outcome Goals

It is very important for goals to be set so that an athlete retains as much control as possible over achievement. There is nothing as dispiriting as failing to achieve a personal goal for reasons beyond an individual's control, such as poor judging, bad weather, injury, excellence of other athletes, or just plain bad luck. Goals based on outcomes are extremely vulnerable to occurrences that are beyond the athlete's control.

Instead, athletes should base goals on personal performance targets or skills to be acquired. This allows control over achievement of the goals. It is important to assign dates and times to goals so that achievement can be measured. If goals are left to chance they will only happen by chance. Specific deadlines help to maintain focus and motivation; both are important to achievement.

Set Specific Goals

Athletes should set specific, measurable goals. When all conditions of a measurable goal are achieved, an athlete's confidence will increase, and he or she will be motivated and able to set more difficult goals. If goals are consistently not met, an athlete will have a basis on which to evaluate the reasons for failure and take appropriate action to improve skills.

Set Goals at the Right Level

Setting goals at the correct level is a skill that is acquired by practice. Athletes should set goals that are slightly out of their immediate grasp, but not so far that there is no hope of achieving them. No one will put serious effort into achieving a goal that he or she believes is unrealistic. Personal factors, such as fatigue, injury, stage in the season, and the like, should be taken into account when goals are set. It is best to set goals that raise average performance.

Setting a measurable, attainable goal will help an athlete strive to accomplish it. Setting a goal too high only leads to frustration and possible failure. Conversely, setting goals too low can lead to complacency and mediocrity. The old saying, "Only the mediocre are always at their best," applies here. If an athlete is not prepared to stretch him- or herself and work hard, then he or she is extremely unlikely to achieve anything of any real worth.

Set Short-Term and Long-Term Goals

Goals can be placed into two categories: short-term and long-term. *Short-term goals* are specific outcomes to be reached within a set period of time: a day, a week, a month, or perhaps even a few months. Any time period of longer than a few months puts the goal into the long-term category. Short-term goals should be perceived as immediate and attainable. An example is an athlete who sets a goal to increase the amount he or she can bench-press by 10 pounds within three weeks. This goal specifies the amount of gain and the time frame within which it must be attained.

Long-term goals are those that one strives to reach in the more distant future. To attain these goals, an athlete must work consistently and reach numerous short-term goals along the way. Long-term goals must be written down, reviewed periodically, and reevaluated as needed.

Imagery and Simulation

Imagery is a training process done purely within the mind. This imagining helps create, modify, or strengthen neurologic pathways that are important to the coordination of the muscles. Imagination is the driving force of imagery.

Imagery is based on the important principle that anyone can exercise parts of the brain with inputs from the imagination rather than from the senses. Imagery allows an individual to practice and prepare for events and eventualities an athlete can never expect to train for in reality. This allows an athlete to pre-experience the achievement of goals.

Practicing with imagery can help "slow down" complex skills so that an athlete can isolate and feel the correct component movements of the skills, and isolate where problems in technique lie. For example, if a discus thrower is having trouble with the release, he can practice the correct technique over and over again in his mind. This can be done anywhere, at any time. He can only physically practice throwing the discus a limited amount of time each day. Through the use of imagery, an athlete can move closer to preparing for the "95 percent mental" part of the game.

Simulation is similar to imagery in that it seeks to improve the quality of training by teaching the brain to cope with circumstances that would not otherwise be encountered until an important competition. Simulation is carried out by making the physical training circumstances as close as possible to the real competition. An example is having training sessions timed or judged, or bringing in spectators to watch the practice performance.

In many ways simulation is superior to imagery as a training technique. The stresses introduced in simulation are more vivid because they exist in reality. However, simulation requires much greater resources of time and effort to set up and implement, and is less flexible in terms of the range of eventualities that can be practiced for.

Strategies to Cope with Stress and Disappointment

Stress from athletics comes in many forms. The proper amount of stress can be healthy and help to improve performance. Stress can help an athlete increase awareness, maintain a clearer focus, increase motivation, and filter out distractions that could have a negative effect on performance. Too much stress can hinder performance and lead to problems in other areas of life. Some situations that can cause excess stress are discussed here.

Transitional Stress

When an athlete makes a transition between levels in a sport, he or she may experience a great deal of stress from being faced with the unknown. These unknowns may include increased competition, new teammates, or simply a change from the level of competition he or she has grown accustomed to. An example of this is the highly talented high school athlete who goes to college on an athletic scholarship and fails to live up to his or her potential. Transitional stress in athletes typically occurs when

- beginning a new sport
- going from high school to college

- changing leagues
- changing levels of competition
- going from junior high to high school
- going from college to professional
- retiring from athletics.

Injuries

Injury can be devastating to a motivated athlete. Not only does an injury take an athlete out of competition, but it also sets him or her back in training and performance goals. Understanding that injuries are a part of competitive athletics will allow an athlete to modify goals when injuries do occur. Support from other athletes, family, and friends will help an athlete cope with the stress of the injury itself and what it has done to his or her competitive life.

Burnout

Burnout is both physically and mentally challenging. Pressure to win, along with criticism from coaches, parents, and other teammates, can create excess stress and anxiety (Figure 11-3). **Burnout** often manifests as dropping out of a sport or quitting an other activity that was once enjoyable. An example is a highly competitive gymnast or swimmer who began the sport very early in life. After a while, the stress of early and late practices, coupled with the lack of a normal social life and pressure from parents and coaches, causes the athlete to quit the sport. These athletes are usually excellent at their sport, but mentally they simply cannot continue.

According to the *Georgia Tech Sports Medicine & Performance Newsletter* (2000), experts say there are steps adults can take to encourage a healthy interest in sports among young people. As many as 70 percent of children who participate in youth sports drop out of athletics by the time they are thirteen. This is true of a variety of sports popular throughout the country. There are several reasons for this dropoff in interest among teens. In some cases, children begin participating in sports too soon. Athletes can become frustrated and quit when parents enroll them in highly competitive situations before they fully understand how to play particular sports.

The Olympics also pose a problem. The games often highlight and promote top athletes who begin training at young ages. This sometimes sends the message that children must have an early start in a specific sport if they are to excel.

• Did You Know? •

As many as 70% of children who participate in youth sports drop out of athletics by the time they are 13.

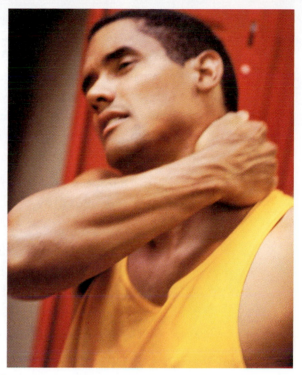

FIGURE 11–3
Athletes must be able to deal with stress and disappointment. It is important that short-term disappointment not be permitted to translate into long-term failure. (Courtesy of Photodisc)

Experts also say that some young athletes achieve success too early. If by the age of twelve a child has won, lost, traveled, attended awards ceremonies, and earned a variety of trophies in a particular sport, he or she might wonder if there is any point in playing for another four or five years.

There are other causes for concern, too. Parents and coaches sometimes emphasize sports performance and winning above enjoyment of the game, especially as they get caught up in wins, losses, and statistics. Young athletes who limit themselves to one sport often face early burnout; most elite athletes enjoy participating in multiple sports during their youth, and some teams and leagues practice and play too much or too often, leaving children exhausted or overextended.

Experts tell parents that they should encourage children to play multiple sports. They should let children eventually specialize in one or two sports they like. No child should be rushed into organized sports before she or he is ready to play. Finally, parents, coaches, and athletes must keep sports in perspective. Participating in sports should be fun, not a profession or a mission with the goal of earning a college scholarship or a professional contract.

• KEY CONCEPT •

Burnout can make an athlete who excels in his or her sport turn away from competition and sports altogether. Burnout can be caused by increased pressure to win, beginning a sport too early, not being involved in other activities, and gender differences.

Gender differences can lead to stress in athletic involvement. The benefits and positive outcomes of sport involvement for both male and females are many. Problems occur when females are involved in sports in which bodily contact and great physical exertion are present and characterized as being masculine. Many girls and women see this as too problematic and decide not to participate. Men and boys who participate in sports and activities that are expressive and artistic in nature (ballet, ice dancing) often have to overcome similar barriers.

The European Federation of Sports Psychology makes the following recommendations (1998):

- Organizations should work toward making all sporting opportunities available to all individuals, regardless of gender. This should not be taken to mean that all sporting contests should be mixed; providers of sport and recreation facilities should recognize that there may be occasions when men and women need to participate in single-sex groupings.

- All involved with the provision and promotion of sport opportunities should recognize the possible existence of psychological barriers and work toward overcoming them.

- All involved with media presentation of sports should work to produce positive images of athletes, regardless of gender.

- Resource allocation in sports should show evidence of gender equity.

- Opportunities for employment and professional development in coaching, management, and sports science should be equally available to all individuals, regardless of gender.

- Organizations should work toward giving all individuals the choice to be coached or advised by someone of their own gender. This includes sport psychology consultants.

- Those involved in sports should recognize that the needs of male and female sports participants may differ in some respects and be similar in others.

- Providers of sport should recognize that participation is influenced by the range of activities available, and should make every effort to promote activities that meet the needs of both men and women.

- Research is fundamental and should not be gender-blind. It should take into consideration the needs and aspirations of girls and boys, men and women.

Managing Stress

The negative effects of stress can interfere with judgment and fine motor control. Stress can also cause competition to be seen as a threat rather than a challenge. This may lead the athlete to think negatively and lose self-confidence. The more stress an athlete has, the more of his or her mental energy it will consume.

One of the best ways to manage stress is through goal setting. Athletes who program their workouts and competitions tend to be better prepared for unforeseen situations. When an unexpected situation does arise, these athletes are more likely to be able to handle it in a positive way. Other ways to handle stress are through meditation, positive thinking, time management, talking with friends, and taking breaks.

The following quiz was designed to be an initial step in understanding and combating the harmful effects that stress has on athletic performance. It was developed by Mick G. Mack of the University of Northern Iowa. Answers appear at the end of the chapter.

STRESS AND ATHLETIC PERFORMANCE QUIZ

True or False?

1. Under high levels of stress, athletes typically have a broad attention span.

2. The clammy feeling we often get when stressed is caused by our body's natural defense against bleeding to death.

3. Elite-level performers have fewer nervous reactions to stress than do non-elite–level performers.

4. High levels of stress make it more difficult to think clearly.

5. Getting sick to your stomach and throwing up when nervous is your body's way of telling you that you are overstressed.

6. Caffeine exaggerates the physical and mental effects of stress.

7. The body's stress response, which is commonly referred to as the fight-or-flight response, allows us to do superhuman feats.

8. The only time stress is good is when there is no stress.

9. Sighing as you exhale is more relaxing than not sighing.

10. Under stress, athletes often revert to their most well-learned behaviors.

Reprinted with permission of Mick G. Mack of the University of Northern Iowa.

Self-Confidence

Self-confidence is arguably one of the most important attributes an athlete can have. Self-confidence reflects an athlete's assessment of his or her own self-worth, and plays a large part in determining the athlete's happiness through life.

Participation in athletics can be enormously positive in improving self-worth and highly negative in damaging it. When sports are used creatively, with emphasis on enjoyment, effective goal setting, and monitoring the achievement of goals, self-confidence builds as targets are reached and improvement in performance is noted. Self-confidence allows athletes to take risks, because they have enough confidence in their own abilities to be sure that if things do go wrong, they can put things right.

When children are compelled to participate in a sport in which they have no interest or aptitude, it can be destructive to self-confidence. Consistent failure can lead to a lack of self-esteem.

The way in which an athlete approaches self-confidence is important: if an athlete is underconfident, he or she will not take the risks that should be taken. Overconfidence can lead to a decrease in performance because the athlete is not trying hard enough.

Confidence should be based on observed reality—that is, on the achievement of performance goals. Athletes should be confident that they will perform up to their current abilities. Good self-confidence comes from a realistic expectation of success based on well-practiced physical skills, thorough knowledge of the sport, respect for one's own competence, adequate preparation, and good physical condition (Figure 11-4). The success attained should be measured by achievement of personal performance goals, not outcome goals such as winning.

Persons who are underconfident commonly suffer from fear of failure (which will prevent them from taking risks effectively), self-doubt, lack of concentration, and negative thinking. Use of imagery and effective goal setting will help improve self-confidence and self-image.

Overconfidence is dangerous because it can lead to situations that an athlete is not able to get out of. It can set an athlete up for serious failure that can devastate the self-confidence she should have. *Overconfidence* is confidence that is not based on ability. It may be a result of parents or coaches who try to help without understanding an athlete's abilities; vanity or ego; or positive thinking or imagery that is not backed up by ability.

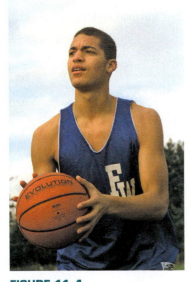

FIGURE 11–4
Confidence leads to success. Athletes should be confident that they will perform up to their current abilities. (Courtesy of Photodisc)

Goal setting is probably the most effective way of building self-confidence. By setting measurable goals, achieving them, then setting new goals and achieving them, an athlete builds self-confidence. This increases the chances for success and allows reasonably accurate assessment of an athlete's real abilities.

Careers in Sports Psychology

The world's first sports psychology laboratory was founded by Carl Diem at the Deutsche Sporthochschule in Berlin, Germany, in 1920. Five years later, in 1925, A. Z. Puni opened a sports psychology laboratory at the Institute of Physical Culture in Leningrad. That same year, Cloman Griffith of the University of Illinois established the first sports psychology laboratory in North America. Griffith had begun his research into psychological factors that affect sports performance in 1918, and in 1923, he offered the first course in sports psychology. Griffith was interested in the effects on athletic performance of factors such as reaction time, mental awareness, muscular tension and relaxation, and personality. Because of the financial constraints that came with the Great Depression, Griffith's laboratory closed in 1932.

In North America, little or no research in sports psychology took place between the closing of Griffith's laboratory and the 1960s. Then, rather quickly, physical education departments in many institutions began to offer courses in sports psychology, and graduate programs began to appear.

The first scholarly journal devoted to sports psychology, the *International Journal of Sport Psychology*, was established in 1970, followed in 1979 by the *Journal of Sport Psychology*. Increasing interest in conducting sports psychology research in settings outside the laboratory triggered the formation of the Association for the Advancement of Applied Sport Psychology (AAASP) in 1985, and focused attention more directly on applied psychology in both the health field and sports contexts.

Sports psychology is a fast-growing field with many career opportunities. It is a very interesting and intriguing area. There are three tracks that a student of sports psychology can pursue:

- Educational sports psychology, which emphasizes working with athletes in an athletic environment
- Clinical sports psychology, dealing with athletes in a clinical setting
- Academic sports psychology, which focuses on research and teaching

For a listing and description of all programs, check out the *Directory of Graduate Programs in Applied Sport Psychology*, available from AAASP.

Chapter Summary

Sports psychology is the study of the mental factors influencing performance in sport and exercise. Sports psychologists apply psychological principles and a number of different techniques to the field of sport and exercise, all aimed at improving performance and positive self-image.

Goal setting can help an athlete attain greater success by focusing his or her energy in a positive, measurable way. By setting goals and measuring their achievement, athletes can see what they have accomplished and discover how much they are capable of achieving.

Chapter Review Questions

1. List several techniques that an athlete can use to increase performance and boost positive self-image.

2. What are the advantages of goal setting?

3. What guidelines apply to setting effective goals?

4. What is the difference between a performance and outcome goal?

5. Compare and contrast imagery and simulation.

6. How can stress be beneficial? Harmful?

7. After taking the stress quiz what did you learn?

8. What are the dangers of being over confident?

9. Who founded the world's first sports psychology laboratory? Where was it located? When was it founded?

10. List the three career tracks a student of sports psychology can pursue.

Projects and Activities

1. Find a sports psychologist practicing in your area. Arrange an interview and ask these questions, plus others.

   a. How did you become interested in this field?

   b. How difficult is it to become a sports psychologist?

   c. What difference do you think you make in the lives of the athletes you work with?

d. What is the most difficult part of your job?

e. Are career opportunities expanding? Will there be opportunities when I graduate from college?

f. How much does a sports psychologist earn?

g. If you had to do it all over again, would you choose this field?

2. Using the information presented in this chapter, establish a personal goal-setting program. List both short-term and long-term goals. Use the worksheet at the end of this chapter.

3. Write a two-page paper on the following: How has stress affected your life? What strategies do you use to manage stress in a positive way?

4. Assume you have decided on a career in sports psychology. Research what you need to do to become a sports psychologist.

5. Meet with the coach you admire most and ask the coach how he or she uses sports psychology in motivating athletes. Report back to class.

Website Resources

- Visit the website www.peaksports.com and see what this mental game coach has to say about motivation and sports psychology.

- Browse the resources and articles at www.topachievement.com and discover some tools and techniques for motivation and goal setting.

- Learn more about careers in sports psychology by visiting the website of the Association for the Advancement of Applied Sport Psychology, www.aaasponline.org.

Answers to Stress Performance Test

1. False. Under high levels of stress, athletes tend to have a narrow attention span, often referred to as tunnel vision. Attention may also focus on the athlete's internal thought process, which can lead to "choking" under pressure.

2. True. One of the physical responses of the body to stress is to divert blood away from the small vessels near the skin. This provides a defense against bleeding to death from wounds, but gives the skin a cold, clammy feeling.

3. False. Elite-level performers have just as many nervous reactions to stress as any other type of performer. However, elite athletes often interpret these reactions as being more positive and beneficial than do other athletes.

4. True. Clear thinking is more difficult in pressure situations. This is why coaches and athletes must constantly practice what they are going to do and how they are going to respond in pressure-packed situations.

5. False. So that more blood will be available to the large muscles of the body in preparation for strenuous physical activity, such as fighting or running away, the digestive system shuts down. During this shutdown, the acid in your stomach makes you feel nauseated, which sometimes results in throwing up. This is a normal reaction to stress.

6. True. Caffeine tends to exaggerate the physical and mental effects of stress. Knowing this, coaches and athletes should avoid caffeinated products before entering potentially stressful situations.

7. True. Under stress, the body produces adrenalin, which provides a powerful, quick burst of energy that sometimes results in superhuman feats.

8. False. There are a number of stresses that are good. For example, being elevated to the starting team brings additional stress that most athletes would enjoy. Another example of positive stress is physical and mental training. All athletes are under stress when, during training, they push themselves to the edge so that their bodies will adapt to the demand and get stronger.

9. True. For some reason, letting out an audible sigh as you exhale is very relaxing. There are a number of additional relaxation techniques that involve breathing exercises.

10. True. In stressful situations, athletes often revert to behaviors they are familiar and comfortable with. This is one of the reasons why athletes should try to learn and perfect new skills and techniques in the off-season.

WHAT ARE YOUR GOALS?

Use the chart below to record your personal, educational, professional, and community goals. Remember to classify goals as either short-term (one year or less to accomplish), intermediate-term (one to five years), or long-term (more than five years to achieve). You may have more than one goal or no goals in a particular category.

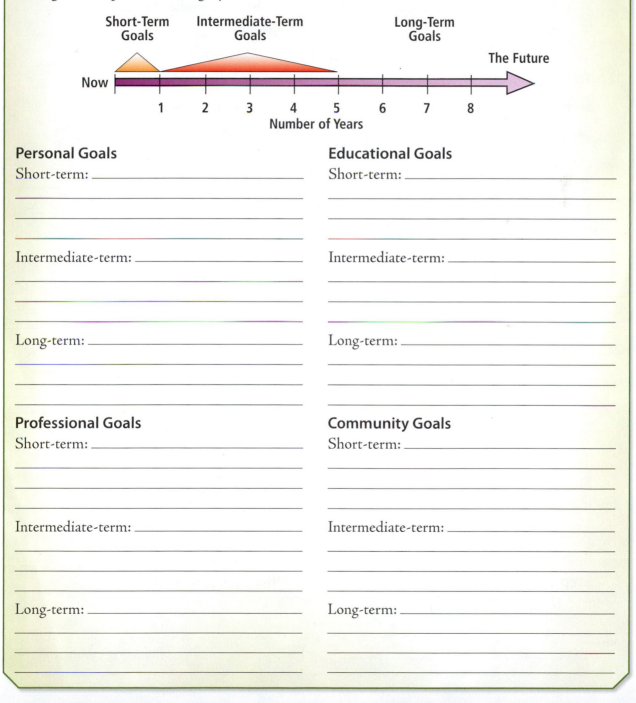

Personal Goals

Short-term: _____

_____

_____

_____

Intermediate-term: _____

_____

_____

Long-term: _____

_____

_____

Educational Goals

Short-term: _____

_____

_____

_____

Intermediate-term: _____

_____

_____

Long-term: _____

_____

_____

Professional Goals

Short-term: _____

_____

_____

_____

Intermediate-term: _____

_____

_____

Long-term: _____

_____

_____

Community Goals

Short-term: _____

_____

_____

_____

Intermediate-term: _____

_____

_____

Long-term: _____

_____

_____

ACTION PLAN: INTERMEDIATE- OR LONG-TERM

1 Intermediate- or long-term goal:

_____

To be accomplished by: _____

Step 1: _____

Results needed:

_____

To be accomplished by: _____

Step 2: _____

Results needed:

_____

To be accomplished by: _____

Step 3: _____

Results needed:

_____

To be accomplished by: _____

Step 4: _____

Results needed:

_____

To be accomplished by: _____

2 Intermediate- or long-term goal:

_____

To be accomplished by: _____

Step 1: _____

Results needed:

_____

To be accomplished by: _____

Step 2: _____

Results needed:

_____

To be accomplished by: _____

Step 3: _____

Results needed:

_____

To be accomplished by: _____

Step 4: _____

Results needed:

_____

To be accomplished by: _____

3 Intermediate- or long-term goal:

_____

To be accomplished by: _____

Step 1: _____

Results needed:

_____

To be accomplished by: _____

Step 2: _____

Results needed:

_____

To be accomplished by: _____

Step 3: _____

Results needed:

_____

To be accomplished by: _____

Step 4: _____

Results needed:

_____

To be accomplished by: _____

(Throop & Castellucci, 1999)

Administration and Management in Sport and Physical Education

Risk Management in Sport and Physical Education

Objectives

Upon completion of this chapter, the reader should be able to:

- Explain the principles of risk management in sport and physical education.
- Define the legal duties associated with coaching and teaching.
- Understand what is meant by ethical responsibility.
- Develop a management plan for practice and game facilities, as well as equipment, supervision, travel, and response to injured athletes.

Key Terms

Ethical responsibilities

Liability

Mission statement

Risk management

Supervision

Risk Management in Sport and Physical Education

Risk management is the course of action taken to reduce potential legal **liability**. It seeks to address potential problems before they occur, and aims to be proactive rather than reactive in creating a safer environment. Physical education instructors and coaches have more liability concerns than academic faculty because of the nature of their work. Understanding risk management and legal liability concepts associated with their profession will help coaches limit liability and create a safer working environment. Although this chapter explains various responsibilities and liability concerns from the coaching perspective, its content has direct implications for the physical education teacher because their job duties are often intertwined (Figure 12-1).

Legal Responsibilities and Risk Management for Coaches

• KEY CONCEPT •

Risk management is the course of action taken to reduce potential legal liability.

Coaches at all levels experience the pleasure of watching young people develop their sport skills and contribute to successful teams. However, coaches also have important legal and ethical obligations to their schools and their athletes. Many of these obligations are natural extensions of the mission and goals of the high school athletic program. Others are derived from laws or from society's expectations. Coaches planning their risk management philosophy should begin by composing a risk management policy statement.

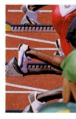
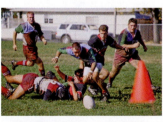
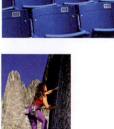
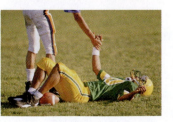

FIGURE 12–1
Risk management involves all aspects of the athletic program. (Courtesy of Photodisc)

Risk Management Policy Statement

This policy statement should describe the coaching staff's commitment to protecting the health and safety of the participants. The statement may contain positive messages (we commit to ensuring participants' safety) or negative ones (we do not tolerate practices that place participants in a position to sustain injuries from causes that are not inherent in the sport). The policy statement must have the commitment of the athletic director and school principal, and must be implemented in practice.

Legal Responsibilities

Legal responsibilities are usually well defined and are often points of emphasis in coaching certification programs. State athletic associations, departments of education, and other government organizations determine the range of legal responsibilities for a coach. These responsibilities usually are formulated to maintain the safety and well-being of the athletes and to maintain the educational focus of the athletic program. Mandatory child-abuse reporting is a legal responsibility of coaches in many states and is a good example of a coach's duty that is mandated by a governmental body. Court rulings or other legal actions may determine other responsibilities. Providing warnings to athletes and parents of the risks associated with a sport is a responsibility that likely arose after a serious sport-related injury occurred during a practice or game. Failure to perform this duty may put a coach, and even an entire athletic program, at risk of litigation.

Another important source of expectations for a coach is the accepted state and national standards for coaching that are published by professional organizations.

Legal and ethical issues are not mutually exclusive, as many legal responsibilities are based upon societal ethics and doing what is morally right. Preventing discrimination against and harassment of athletes is a legal duty of coaches because these activities are illegal, but this duty is also an ethical expectation of society. Athletes in a coach's care are expected to be safe, both physically and emotionally.

The following list of legal duties of a coach is representative of the many codes of conduct and behaviors recommended for coaches.

1. Conduct practices and games in a safe physical environment.

2. Use current knowledge of proper skills and methods of instruction (Figure 12-2).

> ● KEY CONCEPT ●
>
> Legal and ethical issues are not mutually exclusive, as many legal responsibilities are based upon societal ethics and doing what is morally right.

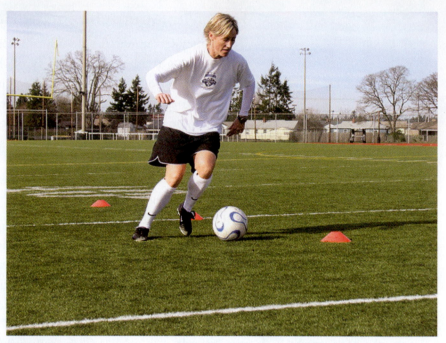

FIGURE 12–2
Former professional soccer great, Justi Baumgardt, demonstrates proper soccer skills.
(Courtesy of Justi Baumgardt)

3. Use safe and appropriate equipment.

4. Conduct proper short- and long-term planning.

5. Match athletes in practices and games according to size, experience, and ability.

6. Provide adequate supervision of athletes.

7. Warn parents and athletes of risks inherent in sport participation.

8. Be sensitive to the health and well-being of athletes under a coach's care.

9. Provide appropriate emergency care.

10. Prevent harassment and discrimination by coaching staff and athletes.

11. Report suspected child abuse to proper authorities.

12. Respect and protect the confidentiality of student personal records.

13. Report breaches of ethics by colleagues.

This list includes many of the legal responsibilities of coaches and physical educators. However, a coach must do more than just what is required by law. There are other **ethical responsibilities** that should also be considered an integral part of a coach's duties. Coaching behaviors that reflect strong ethical conduct should be extensions of the school's **mission statement**. Most schools have a general statement, and many also have a specific mission statement for athletics. It is relatively easy to explore the mission statements of high schools around the country using the Internet. One mission statement that seems particularly relevant to the interscholastic domain and supports many of the ethical responsibilities of coaching is that of West Aurora High School in Aurora, Illinois. We have used excerpts from this statement to illustrate the range of ethical responsibilities that should be part of all youth sport programs.

1. We encourage the development of our youth into productive citizens and hope to develop their abilities and attitudes for further learning and success in life.

2. We encourage participation and would like to involve as many students as possible in a competitive interscholastic experience.

3. All team members, regardless of ability, will be afforded opportunities to develop their work ethic, sense of commitment, and social and athletic skills.

4. The athletic program seeks to educate athletes about community support and encourages them to return that support both now and throughout their lives.

5. The goal is to win, but to win the correct way. Never sacrifice character for wins.

These five excerpts from the West Aurora mission statement illustrate quite well the ethical obligations a coach and athletic program should have to the athletes. It is apparent that although sport is important in the life of the athlete, learning to be a productive citizen with character and social values is even more important. It is a responsibility of every coach to teach and model good citizenship and sportsmanship. This should include showing respect for opposing teams and fans, coaches, parents, and officials. A unique aspect of this mission statement relates to the community focus. Making it a goal to educate the student-athlete about the relationship between the athletic program and the community reflects this program's emphasis on producing not only successful athletic teams, but also caring and concerned citizens of good character.

Another ethical responsibility derived from this mission statement supports the educational value of sports participation. All athletes involved in a sport must be given the attention and time necessary to develop the skills of the sport. The sole focus of a program cannot be the select few elite players on a team. A program should not be so narrowly focused on winning that the educational values of the program are lost. Helping all athletes on teams develop the work ethic, commitment, and social and athletic skills necessary for success in sport and life is perhaps the best test of the educational commitment of an interscholastic sports program.

To summarize the coach's ethical responsibilities, it is useful to list some of the important factors that contribute to the achievement of the educational mission of an interscholastic athletic program.

- Create a healthy and safe emotional environment, free of fear, discrimination, abuse, and harassment. Athletes cannot enjoy their experience without this.

- Teach, and more importantly model, good citizenship and sportsmanship. Athletes must understand your commitment to helping them develop character and moral reasoning.

- Respect the spirit of a rule as well as the letter of the rule. Respect the difficult job officials have in enforcing the rules of any game. Taking advantage of rules to gain an advantage is not ethical. It indicates an unhealthy focus on winning.

- Be fair in the selection of players for teams and in the allocation of practice and playing time. Empathize with the young athletes who are attempting to gain a place on your team.

- Respect the role of sport in the life of a child and the commitment the athlete has to family, friends, and other interests outside of sport. Athletes must be allowed to experience other sports as well as to participate in the arts if they desire. Off-season conditioning activities may be beneficial to a high school athlete, but these activities must be chosen by the athletes and not dictated in such a way that it limits their freedom to participate in other activities of interest.

• KEY CONCEPT •

Helping all athletes on teams to develop the work ethic, commitment, and social and athletic skills necessary for success in sport and life is perhaps the best test of the educational commitment of an interscholastic sports program.

Interscholastic sport is important in the lives of many young people today. In addition, sport's ability to bring a community or school together cannot be overestimated. Our schools and communities would be much less vibrant without it. In order to maintain the importance of sport in the lives of our youth and our communities, it is imperative for sport to contribute to the school's educational mission. If a coach adopts and practices the legal and ethical responsibilities described, here interscholastic sport will grow and prosper and benefit all who participate.

Management of Practice and Game Facilities

All too often the planning of athletic facilities is given serious attention only after the "more important" design of the school is complete (Figure 12-3). After all, they are only P.E. and sports areas. This mistaken approach reflects a lack of understanding of the complex and important relationship these areas have to the total educational program, and the safety and security of students, or of community opportunities for school campus use. At a minimum, those involved in planning athletic sports fields should concentrate on these criteria:

- the overall master plan relationship of the outside areas to the school
- student safety
- access by students from the school during the day and the community at night

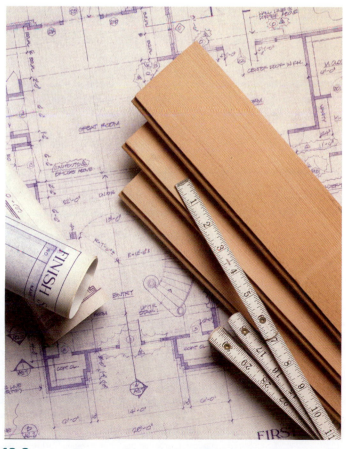

FIGURE 12–3
Management of athletic and fitness facilities begins at the design level. (Courtesy of Photodisc)

- Providing age appropriate equipment and access, particularly for younger students
- Title IX compliance

Conducting a Safe Program: The Field of Play

The field of play, whether indoor or outdoor, should be checked for safety problems before all practices and games. Indoor courts should be clear of any obstacles or obstructions surrounding the out-of-bounds areas. The actual playing surface should be clear, safe, dry, clean, and have proper ventilation, especially in warm climates.

Outdoor facilities should be checked for uneven playing surfaces, including holes, uneven grade, or moisture (Figure 12-4). Out-of-bounds areas should be clear of obstructions, and all boundaries should be clearly marked. Other areas used by players, such as locker rooms and showers, should be reviewed for safety and accessibility. Floors should be properly drained and have non-slip surfaces. Areas utilized by spectators, families, and nonparticipating players should be checked for safety and accessibility. Large, permanent structures such as artificial turf fields and stadium lights should comply with the manufacturer's specifications.

> ● **KEY CONCEPT** ●
>
> Any time the weather conditions jeopardize the health and welfare of the athletes, staff, or spectators, the coach must be willing to cancel or postpone the event.

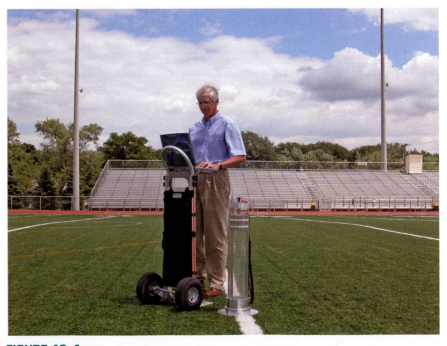

FIGURE 12–4
Even artificial surfaces require frequent safety inspections. (Courtesy of Synthetic Turf Testing Services)

Coaches must also be aware of outdoor weather concerns. Inclement weather includes not just lightning, hail, or heavy rain; but also extremes of heat and cold. Any time the weather conditions jeopardize the health and welfare of the athletes, staff, or spectators, the coach must be willing to cancel or postpone the event.

Conducting a Safe Program: Equipment

Athletic equipment undergoes considerable wear and tear and must be evaluated for safety periodically, if not daily. Athletes must be taught to check their personal equipment (such as shoulder pads and helmets, wrestling headgear, or batting helmets) each time they use it. Other equipment such as hurdles, basketball rims, backboards, and starting blocks for swimming, need only periodic inspections. Athletes need to have the proper equipment for each sport, and it should fit properly. The following areas should be addressed:

- Adequate amount of equipment: All necessary equipment should be available for all practices and events.

- Well-maintained equipment: All equipment should be checked prior to the start of practice or competition. Equipment, whether it is routinely or only occasionally used, should be maintained and checked before each use. Coaches should discard worn or dangerous equipment immediately.

- Proper use of equipment: Manufacturers develop equipment for specific uses. The coaching staff should instruct their players in the correct use of the equipment. Improper use is not only unsafe but may invalidate the warranty.

- Proper size of equipment: Equipment should adhere to the standard specifications designated by the sport.

- Proper fit of equipment: Any equipment used in the context of a sport should be properly fitted to each athlete.

- Proper warranty and safety criteria: Review of the safety criteria and appropriate use guidelines is recommended.

Conducting a Safe Program: Travel

The coaching staff is responsible for all its athletes for the whole time that they are under its care, from the time they arrive at the locker room, to the time they leave or when their parents arrive to pick them up. This is a big responsibility that must be planned for and managed properly.

Before a player travels to a game or competition, the coach should review any special instructions with the player's parents or guardian. The coach should bring written instructions for administering any medications on the trip. Medical staff, such as certified athletic trainers, should be aware of and manage medications and special medical considerations of athletes. Emergency contact information should be readily available, as well as a travel card listing medications taken and any medical concerns that may need to be addressed in an emergency.

Transportation should be adequate for all players; all players should have a seat on a bus, and wear seat belts if traveling by car or van. The mode of transportation should be safe, and follow district transportation rules and procedures. Coaches should inspect cars and vans each time they are used. A strict code of conduct must be enforced while traveling to ensure the safety of passengers, coaches, and drivers.

Weather conditions should be reviewed before leaving for any competition. Traveling should never take place if questionable conditions exist. The head coach is legally responsible for all decisions. The coach should be aware of the opposing team's arrangements for supplies such as water and ice, emergency management plans, and locker room space. Important telephone numbers should be readily at hand.

If the trip involves overnight lodging, safe and accessible accommodations should be secured. Contact information should be given to all parents. Special dietary concerns should be clarified with parents and arrangements made to address them. Parents need to be advised when and where to pick up their students upon return to the school. A plan for a telephone tree should be developed for use in case of an alteration of plans.

Conducting a Safe Program: Athlete Supervision

Insurance companies have seen a large number of claims that allege lack of proper **supervision**. Some experts estimate that 80 percent of athletic injuries result from a lapse in direct or indirect supervision. Supervision is more than just overseeing athletes' activities; it is promoting the health, safety, and well-being of athletes and sports participants. A coach must perform nine legal duties:

1. Properly plan the activity, practice, or game.

2. Provide appropriate instruction.

3. Provide a safe physical environment.

4. Provide adequate and proper equipment, including all prescribed safety equipment for players.

5. Match athletes by ability and age/size.

6. Evaluate athletes for injury or incapacity.

7. Supervise the activity closely.

8. Warn players and spectators of inherent risks.

9. Have an emergency plan and provide appropriate emergency assistance in the event of an accident or injury.

Planning and preparedness are important in developing a successful program. Always have a plan and a backup plan.

Parents can take an active role by helping with supervision. However, parents shouldn't be expected to supervise athletes alone. The degree of liability could actually increase if the supervising parents aren't official members of the coaching staff and have not been through the volunteer/coaching protocol set up by the school district.

Conducting a Safe Program: Injury Prevention, Recognition, and Response

Regardless of the excellence of a risk management program, injuries will still occur. A coach is expected to have basic knowledge as to what he or she should and should not do when an athlete is injured. Most importantly, coaches must know how to implement their emergency plan. Practicing the emergency game plan before an emergency occurs will help everyone know their role and responsibilities (Figure 12-5).

The medical emergency action plan should include meet basic criteria:

1. It should contain information about athletes' preexisting medical problems, such as diabetes, epilepsy, or history of allergic reactions.

2. Signed parental release forms that give permission for medical treatment in case of emergency, should be readily accessible.

3. A well-stocked first-aid kit should be present at all training sessions and competitions.

4. Coaches must be instructed on how to use the materials in the first-aid kit.

5. Should a medical emergency occur at a training site, coaches need to know the location of the nearest telephone to call 911.

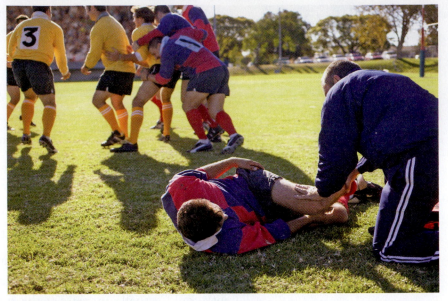

FIGURE 12–5
Injuries unfortunately occur despite the best plan to prevent them. (Courtesy of PunchStock)

6. Should a medical emergency occur at an event or training site, there need to be assistant coaches or volunteers available to stay with uninjured team members while medical emergency procedures are taken.

7. Each coach and volunteer must know the emergency plan: who to contact, location of emergency contact personnel, method of communication, and follow-up procedures.

8. Keys to unlock gates blocking access to the injured athlete must be readily available.

9. Coaches should have a list of athletes' parents'/guardians' names and phone numbers so they may be contacted in the event of a serious injury.

10. The plan should identify the location of the nearest hospital or medical facility.

Coaches should have training in basic first aid and CPR. The school or program should obtain an automated external defibrillator (AED), and make sure as many coaches as possible know how to use it. Maintaining an up-to-date first aid kit and a current set of individual emergency medical forms is a must. Serious injuries require an immediate response by a higher level of medical expertise as quickly as possible after an injury occurs (Figure 12-6).

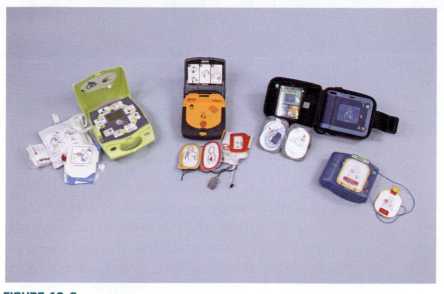

FIGURE 12-6
AED's should be mandatory in all athletic facilities. (Courtesy of the American National Red Cross. All rights reserved in all countries.)

> ● **KEY CONCEPT** ●
>
> Although it sounds simple, parents are less apt to take a coach to court if the coach seems to have been genuinely concerned about the welfare of the student-athlete.

> ● **Did You Know?** ●
>
> Did you know that cheerleading is responsible for 68 percent of injuries to female collegiate athletes?

Report and document all injuries as soon as possible. Accident reports should be factual and to the point. An athlete should not resume practice or competition after an injury without a doctor's written approval.

Other than providing first aid, the single most important thing you can do after an athlete suffers an injury is to show both the athlete and his or her parents that you care. Although it sounds simple, parents are less apt to take a coach to court if the coach seems to have been genuinely concerned about the welfare of the student-athlete.

Another important part of risk management, and one which is the subject of some recent well-publicized court cases, is the coach's role in instructing his or her athletes in a progressive, safe manner. Coaches have a responsibility to develop a sequence of progressive practice sessions and offer competition preparation and strategies that result in a safe experience for athletes.

It is important to put all procedures in writing and to keep accurate records. Documentation should include checklists, practice plans, training plans, medical examination forms, the athletic handbook, consent forms, and return-to-play agreements. Following a written plan lowers the chance that you will forget an issue and demonstrates your professionalism. It will save you a great deal of time in the future. The records you keep on file must reflect what you actually did in a situation. If your school's or program's written rules state athletes cannot practice without passing a physical and then you permit a student to play who hasn't done so, you may be found negligent. Check with your athletic administrator as to how long you should retain these records; typically this is seven years.

LEGAL BRIEF: THE RISK FACTOR

(The following article is reprinted with permission from Dr. Richard P. Borkowski.)

Follow these practical steps to keep your athletes out of harm's way, and your program out of legal hot water. By Dr. Richard P. Borkowski, EdD, CMAA. Dr. Borkowski is a sport safety consultant based in Narberth, Pennsylvania, who served as the Director of Physical Education and Athletics at the Episcopal Academy in Merion, Pennsylvania for thirty three years. His most recent book is titled *Coaching for Safety, A Risk Management Handbook for Coaches,* published by ESD112 (Vancouver, WA). This article initially appeared in Coaching Management, 12.1 (January 2004). Safe Landings

This article is about the most boring subject there is in sports: safety. It's boring, that is, until an athlete gets hurt.

Coaches must know and appreciate their risk management duties. The implementation of solid safety rules will not guarantee your athletes freedom from injury, but it will lower the chances of both common and serious, catastrophic injuries. Lowering the chance of injury lowers the chance of expensive, time-consuming, program-shattering lawsuits.

The following are your legal responsibilities as a coach. They are based on a consensus of opinions by those in athletics, an ongoing review of court cases, and my years of experience as an athletic risk manager. They are also what a good coach does—offer a worthwhile athletic experience that manages the risks of participation.

However, when in doubt about your duties, seek the advice of your school's legal counsel. Do it before an accident occurs.

The Right Attitude

The key to lowering the risk of injury is to make safety important by making it a regular topic of conversation. Explain to your athletes the danger of attempting throws or jumps they haven't been adequately trained in. Correct safety problems immediately. Say, "No, we won't practice," if a situation is hazardous. In addition, talk to your athletes about their responsibility for their own safety and the safety of others. Explain to your throwers what could happen if they leave their shot or discus where someone could trip over them. Show your javelin throwers how to scan the area before starting their practice throws.

When athletes hear you preach safety, they will be less apt to attempt risky behavior. When parents see you take safety seriously, they will trust you and your judgment, even after an injury happens. When you put a priority on safety in your planning, you will be able to spot hazards more easily.

Knowledgeable Coaches

Unlike most sports, track and field is a combination of several events, each of which carries its own level of risk. Therefore, the most significant part of any risk management plan is the hiring of certified and qualified coaches who are intimately familiar with the risks of each event they coach.

Conducting a track and field event when you do not have a coach who is thoroughly familiar with the risks involved creates a major risk. If you don't have a qualified coach for a high-risk event, don't do the event, or send your athletes to specific event centers or to a school with a qualified high-risk-event coach.

Track and field requires at least two, and preferably three, coaches. This is critical because of the numerous and varied events and because of the large area that needs to be supervised. Coaches are required to know the rules of their specific sport and fulfill the requirements of national and state associations. Read the rulebook every season. Attend state and local meetings. Never ignore any regulation that pertains to a safety issue. There is no excuse for not staying current with all rules and regulations. Just as important, follow your athletic department rules and regulations. Talk with your athletic director at least once a year about safety-related issues.

In addition to playing rules, competent coaches know the basic rules of health safety. You are not expected to know all that an athletic trainer knows, but do stay current on the major guidelines. For example, it would be considered a breach of your duty as a coach if you prevented your players from taking water breaks during practice. If you recommend any type of nutritional supplements to your players, be sure there are absolutely no risks involved with taking them. Know about proper warm-up and cool-down.

Warn of Risks

Some coaches feel that if you inform student-athletes of potential injuries, they will stop participating. This has proven to be untrue. In fact, warning and obtaining an informed consent form from players and parents is an established duty, and informing people about the potential risks of participating in any activity actually reduces injuries.

It may seem obvious that an athlete can get hurt in track and field, but informed-consent forms help spell out just what the potential risks are. The form should include pertinent words in large print, such as "Warning," "Attention," and "Please Read." The heading on the form should also be in large print. The form should cover all phases, sites, and timeframes. Your legal counsel should review the informed-consent form. After it has been signed, give a copy to each student-athlete's parents, and keep the original.

It is important that the recipient understands the seriousness of the consent form. Have a parent-information meeting to discuss the risks and benefits of participation. Ask parents and athletes if they have any questions and if they understand what they are signing. They should know that signing the form is voluntary, and that by doing so, they are agreeing to accept the risks that come with participation.

Even after the form has been signed, warnings and reminders should be issued. They should be frequent and given within the context of normal instruction.

Case Study 1

During the first period of a roller hockey game, John slipped while approaching the end dasher boards. His head struck the boards, after which he appeared dazed. Coaches and administrators arrived quickly and provided appropriate care for the immediate situation. As John skated back to the bench, it was clear that his helmet had broken as a result of the impact. A few minutes later, John was observed back in the game with the broken pieces of his helmet taped in place. Other players were observed with mouthpieces hanging loose inside their face shields.

The quality and use of equipment is an essential consideration for both coaches and officials. While equipment review is a game duty of officials, at practice the coach must perform this role and be familiar with both the requirements and the state of equipment during the activity. As described by the case study, the state of equipment may change to the degree that it no longer meets the rules, and coaches and officials must be aware of and enforce proper equipment use. When a bat breaks, for safety reasons both coaches and officials generally do not permit it to be used; the same principle must be applied to all equipment in every sport.

- Health condition of athletes—It is vital that coaches, especially in local sports programs where athletes may not be especially well-conditioned or where there are limited numbers of coaches to supervise a large number of athletes, develop ways to monitor what is happening with their athletes. This is especially important during early season training or where weather conditions may add to the potential for injury or illness.

- Adherence to rules

Case Study 2

Jill was injured when she collided with another athlete during practice. The rules of her sport require that eye protection be worn; however, because this was a practice, neither player was wearing protective eyewear. The eye protection was sitting near the door to the court on a bench. The coach was seated on the same bench and had moved the equipment in order to be able to sit to watch the girl's workout. The same coach is also a referee for the sport, and recently passed a new level of officials' certification. During the last match refereed, he reminded one of the players to put on her required eyewear!

Every sport program should require that all coaches attend rules clinics where it is emphasized that enforcing rules for the safety of the athlete be consistent at all times. This includes rules related to the nature of play and those related to the duties of officials during play. Enforcement of rules is as important during practice as at an event, and the sports organization is open to claims of negligence when it permits activities to be conducted in which the rules of play are ignored.

Risk Management Essentials for Local Sports Programs, David Mair, USOC Risk and Insurance Management.

Chapter Summary

The best defense against injuries and lawsuits is to understand, appreciate, and meet your legal duties as a physical education instructor and as a coach. It's a matter of staying vigilant and caring about the student-athletes for whom you are responsible. It is important to rely on the expertise and help of the principal and athletic director; you may also want to contact the legal department of the school district if questions arise.

Chapter Review Questions

1. What is risk management?

2. What legal responsibilities do coaches and physical education instructors have when dealing with athletes and students?

3. Why is it prudent to have a policy statement for athletics?

4. What are some of the legal duties of a coach?

5. Why should ethical responsibilities be considered in coaching?

6. Explain how you would manage a practice and game facility.

7. What considerations need to be taken into account in the management of outdoor facilities?

8. If a coach wants to take a team on an overnight trip, what procedures should he or she follow?

9. What needs to be considered when supervising student-athletes?

10. What should the coach consider when setting up a medical emergency action plan?

Projects and Activities

1. Visit several college and high school websites and read their risk management statements. Compile a list of common philosophies and procedures.

2. Pay a visit to a local college's department of legal affairs. Ask for and read a copy of the school's mission statement dealing with coaching and athletics. What did you find out?

3. Pay a visit to a local college's department of physical education and department of athletics. Ask for a copy of their emergency management plans and review them. Are the plans the same or different? If different, why?

Website Resources

Guide to Coaching Youth Sports: http://www.guidetocoachingsports.com

Facility and Equipment Planning, Design, and Management

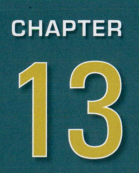

CHAPTER 13

Objectives

Upon completion of this chapter, the reader should be able to:

- Describe the process of planning, design, and management of physical education facilities.
- Describe the unique characteristics and challenges of indoor and outdoor facilities.
- Explain the relevance of community buy-in to school fitness facilities.
- Describe the modern training room facility and its specifications.

Key Terms

Field house

Fitness facilities

Gymnasium

Training room

Weight rooms

Facility and Equipment Planning, Design, and Management

The planning, design, and implementation of physical education athletic and **fitness facilities** (Figure 13-1) are crucial to the overall success of the fitness and athletic programs. Facilities that are well-planned and forward looking have an added benefit: they can adjust to future trends and needs. Physical education instructors need to be intimately involved in all phases of the planning, design, and management of current and future facilities. To be intimately involved, the physical education instructor needs to be an expert in current and future fitness trends and practices. The greater the knowledge, the more informed the instructor can be in developing future facilities and programs.

Indoor Fitness Facilities

Physical education in schools is undergoing extensive change. To keep interest, physical education and athletic departments are taking a lesson from modern consumer health and fitness clubs (Figure 13-2).

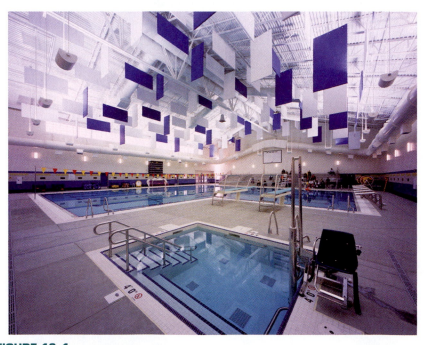

FIGURE 13-1

Mount Tahoma High School Pool, Tacoma, Washington (Copyright 2004 Doug J Scott Photography, Dougscott.com)

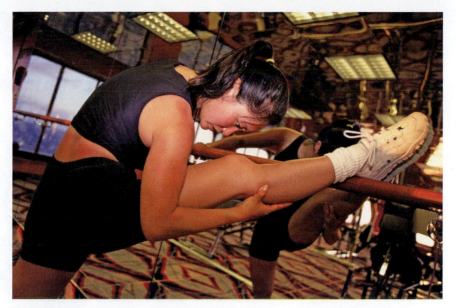

FIGURE 13–2
Indoor facilities allow for year-round fitness activities. (Courtesy of Photodisc)

The current population of under-active children has forced educators to reassess physical education curriculum, looking to establish more realistic and attractive ways to entice students to become and stay fit. The trend is to give students a more consumer-oriented view of physical education, to make physical education more connected to their lives.

Gymnasiums and Field Houses

The predominant indoor activity area with spectator capabilities in a school is the **gymnasium.** (Figure 13-3) Year-round practice schedules and overlapping competitive seasons for both boys' and girls' events place many existing gymnasiums in a constant state of conflict. An existing gymnasium may not meet the current performance and competition criteria for high school athletics. Additionally, its location may limit accessibility for evening and weekend use because of additional security requirements.

The most flexible arrangement of additional athletic space utilizes the **field house** concept. Incorporating multiple activity floors capable of sustaining simultaneous, independent activities with accommodations for spectator seating, a field house provides the most usability for the greatest number of activities. Direct exterior access and security separation from the rest of the school provides added scheduling potential.

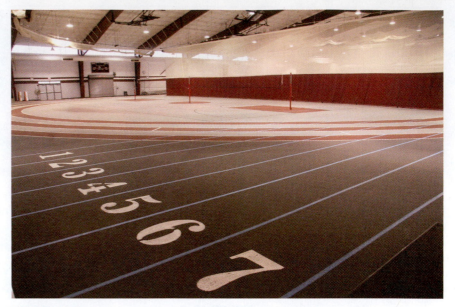

FIGURE 13–3
Argo Community High School, Summit, IL (Courtesy of Argo Community High School)

Expanded athletic programs have created an increased need for offices to accommodate additional coaching staff. Ideally, these offices should be located within locker rooms, facilitating supervision of athletes. However, because the genders of the coaching staff and the team do not always align, the most practical solution is to locate staff offices close to (but not necessarily in) the locker rooms.

There is generally a need for increased parking and access for spectators and participants. This translates into a need for an increased number of restrooms, and concession areas and an overall increase in lobby space.

Weight Rooms

One of the primary changes being made in many schools is the addition of **weight rooms** (Figure 13-4). Weight rooms can be created by renovating existing space or through new construction. While these changes can come with a hefty price tag, most agree the benefits outweigh the cost.

Many schools with weight rooms have created them by converting and equipping existing facilities to meet their needs. Schools have converted portable classrooms, machine shops, and other large areas as space becomes available. Many of these areas are ideal because they offer good ceiling clearance, open floor plans, and ventilation.

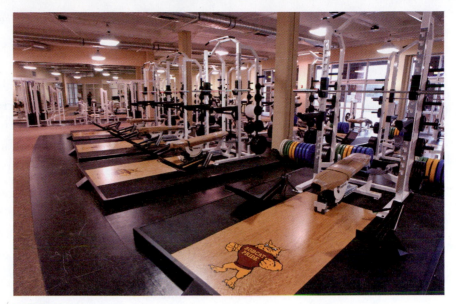

FIGURE 13–4
Texas State University Weight Room Complex

The cost to create a weight room depends on many factors. These factors include whether you are creating or modifying a facility; equipment needs; and anticipated use, which largely determines size and location. If a school already has the space, it can cost $50,000 or more to a equip medium-size space with moderately priced equipment.

When designing a weight training room, numerous factors require consideration. The first step is to determine how the room is going to be used and by whom. The facility coordinator will need to figure in the average number of students per physical education class; the sex and ages of users; the peak number that will use the facility at one time; whether it will be open for community use; and the type of programs for which the room is to be used.

The three types of equipment to consider are cardiovascular, mechanized weights, and free weights. Choices should be ageappropriate for the students, as some machines are not suitable for younger children. Low-tech, high-durability equipment should be purchased if the room is for school use only; slightly higher technology should be purchased if it also is for community use.

One item often forgotten when budgeting for equipment is the cost of maintenance. If the school doesn't have someone on the premises who knows how to repair and maintain the equipment, then buying a service contract with the vendor would be a wise choice. Average maintenance costs can run $2,000 to $5,000 a year, depending on the equipment and the amount of use.

Schools need to have staff knowledgeable in the use of the equipment. This means the staff may need special training. The obvious benefit is that students and athletes are properly trained; the less obvious one is increased equipment life and less maintenance. Most lawsuits result from lack of proper, knowledgeable supervision.

When choosing an existing space to renovate, look for an area with a minimum of 12 feet of ceiling clearance and no less than 1,000 square feet of open floor space. A 1,500 to 2,000-square-foot space would be better because it would permit creating open areas between equipment and moderate flow. The room should also have good internal and external ventilation and outside windows for natural light. Optimally, the space chosen should be near the school's gymnasium and locker rooms and allow for controlled access and after-hours use.

The weight room itself should include wall mirrors and special rubberized sport-type flooring. This is recommended throughout, since dropped free weights can damage tile or concrete floors. Carpet can be used beneath cardiovascular and mechanized equipment; however, perspiration on carpet can produce sanitation concerns. Machines that are plugged into electrical outlets should be placed over the outlets, eliminating cord safety hazards and reducing maintenance. It is important to plan enough floor space between pieces of equipment to allow for safe operation and access.

Fitness Facilities

Indoor **fitness facilities** can include everything from tennis courts, running tracks, multi-purpose Astro Turf facilities, and swimming pools, to a single facility designed primarily for stationary equipment like treadmills, elliptical trainers, and exercise bikes. A facility's configuration will depend on the school and community buy-in for such facilities and the budget to design, build, maintain, and staff them.

New facilities often inspire schools to consider broadening options in the physical education curriculum beyond resistance training and aerobic classes to include such activities as martial arts, inline skating, and biking. A benefit of these activities is that they support lifelong fitness.

> **• KEY CONCEPT •**
>
> New facilities often inspire schools to consider broadening options in the physical education curriculum beyond resistance training and aerobic classes to include such activities as martial arts, inline skating, and biking.

Across the country, school districts are building new fitness centers or renovating and converting underused sections of existing buildings into bright places that not only promote better health among students, but also lead to healthier relations between local schools and their communities.

One of the most ambitious of these collaborative arrangements is the Center of Clayton, an $18 million multi-use facility just west of St. Louis, Missouri, which opened in 2000. Although it is part of Clayton High School, it is owned and operated by an entity separate from the school district or city.

The Clayton Recreation, Sports and Wellness Commission is made up of six members representing the Clayton Board of Aldermen, the board of education, and the community at large. The facility was funded by a one-half–cent sales tax increase and a school bond issue, which also funded an expansion of Clayton High School.

"When we looked at our resources and the city looked at its resources, there was no way each could accomplish what it wanted to alone," says David Krauss, a member of both the Clayton school board and the center's governing commission.

Krauss agrees that such centers are magnets for seniors and, as a result, can garner more support for public education from a demographic group that tends not to vote for school funding issues. "If you could see this place on a Saturday afternoon," Krauss says, "Elementary school basketball going on, people from age 3 to 85 are here, the pool is busy. We definitely have achieved our goal of providing for the broader community. This will be a model for other schools."

Despite their success across the country, fitness centers, whether designed for community and school use, or primarily for student use only, have been slow to catch on. This is more a problem with funding than inspiration. However, the trend is toward facilities that offer life-long fitness options that students enjoy and will continue with long after school is over.

Athletic Training Room

Today's athletic teams are bigger, stronger, and faster, and the number of outstanding male and female athletes has increased significantly. This translates into a pressing need for new **training room** facilities

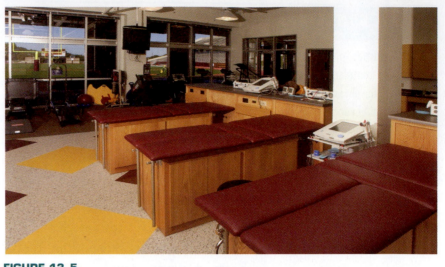

FIGURE 13–5
Texas State University Training Room Complex

(Figure 13-5). As more players put more effort into their sport, the potential for injuries increases. Improperly treated or untreated injuries can become chronic and debilitating conditions that last for years after the initial injury.

Often thought of as an adjunct to the locker room, the athletic training room is an important and vital area that supports the entire athletic department. Special consideration and planning is needed in the design and operation of the athletic department's training room facility.

Design of the Central Training Room

The central training room must be easily accessible to both male and female athletes (Figure 13-6). Depending on the size of the school or facility being served, there may also be a need for a smaller satellite facility. When designing or converting a space for a training room, careful planning is important. Some of the many factors to consider in the planning stage include size, lighting, plumbing, electricity, ventilation and heating, telephone access, storage, office space, wet area, taping area, treatment area, and exercise and rehabilitation areas.

Training Room Dimensions

The industry rule of thumb for college and universities allots 80 square feet per training table, with 3 feet between tables for modality carts and other equipment. That comes down to 6–8 feet per athlete. Boston

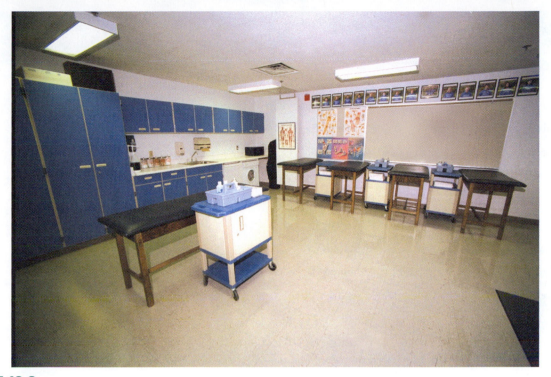

FIGURE 13–6
The central training room

College currently offers 4,000 square feet for their 750 athletes. Athletic trainers at Ohio State University use 13,000 square feet to accommodate their 900 athletes. However, training room facilities at high schools have to make do with much less floor space. This often means a space in the 400–800 square foot range. The optimum training facility size for any high school will be based on the size of the school and the number of athletes served. High schools with a population of 1,500–2,000 students will have approximately 375 athletes, or roughly 25 percent of the school population. The minimum recommended floor space for high schools of this size should be approximately 1,200 square feet. Table 3-1 gives a typical breakdown of sports offered each season and the number of participants that may be on each team for a school of this size.

Outdoor Physical Education Facilities

Physical education facilities are a major part of school campuses. During the past ten years, the importance of athletic facility performance in secondary schools has dramatically increased. With the rise in the number of

TABLE 13-1 Sports by Season with Anticipated Number of Athletes Competing

Fall	Winter	Spring
Football (V) 45	Basketball, Boys (V) 12	Baseball (V) 20
Football (JV) 35	Basketball, Boys (JV) 12	Baseball (JV) 20
Football (C) 50	Basketball, Boys (C) 20	Baseball (C) 20
Cross Country, Boys 35	Basketball, Girls (V) 12	Fastpitch/Softball (V) 25
Cross Country, Girls 35	Basketball, Girls (JV) 12	Fastpitch/Softball (JV) 25
Volleyball (V) 12	Basketball, Girls (C) 20	Fastpitch/Softball (C) 25
Volleyball (JV) 12	Gymnastics 35	Soccer, Boys (V) 20
Volleyball (C) 18	Swimming, Boys 40	Soccer, Boys (JV) 20
Soccer, Girls (V) 20	Wrestling (V) 14	Soccer, Boys (C) 20
Soccer, Girls (JV) 20	Wrestling (JV) 40	Track and Field, Boys 45
Soccer, Girls (C) 20	Wrestling (C) 40	Track and Field, Girls 45
Swimming, Girls 40		Golf, Boys 10
Tennis, Boys 16		Golf, Girls 10
		Tennis, Girls, 16
Cheer team 24		
Drill/Dance team 45		
Sports: 14 Athletes: 427	Sports: 11 Athletes: 326	Sports: 11 Athletes: 390

This table is based on a high school of 1,500–2,200 students grades 9–12.   (V) Varsity   (JV) Junior Varsity   (C) Sophomore or Freshman and Sophomore

female athletes and the demand for gender and/or sport venue diversity, the pressure for facilities to be better, larger, and more comprehensive has exceeded some schools' capabilities. Add to this the multiple feeder programs that incorporate a community's club sports, and the availability of local school athletic facilities for their programs, and it's easy to see that an existing venue may not be able to keep up with the increased demand (Figure 13-7).

School boards are faced with fiscal responsibilities that limit their ability to expand current facilities. Their task is to look for ways to optimize and upgrade current buildings, while creating a flexible environment that allows for broader usage. Often, this involves reconfiguring

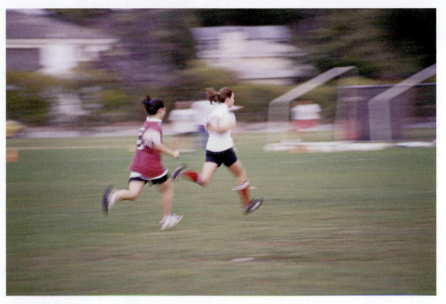

FIGURE 13–7
Outdoor facilities must be adequate to allow for many different activities. (Courtesy of Photodisc)

existing spaces for more suitable functions and/or reorganizing existing spaces to allow for simultaneous use.

Operational costs play a significant role in the life of any facility, especially one that needs to absorb the usage and wear and tear of athletes and their fans. The balance of the operational costs include janitorial services, maintenance, and repairs, as well as administrative and security personnel. Usability and projected life span of the renovated space should be judged in terms of decreased maintenance and increased serviceability. It is important to begin the upgrading process with a solid understanding of the goals for the facility and assume that no current function area or support facility is fixed in its location.

CASE STUDY: THE NEW P.E. CURRICULUM

Every student at Madison Junior High completes a computer-based fitness test. For most of us, P.E. class isn't exactly the first subject that comes to mind when we consider the benefits of integrating technology into the curriculum. But Phil Lawler, head of the Physical Education Department at Madison Junior High in Naperville, Illinois, has seen first-hand how high-tech tools can help to bring a healthier, more balanced approach to physical education.

From the heart-rate monitors that students wear during their weekly 12-minute run/walk (a healthier version of the traditional one-mile run), to a comprehensive computer-based fitness station where students measure everything from strength and flexibility to cholesterol levels, Madison Junior High has embraced the use of state-of-the-art tools to support the physical health and education of its adolescent students. To date, the Naperville School District has spent $450,000 on high-tech P.E. tools for junior and senior high school students.

Included among Madison's unique P.E. facility is a complete fitness center (dubbed the Madison Health Club), which looks more like a neighborhood health club than a junior-high workout room. There's also a rock-climbing wall and a series of computer-enabled fitness test stations, where students create a total health portfolio that will eventually follow them from sixth grade through high school graduation.

The fitness testing system, which measures flexibility, blood pressure, body composition, upper body strength, and cardiovascular health, is integral to Madison's commitment to emphasizing fitness over raw athletic ability—long the emphasis in P.E. classes throughout the country. Once in the fall and then again in the spring, students work their way through a series of "smart" workstations: One test measures flexibility, as students bend and stretch while holding a cord attached to a computer. As they stretch, the cord becomes more taut, and the computer records the results. At another station students perform repetitions of bicep curls and watch as a graph on the computer monitor reflects their efforts. Beginning this fall, parents will be able to enter a PIN number to access their child's fitness test results from the school website.

Lawler, who in addition to his job at Madison coordinates the P.E. program for the entire Naperville Community Unit School District, has been advocating what you might call an enlightened approach to physical fitness for nearly thirteen years. He points to two seminal reports—"Healthy People 2000" (now "Healthy People 2010") and "The Surgeon General's Report on Youth Fitness"—as the impetus for his department's switch from an old-style P.E. curriculum—where speed and ability were paramount—to a program that emphasizes fitness and well-being, not athleticism.

"There's been a major paradigm shift in the teaching of P.E.," says Lawler, whose program has been highlighted in the state and national media and has been identified by the Centers for Disease Control as a national model. "The old-style P.E. met the needs of just 30 percent of our students." Everyone else, he adds with regret in his voice, was often left with a "lifetime of bad memories and demeaning experiences," like being picked last for basketball scrimmage or being ridiculed by teachers and fellow students for being too weak or too slow.

Today, P.E. classes at Madison Junior High are more about developing a healthy lifestyle than they are about learning to throw a baseball or make a jump shot. As part of a statewide effort to encourage physical fitness, students at Madison (and in all junior and senior high schools in the Naperville School District) attend P.E. classes five days a week. One day is devoted to using the state-of-the-art fitness center; another is spent participating in a cardiovascular run/walk; and the remaining three days are devoted to individual and team sports.

But if any of the activities sound familiar, think again. Classes at Naperville couldn't be more different from the P.E. classes you knew as a kid. Data from heart-rate monitors can be printed out and then analyzed by students and teachers. Whether they're working out on the fitness machines or participating in the cardio run/walk, students wear heart-rate monitors, giving both themselves and their instructors an accurate picture of the intensity of their workout. Students routinely talk about being "in their target zone," signifying that they're maintaining a healthy heart rate while exercising.

"Every student now gets credit for what they do, not how fast or how far they run," says Lawler, who recalls one female student who was among the last in her class to complete a mile run. "She was jogging very slowly," says Lawler, and an observer might have thought she wasn't "giving it her all." After the run ended, though, Lawler read the computer-generated printout from her heart monitor and realized that the girl had been working well above her target zone. "In the old days, I might have told her to work harder, but with the heart-rate monitors, I was able to tell how hard she was working—too hard, in fact."

Although he taught P.E. for years without the benefits of heart-rate monitors and other high-tech equipment, Lawler is convinced these tools are not only beneficial to kids, they're necessary. "It's like driving a car without a speedometer. Without the heart-rate monitor, we just can't know how hard kids are really working. Not only is it unfair to some students, it can also be dangerous." Students also wear the monitors when they're playing team sports, providing Lawler and his colleagues with a handy way of making sure everyone gets a good workout. Madison Junior High students spend one day a week in the school's state-of-the-art fitness center, dubbed "The Madison Health Club."

None of the changes at Madison would have been possible, says Lawler, without the commitment of his staff and the school and district administrators to ongoing professional development. In addition to taking courses and attending local and national conferences, once a year Naperville physical education instructors participate in a daylong physical education institute, complete with guest speakers, workshops, and product information. When the program started 15 years ago, there were 8 speakers and 100 attendees. Today, 1,500 P.E. instructors from throughout the county attend the annual event, a testament to what Lawler calls "a hunger to learn about the new P.E." But Lawler isn't content with just advocating change at the local level. Each year, he and his staff welcome visitors from schools throughout the country that, like Madison, are embracing the "new P.E." concept.

Lawler and his Naperville colleagues also work to educate parents on the importance of a healthy, active lifestyle. Last year, for example, one of the high school P.E. instructors lent out pedometers to several parents, encouraging them to keep track of how many steps they took in a day (the surgeon general recommends an average of 10,000 steps a day for a healthy adult). The experience was enlightening, to say the least. One parent returned the pedometer after having taken just 1,000 steps in a day. Few had taken more than 5,000 steps.

"What it all boils down to is information," says Lawler. "We want to provide students [and, he might add, their parents] with the tools and the information they need to live healthy, active lives."

Chapter Summary

The planning, design, and implementation of physical education and athletic facilities is often as important to the community as it is to the school itself. The community can not only benefit from the use of well-designed facilities, but can help to fund and maintain these facilities. Community support and use of fitness facilities has been shown to translate over to positive reviews for their school districts as a whole.

It is important for the physical education instructor to have a good knowledge base regarding facility needs and future development. Planning for new facilities requires expert advice from physical education instructors, and sound goals for achieving the desired outcome.

Chapter Review Questions

1. What is the role of the physical education instructor in facility planning, design, and management?

2. What unique characteristics and challenges do indoor facilities present?

3. What are the differences between a traditional gymnasium and a field house?

4. Why is it important to include well-equipped and designed weight rooms in schools today?

5. What are the anticipated costs associated with maintenance of weight room facilities?

6. What is the difference between a weight room and a fitness facility?

7. Why should the community be involved in the design, use, and maintenance of fitness facilities within the school?

8. What are the most important components of the athletic training room?

9. Explain the guidelines and specifications that are important for operation of the athletic training room.

Projects and Activities

1. Design a weight room facility for a student body of 1,500. All aspects of the facility should be included.

2. Meet with the superintendent of a school district nearby. Ask the superintendent about community partners for fitness facilities in their district. If this isn't a part of the school district's plan, ask how partnerships of this type can develop.

3. Design the optimum athletic training room facility for a high school with a population of 1,500. Include a detailed floor plan and explain each aspect of your facility.

Website Resources

American Association of School Administrators: http://www.aasa.org

North American Society for Sport Management (NASSM): http://www.nassm.com/

School Planning & Management magazine: http://www.peterli.com/

Athletic Administration

Objectives

Upon completion of this chapter, the reader should be able to:

- Describe basic job responsibilities of the athletic director.
- Explain the educational requirements to gain entrance into this field.
- Discuss employment opportunities and requirements.

Key Terms

Academic eligibility

Athletic administration

Certified athletic administrator (CAA)

Certified master athletic administrator (CMAA)

Corporate sponsorship

Registered athletic administrator (RAA)

Student-athlete

Athletic Administration

Athletic directors have a significant impact on school climate and community relations and assist the principal and district administrators in promoting the vision of world-class schools. This is often accomplished while the large majority of school athletic directors serve as teachers on special assignment—an assignment that combines two of the worst things about the job: administrative expectations and teacher pay (Figure 14-1).

The job of the athletic director has become increasingly visible with the tremendous interest in high school and college sports. School officials are more likely to be approached by adults in their community over matters concerning sport teams and coaches than about any other aspect of the educational program. Even so, most athletic directors feel that their job has many rewards, including the opportunity to develop special relationships, the experience of amateur athletics, the opportunity to influence the development of young people, and the ability to make a difference in someone's life.

> **• KEY CONCEPT •**
>
> School officials are more likely to be approached by adults in their community over matters concerning sport teams and coaches than about any other aspect of the educational program.

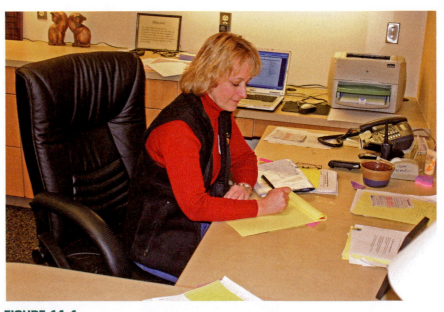

FIGURE 14-1
The athletic director must manage many different tasks simultaneously.

Job Responsibilities

Athletic directors are responsible for all aspects of the athletic program. They are responsible for developing the athletic program within their school and assisting the principal in duties pertaining to athletics. These duties include, but are not limited to:

- Facility planning and management
- Evaluation of athletic and activity programs
- Evaluation of coaches
- **Student-athlete** eligibility
- Rule compliance
- Management of athletic budgets
- Assisting the principal in the hiring and dismissal of coaches
- Monitoring fundraising
- Public relations
- Booster club management
- Communication with students, coaches, parents, teachers, and the administration
- Program recognition

As shown above, the athletic director's job is very complex and diverse. Of all the responsibilities that fall under the purview of the athletic director, there are four basics that athletic directors must master:

- Program success vs. competitive success
- Academic success of student-athletes
- Fiscal responsibility
- Rules compliance

Program Success vs. Competitive Success

Athletic directors are required to guide student-athletes, coaches, and staff to reach the height of their personal potential. Athletic directors are responsible for hiring coaches who will motivate student-athletes and bring continued success and discipline to athletic programs.

The life lessons learned through participation in athletic competition are what makes athletics a special learning environment unlike any other. The experiences of working cooperatively toward a common purpose, learning the value of teamwork, and developing the concept of fair play, help young student-athletes prepare for their future beyond school.

While everyone involved with athletics takes great pride in winning, the athletic director must encourage everyone not to condone the "winning at any cost" mentality, and should discourage any pressures that might cause athletes to neglect good sportsmanship and good mental health. The athletic program must be conducted in such a way as to justify it as an educational activity. The educational side of athletics is that students can benefit from the lessons learned through participation. While winning is usually more fun, the lessons learned from losing are often beneficial.

In winning as in losing, the long-range value of the experience is promoted under certain conditions. An undue emphasis on winning can easily leave the false impression with student-athletes that their athletic activity has value only if the competition results in a win. A "winning is everything" approach leads directly to unsportsmanlike behavior and cheating, and translates to unacceptable ethics and lifelong values. In an educational environment, it is important to emphasize preparing to be competitive, and to focus on doing one's best rather than simply on winning.

> **• KEY CONCEPT •**
>
> The athletic program must be conducted in such a way as to justify it as an educational activity.

Academic Success of Student Athletes

There were more than seven million boys and girls throughout the United States participating in high school sports during the 2005–2006 academic year. Today, with the number of states turning to stricter requirements for high school graduation and the emphasis on preparing students for life, it is important that coaches work to positively impact the student-athlete's ability to succeed academically (Figure 14-2).

According to many physical education professionals, sports play an integral role in the development of students and contribute to the value of traditional educational programs. Proponents of physical education courses view values such as sportsmanship, hard work, and moral character as beneficial aspects of sports. Given the significant amount of time coaches spend with student-athletes, logic indicates that coaches inherently play a large role in the development of student-athletes.

School systems and society view extracurricular activities in American schools in two different ways. The first view is that schools exist

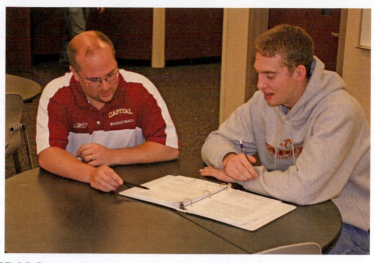

FIGURE 14-2
Athletic director helping student athlete with homework.

primarily for the pursuit of academic excellence and that schools should focus on the teaching of formal knowledge. Proponents of this view assert although athletics are fun, they are not an important aspect of education. The other view suggests that experience gained through sports, in terms of personal development, is a vital part of the educational process.

Athletics support academic objectives and are valuable because they can help student-athletes develop self-respect, self-esteem, self-confidence, teamwork, and the competitive spirit. Furthermore, athletics prepare student-athletes for the world after high school, regardless of whether or not the student will attend college.

Many studies have focused on various aspects of the academic achievement of student-athletes. These studies concluded that interscholastic athletic programs reduced discipline problems, increased academic achievement, and contributed to higher graduation rates. The U. S. Department of Education published two reports, entitled Schools That Work (1987) and Schools Study (1977), which indicated that the school-reform movement was ignoring the potential of athletics to improve education.

Athletics' Responsibility to Academic Achievement

Academic eligibility for student-athletes in public high schools across America has many variations, and has been changing over the past twenty years. The term "student-athlete" implies that the person in question is both a good student in the classroom and an active and effective participant on an athletic team. As school districts and athletic directors work to show accountability to the parents and taxpayers in their respective communities through the revision of athletic codes, it is important to address the issue of student-athlete academic performance.

Efforts to reform academic eligibility for high school athletes began in 1983, amid strong resistance from coaches, parents, and others. The Los Angeles Unified School District instituted a rule that stated, "To be eligible for participation in extracurricular activities students must maintain a C average in four subjects and have no failures." In 1984 the state of Texas introduced a "No Pass, No Play" rule that stated that athletes could not have any failing grades if they were to participate in a sporting activity. Initially, a large group of students became ineligible to compete, and there was strong opposition from coaches and parents. But in a matter of two years, in both of these instances, the percentage of students who were declared ineligible was the same as before the rule was enacted.

Many school districts throughout the United States have begun to institute minimum academic requirements for athletic participation. The requirements for a student's grade point average (GPA) range from no requirements to a minimum of a 2.5 GPA. Some school districts require a minimum of a 2.0 GPA, with no failing grades, in order for a student to be eligible to participate in the interscholastic athletic program. All states require that students be enrolled in a minimum load of courses in order to even participate in athletic programs (Figure 14-3).

> **● KEY CONCEPT ●**
>
> The term "student-athlete" implies that the student in question is both a good student in the classroom and an active and effective participant on an athletic team.

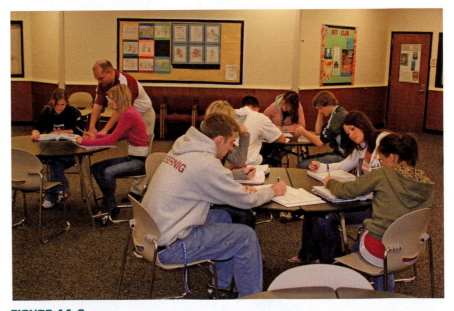

FIGURE 14–3
Study tables allow athletes from all sports to get extra help needed in their classes.

After grade point average, the most popular criterion for athletic eligibility, in many schools is a limit on the number of Fs a student-athlete can earn per semester. This limit can range from no Fs (no pass, no play) to three; most commonly, a student-athlete is limited to one F.

All state athletic associations recommend some form of academic eligibility requirements for student participation in interscholastic sports. These requirements range from enrollment in a minimum number of courses, to a combination of a minimum number of courses, no Fs, a minimum grade point average (GPA), and an attendance policy. Only six state associations currently recommend or require that a minimum GPA be included as part of the academic criteria for athletic eligibility. In Ohio, association guidelines recommend that individual schools should set their own GPA requirements.

In schools that have strong academic requirements, athletic directors reported that students adjusted to the requirements once they were set, and that the requirements had minimal impact on student participation in sports.

Fiscal Responsibility

Athletic directors are responsible for maintaining their programs on a budget allocated by the school's governing board of education. Athletic budgets are complicated and require knowledge of each sport and its associated costs. Funding for athletics generally comes from gate receipts, student-body funds, and district budgets (Figure 14-4).

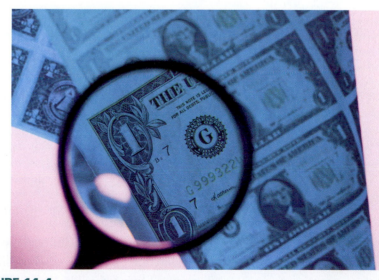

FIGURE 14–4
Athletic programs must always keep a balanced budget. (Courtesy of Photodisc)

The greatest expense is funding salaries for coaches and support staff. These expenses are generally covered by district funds. Transportation is the next category of expense. Most school districts pay for transportation; however, some districts require individual schools to fund part or all of transportation costs. Uniforms and equipment are next in line, and are normally an expense of individual sport budgets. The athletic director is responsible for these budgets, and for oversight to ensure judicious spending.

Corporate Sponsorship

Sponsorship of scholastic athletics represents one of the fastest-growing areas in all of corporate marketing, and involves many Fortune 500 corporations. Estimates of corporate spending on high school sports nationwide exceed $15 million a year, and that number is is growing fast. "This is something that is growing exponentially," says Rick Horrow, visiting professor of sports law at Harvard University. "I'm not sure anybody has a firm handle yet on an aggregate amount of spending, but it's getting very, very big. A targeted, tasteful program that reaches high school purchasers and, by connection, their parents, can be a very efficient corporate play and will be a key part of many future corporate strategies."

Shoe companies such as Nike and Adidas have sponsored basketball camps and supported powerhouse programs for years. But the rising and more universal corporate interest in prep sports is due primarily to three factors: cost, availability, and exposure.

Corporations sponsor high school sports to the tune of several thousands of dollars a year per school. Typically this sponsorship is provided in the form of in-kind contributions of shoes, uniforms, and other gear. Professional and major college shoe deals, ballpark signage, and stadium and event-naming rights have become commonplace fixtures to the teenage athlete.

In Tennessee, the prep championship football game is named The Blue Cross Bowl; ShopRite Gymnasium is an elementary school gym in New Jersey; an award honoring overall excellence in Virginia high school sports is called the Wachovia Cup; and the community football stadium in Sumner, Washington, Sunset Chevrolet Stadium, is named after a city car dealership. A ten-year, $4 million deal between Dr. Pepper and Grapevine High School in Dallas, Texas, a national prep football power,

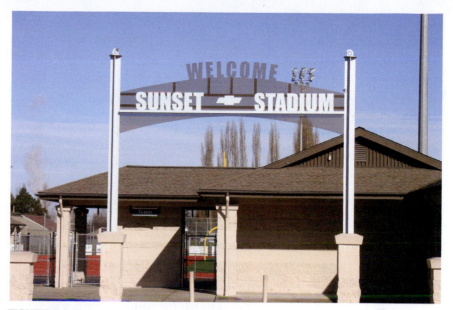

FIGURE 14–5
Sunset Chevrolet Stadium, Sumner School District, Sumner, Washington

is seen as one of the most lucrative in high school sports. The deal includes Dr. Pepper logos on the roofs of school buildings, which are visible to planes taking off and landing at nearby Dallas-Fort Worth International Airport (Figure 14-5).

There are still thousands of schools untouched by corporate America. Sponsorship represents an opportunity for companies to gain an advantage over rivals. High school sports are gaining more exposure through cable television and the Internet, heightening the marketing value for the sponsoring companies.

"It's something that has been very effective and beneficial for us and the schools," says Travis Gonzolez, spokesman for Adidas. The athletic shoe giant provides free sneakers and other gear for more than a hundred high school basketball teams. "There was a stigma out there before, a lot of schools didn't want to be perceived as selling out. But if we and other companies who are committed to high school sports can come in with the same goals and save the school districts money, why shouldn't we be involved?"

Corporate sponsorship of high school athletics is causing major debate among school boards from coast to coast. Critics of corporate involvement say it violates the basic tenets of high school athletics and fosters unhealthy efforts to field winning, high-visibility teams attractive to more companies. "This professionalizes high school sports, and that's a direction exactly opposite of where it needs to go," says David Shields, codirector of the University of Notre Dame's Mendelson Center for Sport, Character and Culture. "There's more pressure on the kids to win; there's more pressure on the administrators to keep winning and justify the investment. Where does it end?"

Many school districts have resisted this trend, although most have accepted funds toward new scoreboards and from more general initiatives, such as placement of soda machines in schools. Other districts facing shrinking budgets have chosen to accept corporate dollars rather than do away with sports programs. "Schools never want to cut programs if they don't have to," says Judy Thomas, marketing director for the National Federation of State High School Associations. "So if you need to rely on corporations, that's what you need to do." The oversight group, best known for compiling rules of play for high school sports, has developed its own sponsorship program that includes credit-card giant MBNA Corporation and Red Roof Inns.

Rules Compliance

Athletic directors are responsible for completing growing amounts of paperwork, primarily to ensure that their school district complies with their athletic governing bodies. Eligibility and rules compliance have four main areas of emphasis: student eligibility requirements, school district requirements, league rule compliance, and state association compliance. These four areas are somewhat tied together, yet can be very different depending upon the governing body.

Student Eligibility Requirements

Eligibility requirements for student athletes consist of many items that may differ from one school district to the next. Most school districts require

- passing a physical evaluation, showing proof of accident insurance, purchasing an associated student body (ASB) card

- obtaining written parental permission

- meeting academic class and grade requirements

- completing an emergency contact/medical card

- adhering to the district athletic code

- complying with all local, league, and state rules.

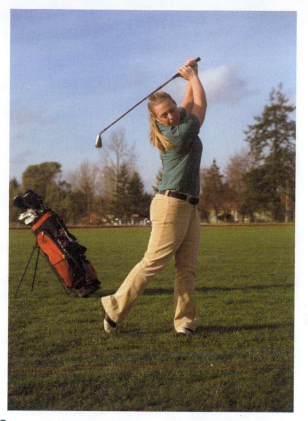

FIGURE 14-6
All schools require athletes to pass certain criteria to be eligible for competition.

In addition, many school districts are now charging students to participate in school sports. This fee can range anywhere from $25 to $150 per sport season (Figure 14-6).

School District Requirements

Each school district across the United States has its own requirements for athletic participation. These rules normally revolve around academics, with the rest of the regulations being taken care of by league and state governing bodies. The academic requirements that most school districts adhere to are listed earlier in this chapter under "Athletics' Responsibility to Academic Achievement."

League and State Regulations

League requirements for participation normally follow district and state guidelines. League rules and procedures pertain to athletic competition, supervision, and sportsmanship. State association guidelines are far-reaching and cover items such as:

- academic progress
- maximum age requirement
- valid physical examination
- residence
- transfer rules between schools and districts
- amateur status
- concurrent sports limitation
- training rules such as alcohol, tobacco, steroids, and drugs

Local, league, and state guidelines ensure fairness in athletics, safety of athletes, and academic rigor for future success.

Employment Opportunities

The Bureau of Labor Statistics projected that the number of entry-level and high school athletic director positions would grow faster than average for the years 2006–2016. Positions with colleges and universities will continue to grow slower than average.

Earnings

The typical starting salary for an athletic director ranges from $40,000 to $100,000, depending on the school district and the funds available for athletics. Many school districts use stipends to compensate their athletic directors. A stipend is typically paid in addition to the salary the athletic director receives for other job responsibilities, such as teaching, coaching, or administration. Stipends can range from $3,000 to more than $20,000 per academic year. College and university athletic directors may earn in excess of $200,000.

Advancement Opportunities

The opportunities for advancement vary. College athletic directors usually stay for long terms. However, the turnover in high school athletic administration is alarmingly high. The national average is 30 percent; some states report a turnover rate as high as 40 percent. The primary reasons for turnovers are long hours and inadequate compensation.

Education

Educational requirements typically include a bachelor's degree in education, with a master's degree often preferred. Most schools require a valid teacher's certificate. These requirements should continue in the future. Majoring or minoring in athletic administration is especially helpful for entry-level positions. Prior experience as a coach (head coaching experience preferred) is normally assumed. Three levels of certification exist nationally: **registered athletic administrator (RAA)**, **certified athletic administrator (CAA)**, and **certified master athletic administrator (CMAA)**.

College athletics has recently discovered the means to help underrepresented groups gain advancement opportunities in college programs. The NCAA has been proactive in recent years, forming special committees to research problematic areas that have prevented women from advancing in athletic administration. The NCAA has helped create internship opportunities for women and minorities to help with training and has also funded several developmental programs, such as the fellowship program and NACWAA's Executive Institute. Division I conferences have also recognized the need to enhance the education and experiences of women in intercollegiate athletics, and have assisted in funding the Women's Leadership Symposium.

The gender and minority gap in leadership positions in intercollegiate athletics should not widen, given the national attention of powerful organizations such as the NCAA, the Women's Sport Foundation, the Black Coaches Association, and NACWAA, all of which are committed to recognizing the need to place more women and minorities in leadership positions. To move ahead with the goal of closing the gender and racial gap in the hiring and promotion of women and minorities in leadership position in athletics, it is paramount that women and minority students recognize athletics as a viable career option. If more women and minorities can obtain entry-level positions, there will be more women and minorities to select from once they have gained the experience and training necessary to assume leadership positions.

Essential Skills and Traits

Athletic directors should be well-rounded individuals who possess a love of athletics and the desire to see student-athletes succeed. A strong sense of teamwork, communication, a willingness to adapt to change, problem-solving skills, strong listening skills, public speaking skills, good resource management skills, and an achievement-oriented attitude are helpful in this career. A typical day may include meetings with coaches, athletes, and other staff members. However, a large part of the day of an athletic director consists of paperwork. The hours for this position are long, and may involve 65-hour weeks, as well as weekend work.

Job Locations

Virtually every school district, college, or university has a need for athletic directors. Rural areas, small school districts, and inner-city school districts experience the greatest turnover, and therefore have the greatest need for athletic directors. Athletic directors should examine the community they wish to work in, and consider the community's support of existing athletic programs, before accepting a position.

Hiring Process

Applicants for athletic-director positions typically must submit a formal letter of application and go through an interview process with a panel of current employees of the school district. The following case study describes a day in the life of an athletic director.

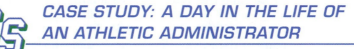

CASE STUDY: A DAY IN THE LIFE OF AN ATHLETIC ADMINISTRATOR

OK, I have to admit that being an obsessive-compulsive athletic administrator is an oxymoron. Every night I leave my office with a list of twenty or so items that need attention, and every next day at noon, not one is crossed off. It's not that I'm lazy or thirsty to be near the water-cooler; rather, the job is that spontaneous.

And everyone's got issues—from parents with important issues (after all, when it's your kid, all concerns are serious), to teachers with important issues (after all, when it's your student, all concerns are serious), to the transportation dispatcher with issues (after all, when you have a schedule the team has to be ready on time). You need an appointment to see a doctor or dentist. Not so the athletic director—just come on in fuming, and I'll be right with you.

After my first year as an athletic administrator, I learned to multitask, gained insight into how valuable a sports program is for kids and community, and put on twenty pounds. So here it is: a typical day at Decatur High School.

At 7:00 a.m. I open the door to my office with nonfat latte in hand, glancing at the red message light on my phone and hoping, against odds, that it is not shining. I sit and turn on the Gateway to check e-mail, with my "to do" list neatly placed on the left corner of the desk. Lastly, I take the two-way radio out of the charger and reluctantly (because as any administrator can tell you, "there's always trouble at the end of the radio") turn it on. And, after a big caffeine hit, my day begins.

When I left last night after the basketball game, there were no messages. This morning there are only four: a lost shooting shirt; a reporter needing the score; the night custodian complaining about a pop spill under the bleachers; and, darn it, a parent complaint about our lousy coach. I make Post-It notes, put them on top of the "to do" list, and delete the messages. On to the eight e-mails: three advertising ploys; a couple of answers to my previous e-mails; an all-staff message from an assistant principal; and a "see me" from the principal, who got the same message about our lousy coach. I print the e-mails that need attention and put them on top of the Post-Its. I delete the e-mails, tuck the radio in the back of my pants, and go see the boss.

Going to the main office is always a challenge, because I have to go by the room of the dance team advisor, who wants to be called a coach. Rarely do I get by without an "I need to talk to you." Today is no exception. After promising to find some practice space after school, I'm back on track to the office, where the secretary is waiting to tell me that the AAU team did not fill out the facility request properly. I finally make it to the principal, who wants me to set up a meeting with our disgruntled and levy-voting parent.

On my way out of the office, I check my mailbox and throw the catalogues in the recycle bin. I put mail that should go to the baseball and soccer coaches in their boxes, take the rest back to my office, and put the pile on top of the printed e-mails. Just as I settle down with the first letter, either the radio or a fire alarm will undoubtedly go off. (My hope is that it will be the fire alarm, as I'm getting too old to get in the middle of "respect" arguments.) After a couple of phone messages and e-mails, which I put on top of the letters, it's time to call the unhappy parent.

Conversations with concerned parents usually have a buzzword motif: *Many* parents are concerned. *Scholarships* are on the line. The coach plays *favorites*. This is *unacceptable*. What are *you* going to do about it? I'm going to (take your pick) the principal, the school board, the superintendent, the press, or my *lawyer*. The one person the parent rarely talks to is the coach.

Just as I put down the phone and start on my pile, in walks the football coach. Now, Coach is a great guy and doesn't need me to solve his problems; he just wants to talk. And talk. And tell war stories. Thank goodness, the bell rings and Coach has to go to his history class.

I pop open a can of Diet Pepsi and start on the mail. I either put the mail in the wastebasket, the "needs-attention basket," or in the "will-get-to-it-when-I-can" basket, which still has September mailings when I clean it out in June. Once through the mail, I start on the e-mails. After the e-mails come the Post-Its and finally the neatly-placed "to do" list is uncovered.

Right about now, the phone rings, and it's the finance lady saying she cannot sell tickets at tonight's wrestling match. I call her backup but get no answer, so I have to go see her to make sure she can sell tickets tonight. If she cannot then I will. As a matter of fact, as the major filler-inner, I often sell, announce, time, sweep, score, setup—everything but drive the bus—which the football coach used to do.

After the match, I make sure the money gets into the safe, the gym is cleared and locked, and kids have rides; then I head back to my office. I can't leave without listening to any new phone messages and reading any new e-mails. I update the "to do" list and place it neatly on the left corner of my desk.

As I turn off the light, I say to myself, "What a great job."

—Greg Flynn, Athletic Director, Federal Way School District

Chapter Summary

The athletic director is considered the top executive in the athletic department and is in charge of the entire athletic program. Athletic directors oversee budgets, hiring and dismissal of coaches, scheduling of competitions, facility repair and maintenance, and fundraising and Title IX compliance.

Individuals interested in athletic administration should have a good sports background and head coaching experience. Advanced education, such as a master's or doctorate in athletic administration, is a plus. Athletic directors must have excellent communication skills, be well organized, and be willing to work extended hours. The excitement of helping mold the athletic experience for student-athletes, as well as the chance to work with highly motivated coaches, makes this career fun and rewarding.

Chapter Review Questions

1. List the job responsibilities of the athletic administrator.

2. What is the difference between program success and competitive success?

3. How important is monitoring academic success to the athletic director? Why?

4. What is academic eligibility for student-athletes?

5. Have stricter academic requirements for participation in athletics cut down on the number of athletes participating in sports? Why?

6. What are the budgetary concerns an athletic director must address?

7. How has corporate sponsorship changed funding of athletics in some schools?

8. What are examples of rules that the athletic director must adhere to?

9. List the different student eligibility requirements explained in the chapter.

10. How much can an athletic director earn in a year?

11. What are the educational requirements to become an athletic administrator?

12. What is being done by the NCAA to address the need of women and minorities to be better represented in positions of athletic administration?

13. What are the essential skills and traits common to successful athletic administrators?

14. Where are most athletic administration jobs located?

15. How many high school athletic directors change jobs each year?

Projects and Activities

1. Select one of the job responsibilities listed in the chapter and write a short paper detailing what this responsibility entails.

2. Select a high school in the area you live. Meet with the athletic director and ask him or her to evaluate the difference in academic success between non-athletes and athletes in their school. What were your findings?

3. Read the two United States Department of Education published reports titled: Schools That Work (1987), and Schools Study (1977). Both reports talked about the potential of athletics to improve education. How?

4. How many high schools in your state require a minimum grade point average for participation in athletics?

Website Resources

American Sport Education Program: http://www.asep.com

Missouri State High School Activities Association: http://www.mshaa.org

National Collegiate Athletic Association: http://www.ncaa.org

National Assn. of Collegiate Directors of Athletics: http://www.nacda.cstv.com

National Assn. of Collegiate Women Athletic Administrators: http://www.nacwaa.org

Gender Equity and Sport: Title IX

CHAPTER 15

Objectives

Upon completion of this chapter, the reader should be able to:

- Define the difference between gender equity and discrimination in sport.
- Understand the historical events leading up to Title IX legislation.
- Explain Title IX and its implications for sport in America.

Key Terms

Civil Rights Restoration Act of 1987

Equity in Athletics Disclosure Act

Gender discrimination

Gender equity

Office of Civil Rights (OCR)

Title IX

Gender Equity and Sport: Title IX

In sports, **gender equity**, as defined by the NCAA, describes an environment in which fair and equitable distribution of overall athletic opportunities, benefits, and resources is available to both women and men and in which student-athletes, coaches, and athletics administrators are not subject to gender-based discrimination (Figure 15-1). An athletics program is gender-equitable when either the men's or women's sports program would accept as its own the overall program of the other gender.

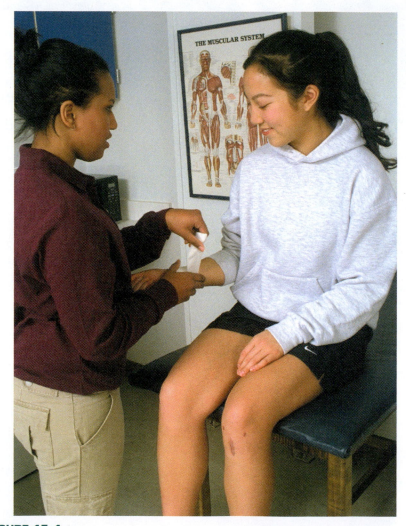

FIGURE 15–1
Title IX has allowed for equal access, facilities, and treatment for women.

Title IX is a law guaranteeing that no person in the United States shall, on the basis of sex, be excluded from participation in, be denied the benefits of, or be subjected to discrimination under any education program or activity receiving federal financial assistance.

Gender Equity and Discrimination in Sport: Pre-Title IX

The following historical discussion was adopted from an article written by Nancy Struna for the Women's Sports Foundation.

Women's sports in the United States has had an enormous influence on women's sports around the world. Title IX, the 1972 federal legislation that has been credited with encouraging much of the growth in women's sports in the United States, has also helped to influence thinking about women's sports elsewhere in the world (Figure 15-2).

Too often, historians present women's sporting experiences as if they were rooted only in modern society, in which they have become increasingly more complex and common. This characterization may be accurate

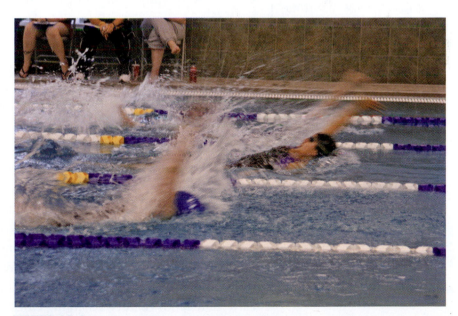

FIGURE 15–2
The advancement of women's sports has been greatly attributed to Title IX legislation. (Courtesy of Federal Way Community Center)

for the twentieth century, but throughout history, women's sporting experiences have been episodic rather than evolutionary. At any given time, women's sports shaped, as much as they were shaped by, the wider web of social, economic, and political experiences. The evolution of women's role in sport in the United States can be divided into three major periods: the colonial era, the transitional nineteenth century, and the age of modern sports.

The Colonial Era: Women and Traditional Sports and Games

Women were far more visible in American sporting life than the portraits of them would suggest, especially prior to the mid-eighteenth century. Around 1600, before Europeans colonized the land that would become the United States, the earliest American sportswomen were Native Americans. Their lifestyle was a traditional one in which sports and other displays of physical prowess were embedded in the rhythms and relations of ordinary life. Religious ceremonies called on women, and men, to dance for hours at a time; rites of passage from maidenhood to womanhood included physical displays and tests. Ball games occurred in the context of women's daily tasks, and the outcomes of these games could affect a woman's place in the family or the village. Even equipment and items for wagering, which women often controlled, came from the material stores of wood, corn, shells, and animal hides.

The migration of colonists from Europe (especially Britain), and Africa began shortly after 1600. These people fashioned a traditional, organic style of life in which sports were interspersed with ordinary tasks and rituals. Initially, there were few women among the colonists, and not surprisingly, there were few opportunities for sports other than hunting and tavern games. After mid-century, the gender ratio gradually evened out, and women assumed their traditional roles as workers in the fields and homes and as producers of community gatherings, fairs, and family events. On warm summer days in New England, husbands and wives fished and sailed together on the numerous waterways. Towns like Boston, Providence, and Hartford offered an even broader variety of sports and recreation, ranging from dances to races to fistfights. By the early eighteenth century, emerging cities were sites for public, commercial, and physical displays, including tightrope dancing by both women and men.

> ● **KEY CONCEPT** ●
>
> By the middle of the eighteenth century, the sporting experiences of women of European and African ancestry, as well as recent immigrants, were far more varied than they had been earlier.

By the middle of the eighteenth century, the sporting experiences of women of European and African ancestry, as well as recent immigrants, had become far more varied than they had been earlier. Enslaved African and African-American women found some solace in their brief respites from work on Sunday evenings, or in the days of celebrating made possible by the observance of holidays. They danced, played simple games, and ran races. Agricultural fairs, initiated by white farmers, planters, and traders, also included contests. Occasionally, women in farming communities raced horses, even against men, and bettors were willing to wager on their skills.

Middle-and upper-class women, especially those who lived in or visited towns and cities, had access to the broadest range of sports and other recreations. In the South, white women who lived on plantations raced horses and went fox hunting. As did their northern contemporaries, southern woman also attended balls, played cards, and attended the increasing array of physical culture exhibitions, which included race walking, tumbling and acrobatic displays, and equestrian shows.

The Nineteenth Century: Domesticity and the Age of Diminishing Returns

The pursuit of active sports by women was not to persist. During the second half of the eighteenth century, a series of complex changes gradually altered gender roles and relations. Enlightenment ideology and the emergent capitalist economy combined to redefine women's place in society. Women moved into the home and away from public activity. This characterization lasted for more than a century and a half. The immediate impact of these changes was the movement of many women from the playing fields into the stands, or out of public view entirely, unless accompanied by men. The trend was especially pronounced in towns and cities among middle- and upper-class people whose lives were increasingly shaped by commercial and industrial tasks. Many people came to believe that women's central role was to bear and nurture children and families.

Slave and free women who continued to live and work on farms and plantations, as well as the increasing number of women who joined in the westward migration, did not experience the full weight of these changes in roles and lifestyles. The experiences of these women in 1850 more closely resembled those of their predecessors in 1750 than those of their urban contemporaries. They remained visible producers and consumers of traditional sports and other displays of physical prowess.

During the first half of the nineteenth century, some people's perceptions and experiences suggested that the health of middle and upper-class women in urbanizing areas was declining. Educators, doctors, and writers of popular magazine articles responded with analyses and prescriptions for improving women's health, including calls for renewed physical exertion via exercises and games. The logic of the health literature was simple and straightforward: if women were to fulfill their roles as caretakers of families and national virtue, they needed to maintain their physical and mental health.

This created a movement to return women to physically active pursuits. This would not, however, occur overnight. Games such as baseball were becoming popular in eastern urban centers at mid-century. Other activities such as skating, croquet, and rowing were also modernizing, acquiring rules, specialized playing spaces, and an organizational base in clubs. Only gradually did women gain access to the new modern sports. In the 1850s, they did so primarily as spectators. At baseball games, male promoters hoped that women would bring their perceived moral superiority to bear on the crowds and thereby ensure social order.

> **• KEY CONCEPT •**
>
> At baseball games, male promoters hoped that women would bring their perceived moral superiority to bear on the crowds and thereby ensure social order.

Challenging Gender Boundaries

Not all middle- and upper-class women were content to remain on the periphery of the action, sporting or otherwise. As of 1848, a feminist movement had formalized at Seneca Falls, New York and elsewhere in the North. Other movements, such as abolitionism, both encouraged women to be social agents and demonstrated that their reappearance in the public domain endangered neither their health nor that of the nation. Moreover, the dynamic events of mid-century, including the Civil War (1861–65), challenged the gender boundaries and expectations that had confined women to the domestic sphere for more than three generations. Middle- and upper-class urban women found and made opportunities in public society during and after the Civil War. Nursing and teaching were precisely such activities, but required additional training. Not surprisingly, some women demanded and received access to colleges. In college, women began to participate in some of the emerging modern sports whose social power was increasing in the aftermath of the Civil War.

At private colleges such as Vassar in New York, and Smith and Wellesley in Massachusetts, women students formed clubs to play baseball and, soon there after, tennis, croquet, and archery. College administrators and faculty responded to the influx of women and their own fears about the negative impact of intellectual work on women students with requirements for medical examinations, exercise and gymnastics regimens, and the gradual absorption of women's sport clubs into the colleges.

Outside of the colleges, middle- and upper-class women were also starting to take advantage of the increasing array of modern sports. Local gymnasiums and armories were turned into playing areas. Hosts of clubs formed as men and women sought new opportunities for a range of sports, from skating and rowing to trap shooting and tennis. Such activities continued to stretch the bounds of activity acceptable to women. They also quieted some of the concerns (held especially by the male-dominated medical profession) about the negative effects that the physical movement required by sports might have on women's biological and reproductive functions.

Another significant challenge to the nearly century-old ideology that placed women in the home and in subservience to men came in the form of a machine: the bicycle. Invented in Europe in the early nineteenth century, early versions of the bicycle had appeared in various forms and had become the object of short-lived fads through the 1860s. Bicycle riding became popular, and the practice afforded women with a means of physical mobility and freedom that they had not known for generations—since the days when horse ownership was common.

> **• KEY CONCEPT •**
>
> Bicycle riding became popular, and the practice afforded women with a means of physical mobility and freedom that they had not known for generations—since the days when horse ownership was common.

The Age of Modern Sports

Historians have labeled the period from the 1890s to World War I as the Progressive Era, largely because "progress" was a common goal during that time, especially among members of the urban middle class. Achievement did not always match rhetoric, but many women did see their positions and the quality of their lives enhanced. Some urban working women earned more pay and experienced improved conditions. Some of the industries that employed women organized calisthenics or physical culture classes, and then team sports to promote personal health and worker efficiency. These programs became more widespread after the turn of the century, and by the 1920s, individual companies and regional industries had multiple teams in sports such as basketball, bowling, tennis, baseball, volleyball, and eventually softball.

Upper-class society also began to provide increasing opportunities for woman to take part in competitive sports. In the 1870s and 1880s, upper-class women had joined clubs, social clubs, country clubs, and then sport-specific clubs. They also engaged in sports at college and, importantly, on their vacations or extended stays in Europe. By 1900, seven of these women had competed in their first Olympics in Paris. Women consistently competed in the Olympic Games thereafter, albeit in small numbers, and in socially acceptable sports such as tennis, archery, and figure skating.

The progressive-era history of middle-class women's sporting experiences is more complicated. Especially before the turn of the century, women experienced considerable latitude in forming sport clubs and organizing competitions. They appeared to gain a degree of physical and personal freedom in sport similar to that enjoyed by their working- and upper-class sisters. Women initially popularized the newly-created sports of basketball and volleyball; it was the rapid spread of such sports, as well as field hockey, cycling, and tennis, that encouraged their teachers and recreation supervisors to form associations and write rules. In men's experience, it was precisely such associations that were critical to the promotion and expansion of modern sports.

Many of the women who came to control sports for girls and adults, especially in institutions such as schools and colleges, had accepted the warnings of the medical profession that unfettered athletic competition would harm female participants physically and psychologically, and detract from or even diminish their femininity. Consequently, in the 1890s, women physical educators began to limit women's sport contests by changing the rules of some games, such as basketball, and eventually by altering the very nature of such contests. By the 1920s, the conservative approach of women physical educators was quite distinct from, and out of sync with, the attitudes and expectations of many other people. The United States was experiencing its first mature burst of popular consumerism, which was buoyed by a fun ethic and a relatively expansive economy. Clubs and teams for women proliferated, in part as more institutions sponsored teams or provided facilities. Improvements in and declining prices of sporting goods, as well as the increasing popularity of sports, spurred the organization of leagues (Figure 15-3).

The Great Depression of 1929 disrupted this sporting boom, but did not end it entirely. In fact, the popularity of industrial sport probably

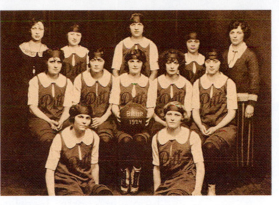

FIGURE 15–3
Girls Varsity Basketball, 1924 (Courtesy of University Archives, University of Pittsburgh)

peaked in the 1930s, and sports such as softball and bowling became extremely popular among women. Women's Olympic competition gained more popular support, in part because of great performances by athletes such as Mildred "Babe" Didrikson. Significantly as well, women continued to enter nontraditional roles outside the sporting world, a trend that became more pronounced as World War II began.

After 1941, more and more women took jobs that had once belonged to the men who went abroad to fight. Even professional baseball opened its doors to women via the All-American Girls Baseball League, financed by Philip Wrigley of chewing gum and Chicago Cubs fame. The All-American Girls Baseball League began play in 1943 in mid-sized cities in the Great Lakes region. (These athletes were not the first professional women athletes in the United States. In the modern era, there had been professional female distance walkers in the 1870s and 1880s, as well as professional female rodeo competitors in the twentieth century.) After 1949, the Ladies Professional Golf Association was organized, offering $15,000 in purse money spread over nine tournaments. Five years later, women golfers could earn $225,000 a year on the LPGA tour.

In the 1940s, an even more significant movement developed in African-American colleges. Track and field teams were training at places such as Tuskegee Institute and Tennessee State; these colleges would produce the athletes that would integrate U.S. women's Olympic teams and revolutionize the contests and the records. By the early 1960s, African-American athletes such as Wilma Rudolph had set records that opened doors for other black women and paved the way for Jackie Joyner-Kersee and Florence Griffith-Joyner, among many others.

The Sixties Boom

A greater revolution in women's sports lay ahead. In the late 1960s, the modern feminist movement, a youth culture, and other sources of social unrest unsettled both the nation as a whole and the sports world in particular. Billie Jean King defied international tennis tradition and authorities at Wimbledon in 1968, when she demanded an end to under-the-table payments. She helped organize the first of several early 1970s professional leagues for women, including the Virginia Slims tennis tour. King symbolized the commencement of the contemporary women's revolution in sports. Legislation, especially Title IX of the Educational Amendments Act of 1972, and the subsequent litigation against unequal opportunities in institutions, has had a great impact on women.

Women's Sport Today

There has been a dynamic and continuing growth of women's sports since the late 1960s. Triathlons, marathons, soccer, aerobics, weightlifting, rugby, skiing, basketball, and even cheerleading are among the many sports available to women. None of these sports existed a century ago, and few of them even existed a generation ago. What remains unknown is the full impact of the generation of women who are now maturing, and who grew up with opportunities that their mothers and grandmothers never dreamed of (Figure 15-4). The experience and involvement of women in

> ### • KEY CONCEPT •
>
> Billie Jean King defied international tennis tradition and authorities at Wimbledon in 1968, when she demanded an end to under-the-table payments.

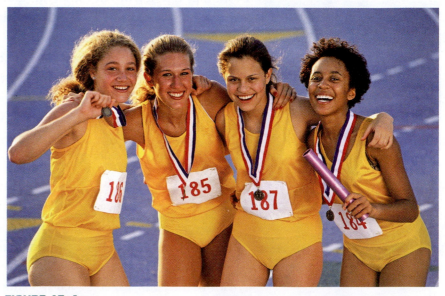

FIGURE 15–4
Female athletes are enjoying greater rewards as a result of equality under Title IX. (Courtesy of Photodisc)

the sporting world, and their demand for equal access to individual participation and to the financial rewards of professional sports, continue to influence the development of women's sports around the world.

Title IX

Title IX of the Education Amendments of 1972 is a federal law prohibiting **gender discrimination** at academic institutions that receive federal funding. Signed into law by President Richard Nixon, it went into effect in July 1975. Title IX states: "No person in the United States shall, on the basis of sex, be excluded from participation in, be denied the benefits of, or be subjected to discrimination under any education program or activity receiving Federal financial assistance." Unfortunately, a concerted move towards gender equity in sports did not begin for another decade. In 1984, the U.S. Supreme Court dealt a blow to women in sports by deciding that only those education programs that received direct federal funding were obligated to satisfy Title IX. Since no athletic departments received direct assistance from federal money, they were exempt from Title IX under this ruling. Fortunately, Congress reversed this decision legislatively by passing the **Civil Rights Restoration Act of 1987**, which asserted that Title IX would be broadly applied to include athletic programs.

Today, athletic departments are often the focus of Title IX litigation. Demonstrating compliance with Title IX generally requires that a school pass one of three tests:

- First, and most commonly, a school can demonstrate that the number of participation opportunities for males and females in athletics is substantially proportional to the percent of males and females in the general student body. For example, a school with a 52 percent female student body should have 52 percent of its athletic opportunities reserved for females. Exact proportionality has typically not been required, with 5 percent differences being considered acceptable in some cases.

- Second, a school can comply with title IX by demonstrating a history of expansion of offerings for the underrepresented gender (almost always the females). In this case, only programs added in very recent years generally warrant consideration.

- The third and most difficult argument for the school to make is to demonstrate that the institution has fully accommodated the interests and abilities of the underrepresented gender. This position cannot be successfully argued when a school is attempting to cut a women's team or to demote one from varsity to club status. Recently, schools have begun to explore the viability of using campus-wide interest surveys to substantiate that the interests of female students are being met, even if the school cannot satisfy the substantial proportionality and history-of-expansion tests.

Satisfying any of these tests, however, does not guarantee that a school is compliant with Title IX. According to the **Office of Civil Rights (OCR)**, there are many areas relative to athletics that can be compared in assessing Title IX compliance at any institution. These include equipment and supplies, scheduling of games and practice time, travel and per diem allowances, tutoring, coaching, locker rooms and other facilities, medical and training services, housing and dining facilities, publicity, support services, and recruitment of student-athletes. Therefore, for example, a school that meets the test of proportionality could still run afoul of Title IX if the women's teams play on lower-quality fields and use older, inferior equipment than do to the men's teams, provided that the women receive no benefits of their own to balance the overall treatment of the genders.

The **Equity in Athletics Disclosure Act** requires coeducational colleges and universities to prepare a yearly report detailing their participation by gender, their staffing, and their revenues, and expenses by men's and women's teams. This report must be submitted to the U.S. Department of Education and is used to provide Congress with a means of assessing college athletics. Middle- and high-school programs are not required to submit such a report. Some states, such as Washington, do require that schools conduct an annual self-evaluation. Otherwise, monitoring compliance is left to the discretion of the local school boards, activists, the courts, or the Office for Civil Rights.

When schools are found to be noncompliant, they generally agree to (or are ordered to) remedy the inequity in a timely manner. Many women's rights advocates would like to see stronger measures used by the Office for Civil Rights. According to Deborah Brake, a University of Pittsburgh law professor, there are no cases in which a school has actually had federal funds withdrawn for a Title IX athletics violation. Currently, Title IX complaints to the Department of Education are far more likely to involve lower-level athletics. Since 2001, the Department of Education has handled five times as many sexual discrimination

> ● **KEY CONCEPT** ●
>
> The Equity in Athletics Disclosure Act requires coeducational colleges and universities to prepare a yearly report detailing their participation by gender, their staffing, revenues, and expenses by men's and women's teams.

complaints involving middle or high schools than to colleges and universities. According to Bob Gardner, the chief officer of the National Federation of High School Associations, "High school is where the Title IX action is. The colleges get all the attention, but Title IX isn't about the nation's elite college athletes. It's about providing a grass-roots gateway to sports that benefit millions" (Figure 15-5).

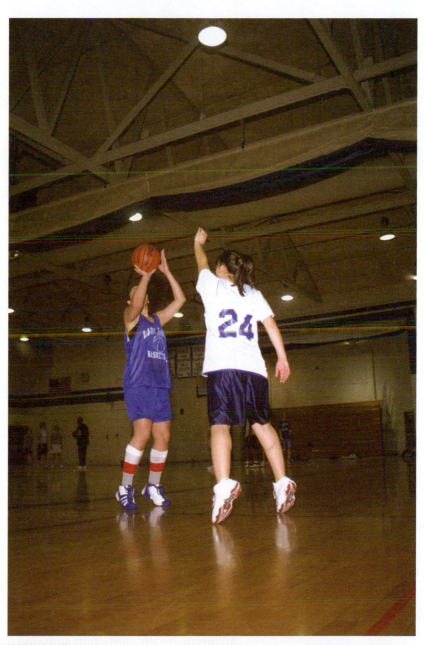

FIGURE 15–5
Athletics allow for greater fitness and personal rewards.

In light of the tremendous growth in sports participation among females since 1972, it is clear that Title IX has had a profound impact. At the time the law was passed, only one in twenty-seven females participated in high school sports. Today, that number is one in three. Studies have shown that if a girl does not participate in sports by the time she is ten years old, there is only a 10 percent chance she will participate when she is twenty-five.

Between 1972 and 1998, the approximate number of women participating in intercollegiate sports increased from 30,000 to 157,000. It is important to note that from 1981 to 1999, the number of male participants in collegiate sports and the number of men's teams also increased, contrary to the widely-believed myth that Title IX is decreasing participation opportunities for men.

Title IX does not require that budgets for sports be equal for each gender. In fact, the law allows schools to take into account the very real differences in outfitting athletes in equipment of comparable quality. Outfitting football players, for example, is more costly than outfitting field hockey players. The criteria for equality of equipment and supplies, then, are to assess the quality, quantity, suitability, maintenance, and availability of equipment for the athletic programs on the whole. Further, schools are allowed to privilege one sport over another, provided that a gender bias does not exist and that the overall quality of opportunities is equal for boys and girls. For example, a school district can choose to provide better facilities for baseball than softball, provided that this gap is balanced elsewhere in the programs (say, by providing outstanding facilities for field hockey). Often, money generated and earmarked for a specific sport leads to an overall imbalance between boys' and girls' sports. When inequity results from gifts given along gender lines, it is the responsibility of the district to correct the inequity by allocation of their own resources.

TITLE IX CASE SCENARIOS

Peter S. Finley of Nova Southeastern University asked twenty Title IX experts via e-mail to share their thoughts for the best practice regarding three scenarios. Each expert had publications in the subject area, participated on panels, appeared as a guest lecturer, and worked as an advocate for women in sport. The scenarios asked the participants to suggest the best way to handle specific situations that frequently challenge athletic directors. The situations were developed through analysis of Title IX cases that have resulted from mismanagement of booster funds. The first scenario dealt with earmarked giving, the second dealt with sport-specific booster clubs, and the third dealt with oversight of the allocation of money raised by a booster club. Six Title IX experts agreed to participate by providing written responses to each scenario.

Participants

- Donna Lopiano is the Executive Director of the Women's Sports Foundation and has been listed as one of "The 100 Most Influential People in Sports" by *The Sporting News.* Dr. Lopiano previously served for seventeen years as the Director of Women's Athletics at the University of Texas.

- Nancy Hogshead-Makar served as President of the Women's Sports Foundation from 1993 to 1994 and has served on its Board of Stewards since 1996. A law professor at Florida Coastal School of Law, Dr. Hogshead-Makar specializes in Title IX law. She became a household name after winning four Olympic medals in swimming at the 1984 Los Angeles Olympiad.

- Donna J. Nelson is an associate professor at the University of Oklahoma, where she has extended concern about equity in education beyond the sports realm to the classroom. Specifically, Dr. Nelson used her Title IX expertise to raise concerns about the underrepresentation of females on college faculties in the science and engineering disciplines.

- Darcy Lees is the Equity Coordination Program Supervisor for the Washington State Office of the Superintendent of Public Instruction. In this capacity, Lees speaks on Title IX law and maintains a website that helps school officials understand all aspects of the law. The site also offers assistance for school officials in the process of evaluating their programs, which is a legal requirement in Washington State.

- Valerie Bonnette is the President of Good Sports, Inc., Title IX and Gender Equity Specialists. She has worked as a Title XI compliance consultant for more than sixty schools' compliance. As a staffer with the U.S. Department of Education's Office of Civil Rights, she co-authored the Title IX investigator's manual.

• Jean Kinn Ashen is Athletic Director at North Salinas High School in Salinas, California. She has been trained by the California Interscholastic Federation to answer questions about and provide practical solutions to Title IX issues for coaches, athletic directors, and administrators in her geographic area.

Scenario One

The baseball and softball teams are wearing old uniforms, but the athletic budget does not allow for their replacement this year. One month prior to the season, a booster offers to buy new uniforms for the baseball team, for which his son plays. He will not, however, give money to the general athletic fund, nor will he give money to the softball team. How would you suggest a new athletic director handle this situation? On its face, this scenario does not necessarily suggest that a Title IX violation will occur should the athletic director accept the donation. As noted, a school can choose to privilege one team over another, provided the difference is balanced in other areas of the athletic program so that the total offerings for males and females are equal. Further, it is remotely possible that the females at this school are the privileged gender and that this gift will, in effect, serve as a remedy for the male participants. However, given the general state of girls' sports relative to Title IX, athletic directors should be cautioned about accepting gifts specifically for boys' teams. Before accepting such a gift, an athletic director should carefully consider whether it will create imbalance and, if so, how the imbalance can be remedied. As such, four of the respondents recommended accepting the donation while exploring creative means for ensuring that it does not cause imbalance in the overall treatment of the male and female participants.

Donna Lopiano suggested that the athletic director should consider moving the baseball team into the slot of a boys' team currently scheduled to receive new uniforms, and move that team into the baseball slot. This would allow the school to benefit from the booster's generosity with minor change to the uniform replacement schedule. Lopiano noted, however, that, "Title IX doesn't require [that] baseball and softball be treated equally. It requires [that] men's and women's participants be treated equally." Donna Nelson suggested that the athletic director use the offer as a challenge grant. She recommended appealing publicly for similar donations from the community to match the booster's gift. Under this plan, the athletic director could publicize the gift, recognize the charity of the booster (which is certainly better than alienating him by rejecting the gift outright), and stimulate the community to show support for softball.

Similarly, Jean Kinn Ashen believes it better to educate and win over parents than to simply turn them away. She wrote, "I would thank the parent and try to involve him in our athletic program. I would ask him to come in and sit down and discuss our athletic program as a whole. I would try to appeal to his parent status . . . [by asking him to] imagine the scenario if he had a daughter and challenge him to find a way to outfit both groups of students. Equity is important and must be taught to our parents and boosters. We are the educators."

Valerie Bonnette wrote, "The athletic director should accept the donation of new uniforms for the baseball team. Administrators need never reject donations." She adds that there are many means for offsetting potential imbalance, such as by giving the females an advantage in another area of the sports program. "If the benefits are of equivalent weight or importance, they may 'offset' each other; in effect complying with Title IX." It is important to note, again, that accepting such earmarked donations can cause Title IX issues, should the athletic director fail to fully assess the impact on the total athletic programs, or fail to carefully plan how equity will be ensured.

Darcy Lees reminded the athletic director to be wary of obligating the school district to make an unplanned expenditure of funds. If accepting the donation is likely to cause inequitable treatment for male or female participants in the total athletic program, "[the] athletic director should not accept the donation unless the district is willing to provide or raise money to provide softball uniforms in a timely manner no later than the following school year."

According to Nancy Hogshead-Makar, "Many schools avoid this situation by prohibiting gifts other than to the athletic department generally. A recipient cannot hide different and discriminatory treatment behind the donor's gift. A recipient cannot say, in effect, 'It isn't me discriminating, it's the donor.' Otherwise, racially segregated schools might never have integrated fully, as school gifts would have had 'white only' earmarks on [them]."

Scenario Two

A recently hired athletic director quickly becomes aware that each team at her new school has its own booster club. The booster clubs for the boys' teams are very active and garner strong community support. Clubs representing girls' sports try very hard to raise funds through a variety of innovative means, but get little support. As a result, the boys' teams have the best equipment available, while the girls' teams wear old uniforms and use questionable equipment. How should this new athletic director proceed?

In this scenario, the new athletic director has inherited a problem common to schools with splintered booster groups. Given that boys' sports have a longer history, receive greater media attention, and have greater numbers of participants (both historically and currently), it should surprise no new athletic director to find that support is more frequently given for boys' sports.

Donna Lopiano suggested several courses of action. First, the athletic director should assemble the booster clubs to explain Title IX law and to describe how it applies to booster clubs. The idea that the actions of the boosters are, in effect, causing discriminatory treatment might be initially rejected. After all, parents in booster clubs are working hard and believe that their children should benefit. They may not understand the deep-seated social issues that make it harder for one club to match the fund-raising potential of another club. Lopiano suggested the athletic director use race as an example. She wrote, "The Civil Rights Act would not permit a separate booster club for white and black athletes . . . why should we send the message that girls and boys be treated differently based on sex?" Lopiano further suggested, "The athletic director should be very positive about the need to be sure our sons and daughters understand that we believe in equality of treatment." From there, the athletic director could form one umbrella booster club that raises funds for the entire athletic program rather than for individual teams. However, in the event that separate clubs are maintained, it is the athletic director's job to ensure the funds do not create inequity. Lopiano suggested the athletic director oversee the expenditure of the funds and that strong relations with the boosters could be maintained by forming an advisory council with representatives from each club so that the athletic director can explain her decisions.

Darcy Lees suggested, "The athletic director may want to personally evaluate the inequities he/she sees and initiate correction . . . which

> ### • KEY CONCEPT •
>
> "The Civil Rights Act would not permit a separate booster club for white and black athletes…why should we send the message that girls and boys be treated differently based on sex?"

may mean using district funds only for improvements of the girls' program in the current year." She also endorsed conducting an annual review related to eight factors of Title IX compliance (interest and ability, equipment and supplies, scheduling, facilities, coaching, publicity, medical and training, and travel and per diem), and then developing a plan to correct inequity. School officials interested in conducting self-analysis of their program should visit http://www.k12.wa.us/equity/AthleticEquity/, which is a well-maintained and thorough resource.

Nancy Hogshead-Makar and Donna Nelson both recommended pairing booster clubs (baseball with softball, for example). This will allow boosters to have greater manpower as they raise funds which can then be more readily divided to promote equity. One problem with the umbrella booster club (one club for all sports) concept is that parents of students in a few sports might then bear the burden for support of students in all sports. This can lead to resentment when funds are allocated to sports for which there is little or no parental contribution to the booster clubs. By pairing teams, a spirit of togetherness can be fostered. Nelson suggested that once booster groups are paired, they should maximize publicity opportunities, including taking photos with the teams and boosters together. Nelson also recommended creation of an "overhead charge" for all donations. A special overhead account would then be created with the express purpose of benefiting the athletic department on the whole at the director's discretion. Nelson recommended that this fund be used to ensure the quality and safety of all equipment in the athletic program. Similarly, this recommendation could be extended to creation of an "equity charge" on gifts, which would be used to address issues of shortcomings in the equity of the programs when they are discovered through annual evaluation.

Valerie Bonnette wrote, "Title IX does not prohibit the existence of booster clubs for each team, and the athletic director should not discourage the great success of the booster clubs that support the boys' teams. The athletic director should explore ways to improve the success of booster clubs that support the girls' teams." Bonnette went on to explain that the athletic director does have the responsibility to remedy disparity, and that several options exist to do so. While the boys' teams receive better equipment, the girls could be given benefits in another area of the program, such as better transportation to away contests. She concluded by suggesting, "Another alternative is to reallocate the school funds to the girls' program that would have been budgeted to the boys' program to provide the girls' program with equipment and supplies comparable to such items provided to the boys' teams." In doing so, the athletic director relies on the boosters to largely fund the boys' programs while concentrating school funds on providing equity for the girls' programs.

Through her position as an athletic director, Jean Kinn Ashen has met the problems presented in this scenario head-on, and is a proponent of having one unified booster club. She wrote, "The Athletic Director must be in control of fund-raising in the community to allow coordination for the boys' and girls' programs. When you have so many different clubs, it is impossible to monitor raising and spending of funds. I have one booster club that supports all sports, plus I can attend the meetings. Each sport is still encouraged to participate in fund-raising, but everything goes through one central control."

Scenario Three

An athletic director has organized parents to form a new booster club to help raise funds for the athletic programs. Parents will oversee door-to-door sales, car washes, a golf outing, concession sales, etc. The athletic director is not sure how to transfer the funds from the booster club to the teams in a way that ensures equity. He calls you for advice. What do you suggest?

Donna Lopiano proposed including parents through the formation of an advisory council with elected representatives. She suggested that the athletic director can then "explain how the decision-making process must comply with Title IX and be fair to all teams." Further, "Decisions should be based on stated policies that conform to Title IX, such as gender-equitable team uniform replacement schedules, or replacement based on equal standards of wear." By including the parents the athletic director will allow the parents to feel ownership and pride, as they will be involved in the allocation of funding and not just its generation. However, in the end, the athletic director will be responsible for Title IX compliance.

Similarly, Darcy Lees recommended creating an advisory committee of parents that can work with the athletic director to establish needs and priorities. She suggested these be based on an annual review of the factors of gender equity discussed in detail on the aforementioned website. A problem inherent in booster clubs is that some parents are likely to participate more than others, and will wish to see their own children rewarded through their work. It is permissible for this athletic director to reward the teams that have the most involved parents, provided that the funds awarded are balanced by gender so that there is no overall inequity between girls' and boys' teams.

Nancy Hogshead-Makar noted, "It is permissible to elevate some teams to some sort of elite status while other teams get bare-boned resources. For example, giving the men's football and basketball teams fancy perks, and then giving the same treatment to the women's crew and soccer teams." If the athletic director wishes to elevate the quality of offerings for all teams, it will be necessary to seek participation from parents representing students in all sports.

Donna Nelson recommended that the new athletic director work to "ensure at the beginning that parents from boys' and girls' teams are both involved in a proportion at least somewhat matching the ratio of boys to girls (or boys' teams to girls' teams) in the overall athletic program." By doing so, it is less likely that there will be squabbling about allocation of money later, since all have fairly worked to raise it. Problems are more likely to arise when parents work hard to raise money then see it go to other sports where no parents lifted a finger in the fund-raising process.

Valerie Bonnette suggested, "The funds should go into a general athletic fund so the athletic director and other administrators may control expenditures for all benefits provided to student-athletes. This approach is not required by Title IX. It simply provides administrators the necessary control to ensure compliance."

Jean Kinn Ashen offered the suggestion that emphasis on sports rotate annually, perhaps by upgrading the softball facilities one season and the baseball facilities the next, so everyone feels important. She also stressed the need for the booster club to have a written constitution and set of bylaws that spells out the procedures that will be used.

Scenario Remarks

Athletic directors can face any number of difficult situations as they work with booster clubs. The job of raising and allocating funds while ensuring gender equity is not an easy one. Despite the challenges of handling earmarked gifts, managing splintered booster clubs, and transferring money from boosters to teams, athletic directors have a clear legal responsibility to provide equitable treatment to those under their charge. These recommendations from the experts can be used as guidance for navigating the dangerous waters that booster-club management can present.

Chapter Summary

Title IX has profoundly influenced the growth of sports for girls and women. Participation in athletics teaches lessons that are required in order to be successful in life. These lessons include teamwork, discipline, dedication, handling success and failure, leadership, and perseverance. When young people prepare for a competitive, globalized society and marketplace, men and women must work together, compete with each other, and lead each other in collective endeavors. Athletics are among several co-curricular activities with the potential to teach these skills, especially since sports figures prominently in the fabric of our society.

Chapter Review Questions

1. What is gender equity, as defined by the NCAA?

2. How have girls and women been discriminated against in athletics?

3. Give a written historical perspective of women's sports in America.

4. What is Title IX?

5. Write a historical timeline of Title IX and subsequent legislation.

6. How does the Civil Rights Restoration Act of 1987 relate to gender equity in sports?

7. Demonstrating compliance with Title IX generally requires passing any one of three tests. Describe each test.

8. What is the Equity in Athletics Disclosure Act? Why is it important?

9. What does a school have to do if it is found to be noncompliant with Title IX?

10. Has Title IX accomplished what it set out to do?

Projects and Activities

1. Compile research on the All-American Girls Basketball League. Write a short essay detailing what you learned.

2. What status does women's sport have in American sport culture today?

3. Research the inequities that still exist between men's and women's sports. Report your findings and analyze them from the perspective of your personal experience.

4. Take time to familiarize yourself with the gender equity resources available at http://www1.ncaa.org/

   In your opinion, which of these materials have the greatest importance.

5. Visit a local high school in your area. Ask the athletic director for their report on Title IX. What did you find out?

Website Resources

Gender Equity/Title IX: http://www.ncaa.org/

Equity Education, Office of Superintendent of Public Instruction, Washington State: http://www.k12.wa.us/

Tournaments and Brackets

CHAPTER 16

Objectives

Upon completion of this chapter, the reader should be able to:

- Explain single-elimination tournaments and their use.
- Explain double-elimination tournaments and their use.
- Explain round-robin tournaments and their use.
- Explain other tournament formats and their application.

Key Terms

Accelerated pairings	Rating
Algorithm	Round-robin tournament
Double-elimination tournament	Seeding
Konrad system	Single-elimination tournament
McMahon System Tournament	Swiss system tournament

Tournaments and Brackets

The creation of tournaments and brackets for the physical educator and coach is a neverending task. Knowledge of which tournaments work best for each sport or situation will make the task of deciding a winner considerably easier, and will result in more support from the coaches and participants. It is important to have a sound understanding of what tournaments work best and what their limitations are (Figure 16-1).

There are a number of computer programs marketed today that make tournament and bracket creation an easy task. With these programs, all the tournament director has to do is plug in the names and click a button (Table 16-1).

Single-Elimination Tournament

A **single-elimination tournament,** also called a knockout or sudden-death tournament, is a type of tournament where the loser of each match is immediately eliminated from winning the championship or first prize in the event. However, it does not always mean that the defeated competitor will not participate further in the tournament: in some such tournaments, consolation or "classification" contests are subsequently held among those already defeated to determine the awarding of lesser places—for example, a third-place playoff.

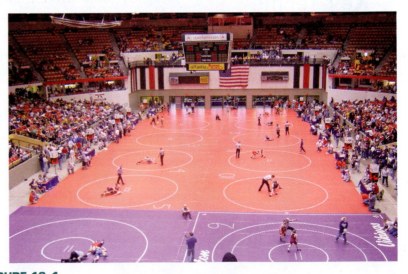

FIGURE 16–1
State Wrestling tournaments draw thousands of spectators. (Courtesy of Wisconsin Wrestling Foundation)

TABLE 16-1 Number of matches that have to be won before winning the final

Number of competitors	Number of matches
2	1
4	2
8	3
16	4
32	5
64	6
128	7
256	8
512	9
1024	10
2048	11
4096	12
8192	13
16384	14

Format

The number of participants in a single-elimination tournament (Table 16-2) is fixed. The full schedule of pairings across all rounds (the bracket) may be allocated before the start of the tournament, or each round may be allocated at the end of the preceding round. Each successive round halves the number of competitors remaining (assuming there are no byes, see below). The round in which only eight remain at the start is generally called the quarter-final round. This is followed by the semi-final round (in which only four are left), the two winners of which then meet in the final, or championship, round. To calculate the number of games in your single-elimination tournament, simply take the number of entries and subtract 1. For example, if you have sixteen teams in your tournament, you will have fifteen games. For a double-elimination tournament, you would multiply the number of teams/competitors by 2 and then subtract 1.

In cases where the number of competitive entities at the start of the tournament is not a power of 2, some competitors may receive a bye in the first round, which entitles these competitors to advance to the second round automatically without playing. Often, these byes will be awarded to the highest-rated competitors in the event as a reward for

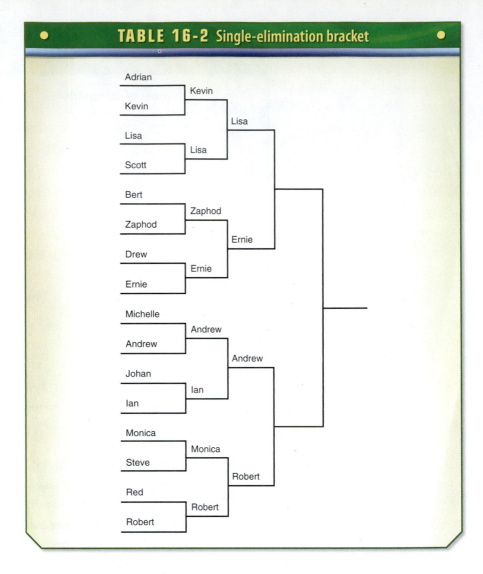

TABLE 16-2 Single-elimination bracket

some previous accomplishment. For example, in some American team sports, most notably professional football, the number of teams qualifying for the post-season tournament will be intentionally set at a number which is not a power of 2, in order to provide an advantage to a high-achieving team in the just-completed regular season.

When matches are held to determine places or prizes lower than first and second (the loser of the final-round match gaining the latter position), these typically include a match between the losers of the semifinal matches, the winner therein placing third and the loser fourth. Sometimes contests are also held among the losers of the quarterfinal matches to determine fifth through eighth places (this is most commonly encountered in the Olympic Games). In one scenario, two "consolation semifinal" matches may be conducted, with the winners of these then facing off to determine fifth and sixth places, and the losers playing for seventh and eighth; or, some method of ranking the four quarterfinal losers might be employed, in which case only one round of additional matches would be held among them, the two highest-ranked therein then playing for fifth and sixth places and the two lowest for seventh and eighth.

Seeding

Opponents may be allocated randomly; however, since the "luck of the draw" may result in the highest-rated competitors being scheduled to face each other early in the competition, **seeding** is often used to prevent this. Brackets are set up, so that the top two seeds could not possibly meet until the final round (should either or both advance that far), none of the top four can meet prior to the semifinals, and so on.

Ideally, the brackets would be set up so that the quarterfinal pairings (barring any upsets) would be the 1 seed vs. the 8 seed, 2 vs. 7, 3 vs. 6 and 4 vs. 5; however, this is not the procedure that is followed in most tennis tournaments, where the 1 and 2 seeds are placed in separate brackets, but then the 3 and 4 seeds are assigned to their brackets randomly, as are seeds 5 through 8, and so on. This may result in some brackets consisting of stronger players than other brackets; since only the top thirty-two players are seeded at all in Tennis Grand Slam tournaments, it is conceivable that the thirty-third-best player in a 128-player field could end up playing the top seed in the first round. While this may seem unfair to a casual observer, it should be pointed out that rankings of tennis players are generated by computers, and players tend to change ranking positions very gradually, so that a more equitable method of determining the pairings might result in many of the same head-to-head match-ups being repeated over and over again in successive tournaments.

Sometimes the remaining competitors in a single-elimination tournament will be "re-seeded" so that the highest surviving seed is made to play the lowest surviving seed in the next round, the second-highest plays the second-lowest, etc. This may be done after each round, or only at selected intervals. In American team sports, for example, both the NFL and NHL employ this tactic, but the NBA does not (and neither does the NCAA college basketball tournament). The NBA's format calls for the winner of the first-round series between the first and eighth seeds (within each of the two conferences the league has) to face the winner of the first-round series between the fourth and fifth seeds in the next round, even if one or more of the top three seeds had been upset in their first-round series; critics have claimed that this gives a team fighting for the fifth and sixth seeding positions near the end of the regular season an incentive to tank (deliberately lose) games, so as to finish sixth and thus avoid a possible match-up with the top seed until one round later.

Evaluation

The single-elimination format enables a relatively large number of competitors to participate. There are no "dead" matches (perhaps excluding "classification" matches), and no matches in which one competitor has more to play for than the other.

The single-elimination format is less suited to games in which draws are frequent. In chess, each game in a single-elimination tournament must be played over multiple matches, because draws are common, and because white has an advantage over black. In soccer, games ending in a draw may be settled in extra time and, eventually, by a penalty shootout (viewed by many fans as an unsatisfactory conclusion to a game) or by replaying the game.

Another perceived disadvantage of the single-elimination format is that most competitors are eliminated after relatively few games. Variations such as the double-elimination tournament allow competitors a single loss, while remaining eligible for overall victory.

Double-Elimination Tournament

A **double-elimination tournament** is a competition in which a participant ceases to be eligible to win the tournament's championship upon having lost two games or matches. It stands in contrast to a single-elimination tournament, in which only one defeat results in elimination.

A double-elimination tournament is broken into two sets of brackets: the Winner's Bracket and the Loser's Bracket (W and L Brackets for short; also sometimes Upper Bracket and Lower Bracket, respectively). After the first round, the winners proceed into the W Bracket and the losers proceed into the L Bracket. The W Bracket is conducted in the same manner as a single-elimination tournament, except, of course, that the losers of each round "drop down" into the L Bracket (Table 16-3). As with single-elimination tournaments, most often the number of competitors is equal to a power of 2 (4, 8, 16, etc), so that there are an even number of competitors at every round.

TABLE 16-3 Double-elimination bracket

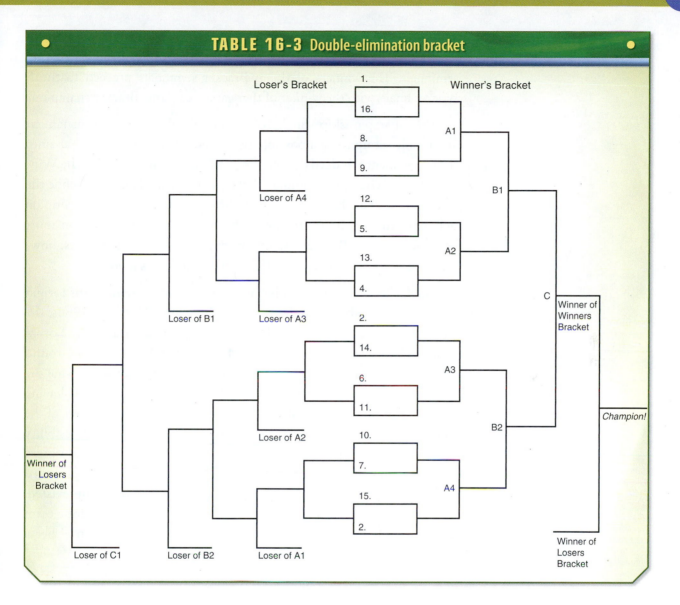

Conducting the Tournament

Each round of the L Bracket is conducted in two stages, the first stage consisting of the winners of the previous stage (or losers of the very first round of competition), and the second stage consisting of the winners of the first stage against the losers of that same round of the W Bracket. This is to allow the losers of each stage of the W Bracket to "filter down" into the L Bracket.

For example, in an eight-competitor double-elimination tournament, the losers of the first round enter the first stage of the L Bracket—the L Bracket quarterfinals—and compete against each other. The losers are eliminated, while the winners proceed to the second stage of the L Bracket—the L Bracket semifinals—to face the losers of the W Bracket semifinals. The winners of the L Bracket semifinals proceed to the L Bracket finals, with the winner of that game being the Bracket champion.

The championship finals of a double-elimination tournament are usually set up to be a possible two games. The rationale is that since the tournament is indeed double elimination, it is unfair to have the Winners' Bracket champion eliminated with its first loss. Therefore, while the Winners' Bracket champion needs to beat the Losers' Bracket champion only once to win the tournament, the Losers' Bracket champion must beat the Winners' Bracket champion twice. In some tournaments, however, this game is winner-take-all, with the unfairness ignored.

The College World Series has frequently tried to modify this format to set up, if possible, a single championship game. Until the 1980s, the College World Series did this by adding an extra round to the Losers' Bracket. What would be the Losers' Bracket semifinals (i.e., the round where the Winners' Bracket semifinal losers dropped down) became the Losers' Bracket quarterfinals, with the Losers' Bracket semifinals having the two participants in the Winners' Bracket final (i.e., the winners of the Winners' Bracket semifinals) drop down. This left open the possibility that the Winners' Bracket champion would pick up a loss in the Losers' Bracket semifinal. If however, the Winners' Bracket champion prevailed in the Losers' Bracket semifinal, the same two-game final setup existed. The CWS subsequently broke up its eight-team field into two four-team double elimination tournaments, with the winners meeting in either a sudden-death final or, currently, a best-of-three final.

Pros and Cons

The double-elimination format has some advantages over the single-elimination format—most notably, the fact that third and fourth places can be determined without the use of a consolation or classification match involving two contestants who have already been eliminated from winning the championship. A common criticism of the double-elimination format is that sometimes the last competitor to remain undefeated (i.e., the winner of the Winners Bracket) can actually lose only once and still be eliminated. However, that competitor does draw two byes during the course of the tournament, which many think compensates for that fact. This complaint is not an issue with full double elimination.

A disadvantage compared to the single-elimination format is that a considerably greater number of matches have to be conducted, since each player has to lose twice, and since the tournament ends when only one player remains. This format still allows a competitor to lose (perhaps multiple times) while still remaining eligible to win the tournament. Of course, having multiple games in each series also requires considerably more games to be conducted.

Another disadvantage is that the double-elimination format is more difficult to understand and explain. However, once it is understood, this then becomes a moot point.

Round-Robin Tournament

A **round-robin tournament,** or all-play-all tournament, is a type of group tournament in which each participant plays every other participant an equal number of times (Table 16-4). The term "round robin" is

TABLE 16-4 Round-robin tournament

ROUND ROBIN TOURNAMENT

SAMPLE

4-Team Schedule								
A	2-1	4-2	4-1					
B	3-4	1-3	2-3					
5-Team Schedule								
A	1-2	3-1	5-3	2-5	4-2			
B	2-3	4-5	1-2	3-4	5-1			
6-Team Schedule								
A	2-1	3-4	6-4	5-3	5-6			
B	4-5	6-1	2-3	6-2	1-3			
C	3-6	2-5	1-5	4-1	4-2			
7-Team Schedule								
A	1-6	4-2	2-7	5-3	3-1	6-4	7-5	
B	2-5	5-1	3-6	6-2	4-7	7-3	1-4	
C	3-4	6-7	4-5	7-1	5-6	1-2	2-3	
8-Team Schedule								
A	5-6	3-4	7-8	7-5	1-3	3-6	8-2	
B	3-8	1-7	6-2	6-1	4-2	4-5	7-3	
C	4-7	8-6	4-1	2-3	5-8	2-7	1-5	
D	2-1	2-5	5-3	8-4	6-7	8-1	6-4	
9-Team Schedule								
A	1-8	5-3	2-9	6-4	3-1	7-5	4-2	8-6	9-7
B	2-7	6-2	3-8	7-3	4-9	8-4	5-1	9-5	1-6
C	3-6	7-1	4-7	8-2	5-8	9-3	6-9	1-4	2-5
D	4-5	8-9	5-6	9-1	6-7	1-2	7-8	2-3	3-4

derived from the French term "ruban" (meaning ribbon). Over a period of time, the term got changed to "robin".

In a pure round-robin schedule, each participant plays every other participant once. If each participant plays all others twice, this is frequently called a double round-robin. The term is rarely used when all participants play one another more than twice, and is never used when one participant plays others an unequal number of times.

In sports with a large number of competitive matches per season, double round-robins are common. Almost all soccer leagues in the world are organized on a double round-robin basis, in which every team plays all others in its league once at home and once away. There are also round-robin chess tournaments; the World Chess Championship is an eight-player double round-robin tournament, where each player faces every other player once as white and once as black.

Evaluation

In a round-robin format, the element of luck is reduced, given that all competitors face the same opponents, and a few bad performances may not decide a competitor's chances of ultimate victory.

Disadvantages of the round-robin format include the existence of games late in the competition between competitors with no remaining chance of success. Moreover, some later matches will pair one competitor who has something left to play for against another who does not. This asymmetry means that playing the same opponents is not necessarily equitable; the same opponents in a different order may play harder or easier matches. There is also no "showcase" final match. The ability to recover from defeats, while rewarding overall consistency, may also be seen as a crutch for competitors who lack the temperament to handle the pressure of a knockout tournament.

Further issues arise where a round-robin is used as a qualifying round within a larger tournament. A competitor already qualified for the next stage before its last game may either not try hard (in order to conserve resources for the next phase) or even deliberately lose (if the scheduled next-phase opponent for a lower-placed qualifier is perceived to be easier than for a higher-placed one). Swiss system tournaments, which attempt to combine elements of the round-robin and elimination formats, provide a reliable champion within fewer rounds than a round-robin, while allowing draws and losses.

Scheduling Algorithm for Round-Robin Tournaments

The standard **algorithm** for round-robin tournaments is to assign each competitor a number, and pair them off in the first round.

Round 1. (1 plays 14, 2 plays 13, …)

Round 2. (1 plays 13, 14 plays 12, …)

Round 3. (1 plays 12, 13 plays 11, …) until you end up almost back at the initial position

Round 13. (1 plays 2, 3 plays 14, …)

If there are an odd number of competitors, a dummy competitor can be added, whose scheduled opponent in a given round does not play and has a bye. The upper and lower rows can indicate home/away in sports, white/black in chess, etc (this must alternate between rounds since competitor 1 is always on the first row). If, say, competitors 3 and 8 were unable to fulfill their fixture in the third round, it would need to be rescheduled outside the other rounds, since both competitors would already be facing other opponents in those rounds. More complex scheduling constraints may require more complex algorithms.

Swiss System Tournament

A **Swiss system tournament** is a commonly used type of tournament in chess and other games where players or teams need to be paired to face each other. This type of tournament was first used in a Zurich tournament in 1895, hence the name "Swiss system."

The Pairing Procedure

The principle of a Swiss tournament is that each player will be pitted against another player who has done as well, or as poorly. The first round is either drawn at random or is seeded according to **rating**. Players who win receive a point, those who draw receive half a point, and losers receive no points. Win, lose, or draw, all players proceed to the next round, where winners are pitted against winners, losers are pitted against losers, and so on. In subsequent rounds, players face opponents with the same (or almost the same) score. However, no player is paired up against the same opponent twice. In chess, it is also attempted to ensure that each player plays an equal number of games with white and black, alternate colors in each round being the most preferable, and definitely not the same color three times in a row.

The basic rule is that players with the same score are ranked according to rating. Then the top half is paired with the bottom half. For instance, if there are eight players in a score group, number 1 is paired with number 5, number 2 is paired with number 6, and so on. Modifications are then made to balance colors and to prevent players from meeting each other twice. The detailed rules of how to do the pairing are usually quite complicated, and often the tournament organizer has access to a computer to do the pairing for him or her. If the rules are strictly adhered to, the organizer has no discretion in pairing the round.

The tournament lasts for a number of rounds announced before the tournament (usually between three and nine rounds). After the last round, players are ranked by their score; if there is a tie, a tie-breaker score can be used.

Analysis, Advantages and Disadvantages

Determining a clear winner (and, incidentally, a clear loser) usually requires the same number of rounds as a knockout tournament, which is the base 2 logarithm of the number of players rounded up. Therefore three rounds can handle eight players, four rounds can handle sixteen players, and so on; however, it is not uncommon to have more players than this, and, if fewer than the correct number of rounds are played, it can happen that two or more players finish the tournament with a perfect score, having won all their games but never having faced each other.

Compared to a knockout tournament, the Swiss system has the inherent advantage of not eliminating anyone. That means that a player can enter such a tournament knowing that he will be able to play in all rounds, regardless of how well he does. The worst that can happen in this respect is being the player left over when there is an odd number of players. The player left over receives a bye, meaning that he does not play that particular round, but receives a full point as if he had won a game. He is reintroduced in the next round and does not receive another bye. However, a Swiss system tournament does not always end with the exciting climax of the knockout's final. Sometimes a player may have picked up such a great lead that by the last round he is assured of winning the tournament, even if he loses the last game. One fairly common fix for this dilemma is to hold single-elimination rounds among the top scorers.

Compared with a round-robin tournament, a Swiss tournament can handle many players without requiring an impractical number of rounds. However, the final rankings of a Swiss tournament are usually more random, depending on the tie-breakers used. Even though the correct player usually wins, and the correct player usually winds up in last place, the players in between are sorted only roughly without a good tie-breaker depth.

Variations of the Swiss System: Accelerated Pairings

The method of **accelerated pairings** is used in some tournaments with far more than the optimal number of players for the number of rounds. This method pairs top players more quickly than the standard method, and has the effect of more rapidly reducing the number of players with perfect scores.

For the first two rounds, players who started in the top half have one point added to their score for pairing purposes only. Then the first two rounds are paired normally, taking this added score into account. In effect, in the first round the top quarter plays the second quarter and the third quarter plays the fourth quarter. Most of the players in the first and third quarters should win the first round. Assuming that this is the case, in effect in the second round the top eighth plays the second eighth, the second quarter plays the third quarter and the seventh eighth plays the bottom eighth. That is, in the second round, winners in the top half play each other, losers in the bottom half play each other, and losers in the top half play winners in the bottom half (for the most part). After two rounds, about one-eighth of the players will have a perfect score, instead of one-fourth. After the second round, the standard pairing method is used (without the added point for the players who started in the top half).

As a comparison between the standard Swiss system and the accelerated pairings, consider a tournament with eight players, ranked 1 through 8. Assume that the higher-ranked player always wins.

Standard Swiss System

Round 1:

1 plays 5, 1 wins

2 plays 6, 2 wins

3 plays 7, 3 wins

4 plays 8, 4 wins

Round 2:

1 plays 3, 1 wins

2 plays 4, 2 wins

5 plays 7, 5 wins

6 plays 8, 6 wins

After two rounds, the standings are:

1   2–0
2   2–0
3   1–1
4   1–1
5   1–1
6   1–1
7   0–2
8   0–2

Accelerated Pairings

Round 1:

1 plays 3, 1 wins
2 plays 4, 2 wins
5 plays 7, 5 wins
6 plays 8, 6 wins

Round 2:

1 plays 2, 1 wins
3 plays 5, 3 wins
4 plays 6, 4 wins
7 plays 8, 7 wins

After two rounds, the standings are:

1   2–0
2   1–1
3   1–1
4   1–1
5   1–1
6   1–1
7   1–1
8   0–2

Variations of the Swiss System: McMahon System

A variant known as the **McMahon System Tournament** is the established way in which European Go tournaments are run. This differs mainly from the Swiss system mainly in that players start at different levels; so the Swiss system is the special case where all players start at the same level. It is named for Lee McMahon (1931–1989) of Bell Labs.

Variations of the Swiss System: Konrad System

In a few tournaments that run over a long period of time, such as a tournament with one round every week for three months, a flexible system called a **Konrad** tournament can be used. A player's final score is based on his best results (e.g., the best ten results out of the twelve rounds). Players are not required to play in every round; they may enter or drop out of the tournament at any time. Indeed, they may decide to play only one game if they wish to, although if a player wants to get a prize, he or she will need to play more rounds to accumulate points. The tournament therefore includes players who want to go for a prize and play several rounds, as well as players who only want to play an off game. This system is used by a few chess clubs in Norway.

Chapter Summary

Athletic tournaments take many shapes and forms, but always attempt to create a way in which a winner can be decided. Different sports require different methods of measuring what individual or team is the best for any given situation. Single-elimination, double-elimination, round-robin, and specialty tournaments all have their advantages and disadvantages, and all have found support for their particular application.

Chapter Review Questions

1. Devise a single-elimination tournament for badminton with twenty-six participants.

2. Devise a double-elimination tournament for basketball with ten teams.

3. Devise a round-robin tournament for golf with twelve participants.

4. Explain the Swiss system tournament, its usage, advantages, and disadvantages.

5. What is meant by accelerated pairings?

Projects and Activities

1. Using the Internet, find and print an example of each of the tournaments explained in the chapter. The tournaments shouldn't be blank: they should be recently completed examples with real teams and/or names.

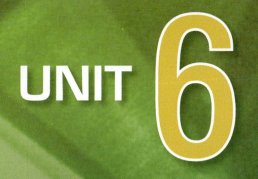

Opportunities and Challenges in Physical Education and Exercise Science

The Future of Fitness and Sport

Objectives

Upon completion of this chapter, the reader should be able to:

- Explain the challenges that face the nation with youth fitness and activity.
- Recite several strategies that are designed to promote lifelong participation.
- Discuss implementation of the ten strategies.
- Describe the five components of fitness.
- Explain *Healthy People 2010* and what it means to the nation's youth.

Key Terms

Body composition

Cardiorespiratory endurance

Flexibility

Healthy People 2010

Muscular endurance

Muscular strength

President's Council on Physical Fitness and Sports (PCPFS)

The Centers for Disease Control and Prevention (CDC)

The National Association for Sport and Physical Education (NASPE)

Title IX

Youth Risk Behavior Surveillance System (YRBSS)

The Future of Fitness and Sport

This chapter is devoted to material written by the National Center for Chronic Disease Prevention and Health Promotion. This material was written and presented to the president of the United States in an effort to highlight and specifically detail the challenges that lie ahead to educate today's youth in the benefits of fitness and sport. The material for this chapter is taken directly from *Promoting Better Health for Young People through Physical Activity and Sports: A Report to the President*.

Executive Summary

Our nation's young people are, in large measure, inactive, unfit, and increasingly overweight. In the long run, this physical inactivity threatens to reverse the decades-long progress we have made in reducing death from cardiovascular diseases and could devastate our national health care budget. In the short run, physical inactivity has contributed to an unprecedented epidemic of childhood obesity that is currently plaguing the United States. The percentage of young people who are overweight has doubled since 1980 (Figure 17-1).

Enhancing efforts to promote participation in physical activity and sports among young people is a critical national priority. Physical activity has been identified as one of our nation's leading health indicators in *Healthy People 2010*, the national health objectives for the decade.

> ● **KEY CONCEPT** ●
>
> Enhancing efforts to promote participation in physical activity and sports among young people is a critical national priority.

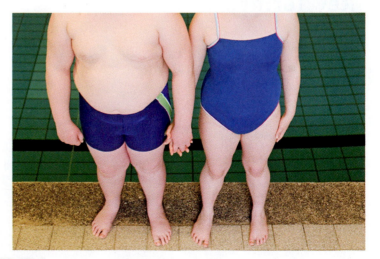

FIGURE 17–1
Obesity has become a national epidemic. (Courtesy of PunchStock)

To increase their levels of physical activity and fitness, young people can benefit from:

- Families who model and support participation in enjoyable physical activity (Figure 17-2).

- School programs (including quality, daily physical education; health education; recess; and extracurricular activities) that help students develop the knowledge, attitudes, skills, behaviors, and confidence to adopt and maintain physically active lifestyles, while providing opportunities for enjoyable physical activity.

- After-school care programs that provide regular opportunities for active, physical play.

- Youth sports and recreation programs that offer a range of developmentally appropriate activities that are accessible and attractive to all young people.

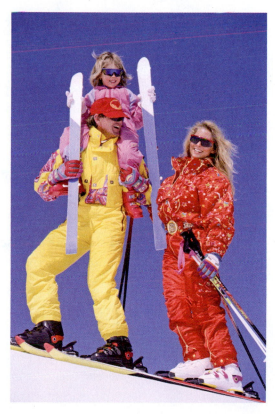

FIGURE 17–2

Families that are active together enjoy a greater degree of fitness than those that are not. (Courtesy of Photodisc)

- A community structural environment that makes it easy and safe for young people to walk, ride bicycles, and use close-to-home physical activity facilities.

- Media campaigns that help motivate young people to be physically active.

Strategies

The following strategies are all designed to promote lifelong participation in enjoyable and safe physical activity and sports.

1. Include education for parents and guardians as part of youth physical activity promotion initiatives.

2. Help all children, from pre-kindergarten through grade 12, to receive quality, daily physical education. Help all schools to have certified physical education specialists; appropriate class sizes; and the facilities, equipment, and supplies needed to deliver quality, daily physical education.

3. Publicize and disseminate tools to help schools improve their physical education and other physical activity programs.

4. Enable state education and health departments to work together to help schools implement quality, daily physical education and other physical activity programs:

   - With a full-time state coordinator for school physical activity programs
   - As part of a coordinated school health program
   - With support from relevant governmental and nongovernmental organizations

5. Enable more after-school care programs to provide regular opportunities for active, physical play.

6. Help provide access to community sports and recreation programs for all young people.

7. Enable youth sports and recreation programs to provide coaches and recreation program staff with the training they need to offer developmentally appropriate, safe, and enjoyable physical activity experiences for young people.

8. Enable communities to develop and promote the use of safe, well-maintained, and close-to-home sidewalks, crosswalks,

bicycle paths, trails, parks, recreation facilities, and community designs featuring mixed-use development and a connected grid of streets.

9. Implement an ongoing media campaign to promote physical education as an important component of a quality education and long-term health.

10. Monitor youth physical activity, physical fitness, and school and community physical activity programs in the nation and each state.

Implementation

Full implementation of the strategies recommended will require the commitment of resources, hard work, and creative thinking from many partners in federal, state, and local governments; nongovernmental organizations; and the private sector. Only through extensive collaboration and coordination can resources be maximized, strategies integrated, and messages reinforced. Development or expansion of a broad, national coalition to promote better health through physical activity and sports is an important first step toward collaboration and coordination. A foundation to support the promotion of physical activity could complement the work of the coalition and play a critical role in obtaining the resources needed to help our young people become physically active and fit. The 10 strategies and the process for facilitating their implementation described in this chapter provide the framework for our children to rediscover the joys of physical activity and to incorporate physical activity as a fundamental building-block of their present and future lives.

Introduction

America loves to think of itself as a youthful nation focused on fitness. But behind the vivid media images of robust runners, Olympic Dream Teams, and rugged mountain bikers is the troubling reality of a generation of young people that is, in large measure, inactive, unfit, and increasingly overweight.

The consequences of the sedentary lifestyles lived by so many of our young people are grave (Figure 17-3).

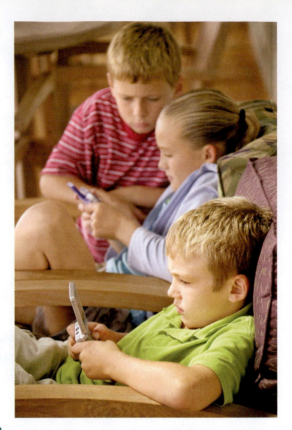

FIGURE 17–3
The more time spent playing video games, the less time being active. (Courtesy of PunchStock)

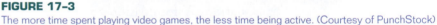

> **KEY CONCEPT**
>
> A physically inactive population is at increased risk for many chronic diseases, including heart disease, stroke, colon cancer, diabetes, and osteoporosis.

In the long run, physical inactivity threatens to reverse the decades-long progress made in reducing death and suffering from cardiovascular diseases. A physically inactive population is at increased risk for many chronic diseases, including heart disease, stroke, colon cancer, diabetes, and osteoporosis. In addition to the toll taken by human suffering, surges in the prevalence of these diseases could lead to crippling increases in our national health care expenditures.

In the short run, physical inactivity has contributed to an unprecedented epidemic of childhood obesity that is currently plaguing the United States. The percentage of young people who are overweight has doubled since 1980. Of children aged 5 to 10 who are overweight, 61 percent have one or more cardiovascular disease risk factors, and 27 percent have two or more. The negative health consequences linked to the childhood obesity epidemic include the appearance, in the past two decades, of a new and frightening public health problem: Type 2 diabetes among adolescents. Type 2 diabetes was previously so rarely seen in children or adolescents that it came to be called "adult-onset diabetes." Now, an increasing number of teenagers and preteens must be treated for diabetes and strive to ward off the life-threatening health complications that it can cause.

Obesity in adolescence also has been associated with poorer self-esteem and with obesity in adulthood. Among adults today, 25 percent of women and 20 percent of men are obese. The total costs of diseases associated with obesity have been estimated at almost $100 billion per year, or approximately 8 percent of the national health care budget.

In January 2000, the nation issued *Healthy People 2010*, its health objectives for the decade. Unlike previous sets of national health objectives, *Healthy People 2010* included a set of leading health indicators: ten high-priority public health areas for enhanced public attention. The fact that the first leading health indicator is physical activity and the second is overweight and obesity speaks clearly to the national importance of these issues.

Enhancing efforts to promote participation in physical activity and sports among young people is a critical national priority. That is why, on June 23, 2000, President Clinton issued a directive to the Secretary of Health and Human Services and the Secretary of Education to work together to identify and report within 90 days on "strategies to promote better health for our nation's youth through physical activity and fitness."

The President instructed the Secretaries to include in this report strategies for

- Promoting the renewal of physical education in our schools and the expansion of after-school programs that offer physical activities and sports in addition to enhanced academics and cultural activities.

- Encouraging participation by private-sector partners in raising the level of physical activity and fitness among our young people.

- Promoting greater coordination of existing public and private resources that encourage physical activity and sports.

Furthermore, the President directed the Secretaries to work with the United States Olympic Committee (USOC) and other private and nongovernmental sports organizations, as appropriate. The President concluded his directive by saying: "By identifying effective new steps and strengthening public-private partnerships, we will advance our efforts to prepare the nation's young people for lifelong physical fitness."

Benefits of Physical Activity

The landmark 1996 Surgeon General's report, *Physical Activity and Health*, identified substantial health benefits of regular participation in physical activity, including reducing the risks of dying prematurely (Figure 17-4); dying prematurely from heart disease; and developing diabetes, high blood pressure, or colon cancer. When physical inactivity is combined with poor diet, the impact on health is devastating, accounting for an estimated 300,000 deaths per year. Tobacco use is the only behavior that kills more people.

The Surgeon General's report made clear that the health benefits of physical activity are not limited to adults. Regular participation in physical activity during childhood and adolescence

- Helps build and maintain healthy bones, muscles, and joints.

- Helps control weight, build lean muscle, and reduce fat.

- Prevents or delays the development of high blood pressure and helps reduce blood pressure in some adolescents with hypertension.

- Reduces feelings of depression and anxiety.

Although research has not been conducted to conclusively demonstrate a direct link between physical activity and improved academic performance, such a link might be expected. Studies have found participation in physical activity increases adolescents' self-esteem and reduces anxiety and stress. Through its effects on mental health, physical activity may help increase

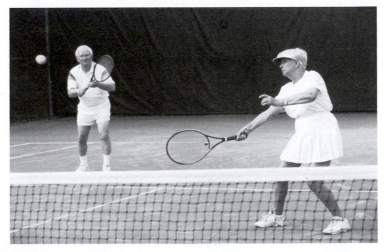

FIGURE 17–4
How old is too old to enjoy an active lifestyle? (Courtesy of Photodisc)

students' capacity for learning. One study found that spending more time in physical education did not have harmful effects on the standardized academic achievement test scores of elementary school students; in fact, there was some evidence that participation in a 2-year health-related physical education program had several significant favorable effects on academic achievement.

Participation in physical activity and sports can promote social well-being, as well as physical and mental health, among young people. Research has shown that students who participate in interscholastic sports are less likely to be regular and heavy smokers or use drugs, and are more likely to stay in school and have good conduct and high academic achievement (Figure 17-5).

Sports and physical activity programs can introduce young people to skills such as teamwork, self-discipline, sportsmanship, leadership, and socialization. Lack of recreational activity, on the other hand, may contribute to making young people more vulnerable to gangs, drugs, or violence.

One of the major benefits of physical activity is that it helps people improve their physical fitness. Fitness is a state of well-being that allows people to perform daily activities with vigor, participate in a variety of physical activities, and reduce their risks for health problems. Five basic components of fitness are important for good health: **cardio-respiratory endurance, muscular strength, muscular endurance, flexibility,** and

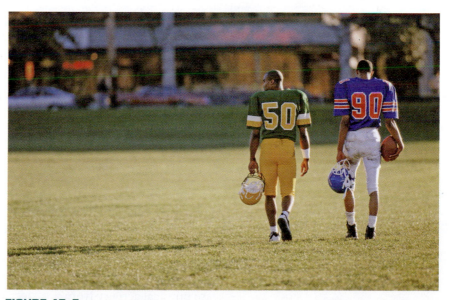

FIGURE 17–5
Athletics helps to promote a healthy lifestyle. (Photodisc)

body composition (percentage of body fat). A second set of attributes, referred to as sport- or skill-related physical fitness, includes power, speed, agility, balance, and reaction time. Although skill-related fitness attributes are not essential for maintaining physical health, they are important for athletic performance or physically demanding jobs such as military service and emergency and rescue service.

How Much Physical Activity and Fitness Do Young People Need?

The Surgeon General's report on physical activity and health concluded that

- People who are usually inactive can improve their health and well-being by becoming even moderately active on a regular basis.

- Physical activity need not be strenuous to achieve health benefits.

- Greater health benefits can be achieved by increasing the amount (duration, frequency, or intensity) of physical activity.

- Rigorous scientific reviews have led to two widely accepted sets of developmentally appropriate recommendations (one for adolescents, the other for elementary school-aged children) for how much and what kinds of physical activity young people need. The International Consensus Conference on Physical Activity Guidelines for Adolescents issued the following recommendation: all adolescents should be physically active daily, or nearly every day, as part of play, games, sports, work, transportation, recreation, physical education, or planned exercise, in the context of family, school, and community activities.

- Adolescents should engage in three or more sessions per week of activities that last 20 minutes or more at a time and that require moderate to vigorous levels of exertion.

The developmental needs and abilities of younger children differ from those of adolescents and adults. **The National Association for Sport and Physical Education (NASPE)** has issued physical activity guidelines for elementary school-aged children that recommend the following:

- Elementary school-aged children should accumulate at least thirty to sixty minutes of age-appropriate and developmentally appropriate physical activity from a variety of activities on all, or most, days of the week.

- An accumulation of more than sixty minutes, and up to several hours per day, of age-appropriate and developmentally appropriate activity is encouraged.

- Some of the child's activity each day should be in periods lasting ten to fifteen minutes or more and include moderate to vigorous activity. This activity will typically be intermittent in nature, involving alternating moderate to vigorous activity with brief periods of rest and recovery.

- Children should not have extended periods of inactivity.

Healthy People 2010, the national initiative that established health objectives for the first decade of this century, includes objectives to increase levels of moderate and vigorous physical activity among adolescents, to increase the proportion of trips made by walking and bicycling, and to decrease the amount of time young people spend watching television.

Furthermore, *Healthy People 2010* includes participation in physical activity as one of the nation's ten leading health indicators. Of the two objectives that will be used to measure progress in meeting this indicator, one targets adolescents: Increase the proportion of adolescents who engage in vigorous physical activity that promotes cardio-respiratory fitness three or more days per week for twenty or more minutes per occasion.

Healthy People 2010 does not specify national objectives related to youth fitness in part because there is no scientific consensus on which of the various existing fitness tests and classification standards to use. However, there is widespread agreement that fitness tests should emphasize health-related fitness components, and that those standards for interpreting test results should be based on the relationship between physical activity and health rather than on the results of other students (i.e., norms). This will give all children and adolescents the opportunity to experience success, reinforce the link between fitness and health, and emphasize that one can be fit without being an elite athlete.

The importance of physical activity is reinforced in the 2000 version of the *Dietary Guidelines for Americans*, which forms the basis of all federal nutrition education and promotion activities. One of the guidelines advises Americans to "be physically active each day"; children and teens are advised to aim for at least sixty minutes of moderate physical activity most days of the week, preferably daily.

How Active and Fit Are Our Children and Adolescents?

Available data indicate that young children are among the most active of all segments of the population, but physical activity levels begin to decline as children approach their teenage years and continue to decline throughout adolescence.

Even among children and adolescents, however, a substantial proportion of the population does not meet recommended levels of participation in physical activity. **The Centers for Disease Control and Prevention (CDC)'s Youth Risk Behavior Surveillance System (YRBSS)** collects data on participation in physical activity from a nationally representative sample of students in grades nine through 12. YRBSS data for 1999 show that, among U.S. high school students:

- More than one in three (35 percent) do not participate regularly in vigorous physical activity.

- Regular participation in vigorous physical activity drops from 73 percent of ninth grade students to 61 percent of twelfth grade students.

- Nearly half (45 percent) do not play on any sports teams during the year.

- Nearly half (44 percent) are not even enrolled in a physical education class; enrollment in physical education drops from 79 in ninth grade to 37 percent in twelfth grade.

- Only 29 percent attend daily physical education classes, a dramatic decline from 1991, when 42 percent of high school students did so.

National transportation surveys have found that walking and bicycling by children aged five to fifteen years dropped 40 percent between 1977 and 1995. More than one-third (37 percent) of all trips to school are made from one mile away or less, but only 31 percent of these trips are made by walking. Although an estimated 38 million young people participate in youth sports programs, participation declines substantially as children progress through adolescence. One study found that attrition from youth sports programs was occurring among ten-year-olds and peaked among fourteen- to fifteen-year-olds.

One factor contributing to low levels of physical activity among young people might be the many hours that they spend doing sedentary

> ● **KEY CONCEPT** ●
>
> More than one-third (37 percent) of all trips to school are made from one mile away or less, but only 31 percent of these trips are made by walking.

activities, most notably using electronic media. A 1999 national survey found that young people aged two to eighteen years spend, on average, over four hours a day watching television, watching videotapes, playing video games, or using a computer. Most of this time (2 hours and 46 minutes per day, on average) is spent watching television. One-third of children and adolescents watch television for more than three hours a day, and nearly one-fifth (17 percent) watch more than five hours of television a day.

Physical inactivity has contributed to the 100 percent increase in the prevalence of childhood obesity in the United States since 1980. According to the National Health and Nutrition Examination Survey (NHANES), between 1976–1980 and 1988–1994, the percentage of U.S. adolescents (aged twelve to nineteen years) who were overweight increased from 5.4 percent to 9.7 percent of girls and 4.5 percent to 11.3 percent of boys. The changes among young children (ages six to eleven) in the same period were similar, rising from 6.4 percent to 11.0 percent of girls and from 5.5 percent to 11.8 percent of boys (Figure 17-6).

The last nationally representative study of youth fitness was conducted in the mid-1980s, but it did not classify students based on whether or not they met health-related fitness standards. However, fitness tests administered throughout California in 1999 found that only about one in five students in the fifth, seventh, and ninth grades met the standards for all health-related fitness components, and that more than 40 percent did not meet the minimum fitness standard for endurance.

How Our Society Discourages Physical Activity

Behavior is shaped, in large measure, by one's environment. Our young people live in a social and physical environment that makes it easy to be sedentary and inconvenient to be active. Developments in our culture and society over the past few decades that have discouraged youth physical activity include the following:

- Community design centered around the automobile has discouraged walking and bicycling and has made it more difficult for children to get together to play.

- Increased concerns about safety have limited the time and areas in which children are allowed to play outside.

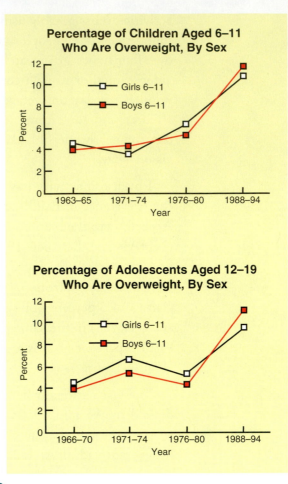

FIGURE 17–6

[1] Data for 1966–70 are for adolescents 12–17, not 12–19 years.

NOTE: Overweight is defined as body mass index (BMI), at or above the sex- and age-specific 95th percentile cutoff points from the revised CDC Growth Chart: United States.

Source: Centers for Disease Control and Prevention, National Center for Health Statistics. Division of Health Examination Statistics. Unpublished data.

- New technology has conditioned our young people to be less active, while new electronic media (e.g., video and computer games, cable and satellite television) have made sedentary activities more appealing.

- States and school districts have reduced the amount of time students are required to spend in physical education classes, and many of those classes have so many students that teachers cannot give students the individual attention they need.

- Communities have failed to invest adequately in close-to-home physical activity facilities (e.g., parks, recreation centers).

Strategies

Children and adolescents in the United States cannot become more physically active and fit if they don't have a wide range of accessible, safe, and affordable opportunities to be active. However, opportunities alone are not enough: In twenty-first century America, physical activity is, for the most part, a voluntary behavior. Our young people, therefore, will not increase their levels of physical activity and fitness unless they are sufficiently motivated to do so. Their motivation to be active will depend on the degree to which they find their physical activity experiences to be enjoyable. Enjoyment of physical activity, in turn, will be influenced by the extent to which young people

- can choose to engage in sports and recreational activities that are most appealing to them.

- are taught necessary skills.

- develop confidence in their physical abilities.

- are guided by competent, knowledgeable, and supportive adults.

- are supported by cultural norms that make participation in physical activity desirable.

To obtain the opportunities and motivation that will enable them to increase their levels of physical activity and fitness, young people can benefit from

- Families who model and support participation in enjoyable physical activity.

- School programs (including quality, daily physical education; health education; recess; and extracurricular activities) that help students develop the knowledge, attitudes, skills, behaviors, and confidence to adopt and maintain physically active lifestyles, while providing opportunities for enjoyable physical activity.

- After-school care programs that provide regular opportunities for active, physical play.

- Youth sports and recreation programs that offer a range of developmentally appropriate activities that are attractive to all young people.

- A community structural environment that makes it easy and safe for young people to walk, ride bicycles, and use close-to-home physical activity facilities.

- Media campaigns that increase the motivation of young people to be physically active.

> ● **KEY CONCEPT** ●
>
> Our young people will not increase their levels of physical activity and fitness unless they are sufficiently motivated to do so.

The strategies presented are all designed to promote lifelong participation in enjoyable and safe physical activity. Special efforts must be made to ensure that programs are responsive to those in greatest need, including girls and racial/ethnic minorities.

Girls are significantly less likely than boys to participate regularly in vigorous physical activity and on sports teams. Among high school students in 1999, 57 percent of girls participated regularly in vigorous physical activity compared with 72 percent of boys, and 49 percent of girls played on a sports team compared with 62 percent of boys. Despite the tremendous gains girls have made in sports participation during the last thirty years, no doubt due in large measure to the 1972 **Title IX** legislation that prohibited sex discrimination in school athletics, the ratio of female to male participants in interscholastic sports is still only 3 : 5. Girls join organized sports programs at later ages than boys and drop out at younger ages.

In its 1997 report, *Physical Activity and Sport in the Lives of Girls*, the **President's Council on Physical Fitness and Sports (PCPFS)** concluded that physical activity has an increasingly important role in the lives of girls, because of both its physical and emotional health benefits. Strategies to increase the amount of physical activity for boys and girls will need to be different, because girls tend to prefer different types of physical activity and pursue it for different reasons than do boys. Since girls are more likely to have lower self-esteem related to their physical capabilities, programs that serve girls should provide instruction and experiences that increase their confidence, offer ample opportunities for participation, and establish social environments that support involvement in a range of physical activities.

Among high school students in 1999, whites were significantly more likely than blacks to report regular participation in physical activity (67 percent vs. 56 percent) and more likely than Hispanics to play on sports teams in and out of school (57 percent vs. 51 percent). Establishing a physically active lifestyle in adolescence is particularly important for African Americans and Hispanics, because African American and Hispanic adults are at increased risk for physical inactivity, obesity, and diabetes; African American adults also are at increased risk for death from heart disease. Resources must be invested in creative, culturally sensitive, linguistically appropriate programs to give all young Americans the opportunities and motivation they need to become more active.

Implementation

Implementing strategies to promote physical activity and sports participation will require the commitment of resources from federal, state, and local governments and the private sector, as well as close collaboration among health, education, and youth-serving organizations. National efforts to implement and sustain activities to promote youth participation in physical activity and sports would benefit from the establishment or enhancement of a coordinating mechanism, such as a national coalition. To measure the progress of a national initiative and guide its management, national systems should be supported to monitor youth physical activity and fitness and programs designed to promote youth physical activity. To help inform policymakers about the importance of this issue, researchers need to document the effects of participation in physical activity and sports on desired public health and social outcomes, particularly improved academic performance and reductions in youth violence.

A Call to Action

Full implementation of the strategies recommended in *Healthy People 2010* will require the commitment of resources, hard work, and creative thinking from many partners in federal, state, and local governments; nongovernmental organizations; and the private sector. Only through extensive collaboration and coordination can resources be maximized, strategies integrated, and messages reinforced.

The following actions should be taken to facilitate the process of implementing the ten strategies identified in this report:

- The federal government will convene a working group to develop a detailed implementation plan to promote physical activity among young people. The Secretary of Health and Human Services, in collaboration with the Secretary of Education, will bring together key players from national, state, and local levels and from the public and the private sectors to work together to achieve the strategies recommended in this report.

- National nongovernmental organizations and the private sector should work together to develop or expand a national coalition to promote physical activity and a foundation to support its efforts.

- National, state, and local leaders should encourage concerned citizens to work together to establish state and local councils or coalitions to promote physical activity among young people.

- The President, the Secretary of Health and Human Services, the Secretary of Education, and the nation's governors and mayors should educate the American public in general, and educational policymakers in particular, about the importance of having all children participate in quality, daily physical education.

The Secretary of Health and Human Services and the Secretary of Education can facilitate progress in efforts to promote youth physical activity by providing annual reports to the President on actions taken to implement the strategies identified in this report.

Development or expansion of a broad, national coalition to promote better health through physical activity and sports is an important first step toward collaboration and coordination. An effective national coalition will draw public attention to the need for action, educate the public and policymakers about the strategies recommended in this report, and develop coordinated initiatives to implement the strategies. A number of national coalitions currently exist to promote physical activity or fitness, and a merger of these, or an intensive expansion of participation in one of them, would initiate a national coordinating mechanism. Among the organizations that should be added to such a national coalition are the USOC and the professional sports leagues. A foundation to support promotion of physical activity could complement the work of the coalition and play a critical role in obtaining the resources needed to help our young people become physically active and fit.

Chapter Summary

Physical activity is crucial to our health, happiness, and well-being. The staggering consequences of decreases in physical activity are clear: soaring rates of obesity and diabetes, potential future increases in heart disease, and devastating increases in health care costs. We now have the opportunity to reshape our sedentary society into one that facilitates and promotes participation in physical activity during childhood, throughout adolescence, and into adulthood. The ten strategies and the process for facilitating their implementation described in this chapter provide the foundation for today's youth to rediscover the joys of physical activity and to incorporate physical activity as a fundamental building block of their present and future lives.

Chapter Review Questions

1. What does *Healthy People 2010* attempt to do?

2. What are the ten strategies that are designed to promote lifelong participation?

3. What are the recommendations for implementing these strategies?

4. What are the consequences of sedentary lifestyles?

5. Explain the percentages of overweight people in the United States today.

6. The Surgeon General explained the health benefits of physical activity. What are they?

7. What are the five basic components of fitness?

8. Explain the fitness guidelines issued by the National Association for Sport and Physical Education for elementary children.

9. Explain the data collected by the Youth Risk Behavior Surveillance System for U.S. high school students on fitness.

10. Over the past few decades, developments in our culture and society has discouraged youth physical activity. How?

Projects and Activities

1. Compile the statistics in this chapter into a database. Research similar data for France, Germany, Japan, and China. What can you conclude from your findings?

2. Research what, (if any thing) corporate America is doing to stem the decline in fitness and obesity.

Website Resources

http://www.cdc.gov/

http://www.census.gov/

Career Perspectives in Physical Education

Objectives

Upon completion of this chapter, the reader should be able to:

- Distinguish different career options for the physical education major.
- Describe job outlook for the different career options explained in the chapter.
- Describe job responsibilities for each career option.
- Describe salary range for each career option.

Key Terms

Camp counselors

Certified athletic trainers

Fitness directors

Fitness workers

Personal trainers

Pilates

Recreation workers

Sport management

Sport psychology

Yoga

Career Perspectives in Physical Education

Career opportunities in physical education and fitness-related fields will continue to attract quality applicants for the foreseeable future (Figure 18-1). As with any profession, applicants need to be knowledgeable, support a quality resume, and have the personal skills that will enable them to work well with young adults. This chapter is designed to help the physical education major narrow his or her scope in securing their first employment in the physical education profession.

Physical Education Teacher

As with most occupations, projections for physical education career opportunities are largely dependent upon future trends and national economic forecasts. The increase in non-teaching job opportunities, coupled with a decrease in the number of available teaching positions, has resulted in a movement away from the traditional physical education teaching major. This trend, in conjunction with cuts in physical education programs due to budget constraints, meant that large numbers of physical education teachers left teaching.

Even though there is still a shift away from the traditional physical education major, it is important to note that students who have already

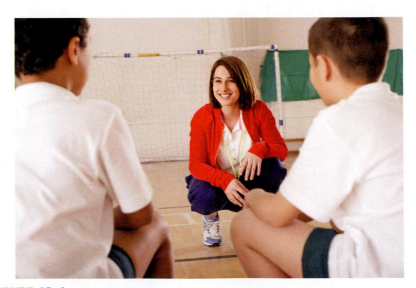

FIGURE 18–1
Careers in Physical Education are rewarding and fast-paced. (Courtesy of PunchStock)

earned a degree are beginning to return to school for teacher education certification. There appear to be three reasons for this. First, the non-teaching exercise and sport job market has become so heavily saturated that job opportunities are not as plentiful today. Second, physical education teachers who have been teaching for twenty or thirty years are beginning to retire, and there will be a gradual increase in the number of physical education teaching positions available. And third, in some non-teaching careers, there is no career ladder. There is potential for a shortage of physical educators as a result of the small pool of students being certified to teach physical education, although this shortage may be keener in specific geographic areas.

The ability to draw knowledge from strong scientific foundations continues to be paramount as students prepare for careers in exercise and sport. Courses such as anatomy and physiology, exercise physiology, kinesiology, and other courses in the study of human movement have provided these scientific foundations. Along with college and university-based professional preparation programs, many professional organizations now provide exercise and sport credentialing opportunities.

The challenge for physical education professionals is to provide the knowledge necessary to be at the forefront of change. Emphasis must be placed on continued study of present trends and forecasts and their relationship to physical activity careers. The public's pursuit of a healthy lifestyle through physical activity will be best served if exercise and sport professionals are leading, rather than reacting to, the latest trends.

Examples of some present trends that may have an impact on curriculum development include: aging of the population, more at-risk children in the school system, and increased use of technology (Figure 18-2). While emphasis has been placed on nontraditional physical education careers, it is also important to continue a focus on traditional teaching and coaching opportunities.

Careers in Teaching

Teachers act as facilitators or coaches, using interactive discussions and "hands-on" approaches to help students learn and apply concepts (Figure 18-3). Preschool, kindergarten, and elementary school teachers play a vital role in the development of children. What children learn and experience during their early years can shape their views of themselves and the world, and can affect their later success or failure in school, work, and their personal lives.

Teachers often work with students from varied ethnic, racial, and religious backgrounds. With growing minority populations in most parts of the country, it is important for teachers to work effectively with a diverse student population. Accordingly, some schools offer training to help teachers enhance their awareness and understanding of different cultures. Teachers may also include multicultural programming in their lesson plans to address the needs of all students, regardless of their cultural background.

Teachers design classroom presentations to meet students' needs and abilities. They also work with students individually. Teachers plan, evaluate, and assign lessons; prepare, administer, and grade tests; listen to oral presentations; and maintain classroom discipline. They observe and evaluate a student's performance and potential, and increasingly are asked to use new assessment methods. For example, teachers may examine a

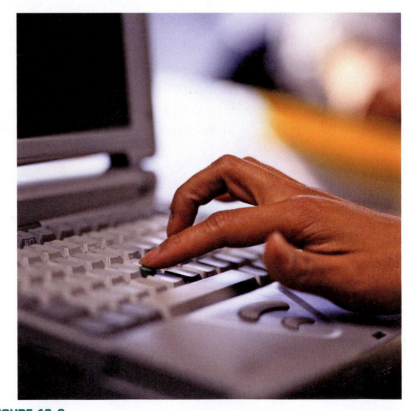

FIGURE 18–2
Today's student is tech savvy. Physical educators will need to keep pace with the newest technology in achieving attractive fitness options. (Courtesy of Photodisc)

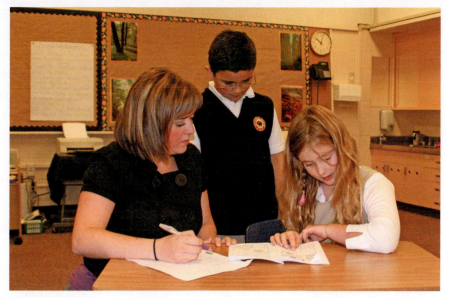

FIGURE 18–3
Teaching can be a wonderful fulfilling career that helps shape a child's future.

portfolio of a student's artwork or writing in order to judge the student's overall progress. They then can provide additional assistance in areas in which a student needs help. Teachers also grade papers, prepare report cards, and meet with parents and school staff to discuss a student's academic progress or personal problems.

In addition to conducting classroom activities, teachers oversee study halls and homerooms, supervise extracurricular activities, and accompany students on field trips. They may identify students with physical or mental problems and refer the students to the proper authorities. Secondary-school teachers occasionally assist students in choosing courses, colleges, and careers. Teachers also participate in education conferences and workshops.

In recent years, site-based management, which allows teachers and parents to participate actively in management decisions regarding school operations, has gained popularity. In many schools, teachers are increasingly involved in making decisions regarding the budget, personnel, textbooks, curriculum design, and teaching methods.

Seeing students develop new skills and gain an appreciation of knowledge and learning can be very rewarding. However, teaching may be frustrating when one is dealing with unmotivated or disrespectful students. Occasionally, teachers must cope with unruly behavior and violence in the schools. Teachers may experience stress in dealing with large classes, heavy workloads, or old schools that are run down and lack many modern amenities. Accountability standards also may increase stress levels, with teachers expected to produce students who are able to exhibit satisfactory performance on standardized tests in core subjects. Many teachers, particularly in public schools, are also frustrated by the lack of control they have over what they are required to teach.

Teachers in private schools generally enjoy smaller class sizes and more control over establishing the curriculum and setting standards for performance and discipline. Their students also tend to be more motivated, since private schools can be selective in their admissions processes.

Teachers are sometimes isolated from their colleagues because they work alone in a classroom of students. However, some schools allow teachers to work in teams and with mentors to enhance their professional development.

Including school duties performed outside the classroom, many teachers work more than forty hours a week. Part-time schedules are more common among preschool and kindergarten teachers. Although some school districts have gone to all-day kindergartens, most kindergarten teachers still teach two kindergarten classes a day. Most teachers work the traditional ten-month school year with a two-month vacation during the summer. During the vacation break, those on the ten-month schedule may teach in summer sessions, take other jobs, travel, or pursue personal interests. Many enroll in college courses or workshops to continue their education. Teachers in districts with a year-round schedule typically work eight weeks, are on vacation for one week, and have a five-week midwinter break. Preschool teachers working in day care settings often work year round.

Most states have tenure laws that prevent public school teachers from being fired without just cause and due process. Teachers may obtain tenure after they have satisfactorily completed a probationary period of teaching—normally three years. Tenure does not absolutely guarantee a job, but it does provide some security.

Licensure

All fifty States and the District of Columbia require public school teachers to be licensed. Licensure is not required for teachers in private schools in most states. Usually licensure is granted by the state board of education or a licensure advisory committee. Teachers may be licensed to teach the early childhood grades (usually preschool through grade three); the elementary grades (grades one through six or eight); the middle grades (grades five through eight); a secondary-education subject area (usually grades seven through twelve); or a special subject, such as reading or music (usually grades kindergarten through twelve).

Requirements for regular licenses to teach kindergarten through grade twelve vary by state. However, all states require general education teachers to have a bachelor's degree and to have completed an approved teacher training program with a prescribed number of subject and education credits, as well as supervised practice teaching. Some states also require technology training and the attainment of a minimum grade point average. A number of states require that teachers obtain a master's degree in education within a specified period after they begin teaching.

Almost all states require applicants for a teacher's license to be tested for competency in basic skills, such as reading and writing, and in teaching. Almost all also require the teacher to exhibit proficiency in his or her subject. Many school systems are presently moving toward implementing performance-based systems for licensure, which usually require a teacher to demonstrate satisfactory teaching performance over an extended period in order to obtain a provisional license, in addition to passing an examination in their subject. Most states require continuing education for renewal of the teacher's license. Many states have reciprocity agreements that make it easier for teachers licensed in one state to become licensed in another.

Many states also offer alternative licensure programs for teachers who have a bachelor's degree in the subject they will teach, but who lack the necessary education courses required for a regular license. Many of these alternative licensure programs are designed to ease shortages of teachers of certain subjects, such as mathematics and science. Other programs provide teachers for urban and rural schools that have difficulty filling positions with teachers from traditional licensure programs.

Alternative licensure programs are intended to attract people into teaching who do not fulfill traditional licensing standards, including recent college graduates who did not complete education programs and those changing from another career to teaching. In some programs, individuals begin teaching quickly under provisional licensure. After working under the close supervision of experienced educators for one or two years while taking education courses outside school hours, they receive regular licensure if they have progressed satisfactorily. In other programs, college graduates who do not meet licensure requirements take only those courses that they lack and then become licensed. This approach may take one or

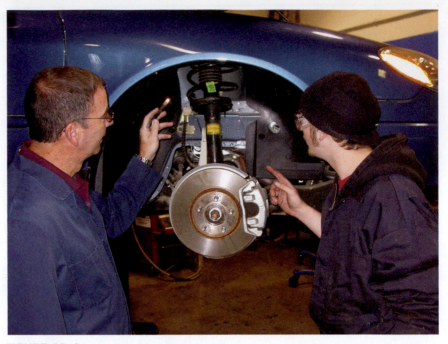

FIGURE 18–4
Vocational programs such as automotive, have different qualification standards for teachers.

two semesters of full-time study. States may issue emergency licenses to individuals who do not meet the requirements for a regular license when schools cannot attract enough qualified teachers to fill positions. Teachers who need to be licensed may enter programs that grant a master's degree in education, as well as a license.

In many states, vocational teachers have many of the same requirements for teaching as their academic counterparts (Figure 18-4). However, because knowledge and experience in a particular field are important criteria for the job, some states will license vocational education teachers without a bachelor's degree, provided they can demonstrate expertise in their field. A minimum number of hours in education courses may also be required.

Licensing requirements for preschool teachers also vary by state. Requirements for public preschool teachers are generally more stringent than those for private preschool teachers. Some states require a bachelor's degree in early childhood education, while others require an associate's degree, and still others require certification by a nationally recognized authority. The Child Development Associate (CDA) credential, the most common type of certification, requires a mix of classroom training and experience working with children, along with an independent assessment of an individual's competence.

Private schools are generally exempt from state licensing standards. For secondary school teacher jobs, they prefer candidates who have a bachelor's degree in the subject they intend to teach, or in childhood education for elementary school teachers. They seek candidates among recent college graduates as well as from those who have established careers in other fields. Private schools associated with religious institutions also desire candidates who share the values that are important to the institution.

In some cases, teachers of kindergarten through high school may attain professional certification in order to demonstrate competency beyond that required for a license. The National Board for Professional Teaching Standards offers a voluntary national certification. To become nationally accredited, experienced teachers must prove their aptitude by compiling a portfolio showing their work in the classroom and by passing a written assessment and evaluation of their teaching knowledge. Currently, teachers may become certified in a variety of areas, on the basis of the age of the students and, in some cases, the subject taught. For example, teachers may obtain a certificate for teaching English language arts to early adolescents (aged eleven to fifteen), or they may become certified as early childhood generalists. All states recognize national certification, and many states and school districts provide special benefits to teachers holding such certification. Benefits typically include higher salaries and reimbursement for continuing education and certification fees. In addition, many states allow nationally certified teachers to carry a license from one state to another.

The National Council for Accreditation of Teacher Education currently accredits teacher education programs across the United States. Graduation from an accredited program is not necessary to become a teacher, but it does make it easier to fulfill licensure requirements. Generally, four-year colleges require students to wait until their sophomore year before applying for admission to teacher education programs. Traditional education programs for kindergarten and elementary school teachers include courses designed specifically for those preparing to teach in mathematics, physical science, social science, music, art, and literature, as well as prescribed professional education courses, such as philosophy of education, psychology of learning, and teaching methods. Aspiring secondary school teachers most often major in the subject they plan to teach, while also taking a program of study in teacher preparation. Teacher-education programs are now required to include classes in the use of computers and other technologies in order to maintain their accreditation. Most programs require students to perform a student-teaching internship.

Many States now offer professional development schools, which are partnerships between universities and elementary or secondary schools. Students enter these one-year programs after completion of their bachelor's degree. Professional development schools merge theory with practice and allow the student to experience a year of teaching firsthand, under professional guidance.

In addition to being knowledgeable in their subject, teachers must have the ability to communicate, inspire trust and confidence, and motivate students, as well as understand the students' educational and emotional needs. Teachers must be able to recognize and respond to individual and cultural differences in students and employ different teaching methods that will result in higher student achievement. They should be organized, dependable, patient, and creative. Teachers also must be able to work cooperatively and communicate effectively with other teachers, support staff, parents, and members of the community.

With additional preparation, teachers may move into positions as school librarians, reading specialists, instructional coordinators, or guidance counselors. Teachers may become administrators or supervisors, although the number of these positions is limited and competition can be intense. In some systems, highly qualified, experienced teachers can become senior or mentor teachers, with higher pay and additional responsibilities. They guide and assist less experienced teachers while keeping most of their own teaching responsibilities. Preschool teachers usually work their way up from assistant teacher, to teacher, to lead teacher (who may be responsible for the instruction of several classes) and, finally, to director of the center. Preschool teachers with a bachelor's degree frequently are qualified to teach kindergarten through grade three as well. Teaching at these higher grades often results in higher pay.

Employment Opportunities

Preschool, kindergarten, elementary school, middle school, and secondary school teachers, except special education, held about 3.8 million jobs in 2004. Of the teachers in those jobs, about 1.5 million are elementary school teachers, 1.1 million are secondary school teachers, 628,000 are middle school teachers, 431,000 are preschool teachers, and 171,000 are kindergarten teachers. The majority work in local government educational services. About 10 percent work for private schools. Preschool teachers, except special education, are most often employed in child daycare services (61 percent), religious organizations (12 percent), local government educational services (9 percent), and private educational services (7 percent). Employment of teachers is geographically distributed much the same as the population.

Job opportunities for teachers over the next ten years will vary from good to excellent, depending on the locality, grade level, and subject taught. Most job openings will result from the need to replace the large number of teachers who are expected to retire over the 2004–2014 period. Also, many beginning teachers decide to leave teaching after a year or two; especially those employed in poor, urban schools, creating additional job openings for teachers. Shortages of qualified teachers will likely continue, resulting in competition among some localities, with schools luring teachers from other states and districts with bonuses and higher pay.

Through 2014, overall student enrollments in elementary, middle, and secondary schools, a key factor in the demand for teachers, are expected to rise more slowly than in the past as children of the baby-boom generation leave the school system. This will cause employment to grow as fast as the average for teachers from kindergarten through the secondary grades. Projected enrollments will vary by region. Fast-growing states in the West, particularly California, Idaho, Hawaii, Alaska, Utah, and New Mexico, will experience the largest enrollment increases. Enrollments in the South will increase at a more modest rate than in recent years, while those in the Northeast and Midwest are expected to hold relatively steady or decline. Teachers who are geographically mobile and who obtain licensure in more than one subject should have a distinct advantage in finding a job.

The job market for teachers also continues to vary by school location and by subject taught. Job prospects should be better in inner cities and rural areas than in suburban districts. Many inner cities, often characterized by overcrowded, ill-equipped schools and higher-than-average poverty rates, and rural areas characterized by their remote location and relatively low salaries, have difficulty attracting and retaining enough teachers.

Currently, many school districts have difficulty hiring qualified teachers in some subject areas, most often mathematics, science (especially chemistry and physics), bilingual education, and foreign languages. Increasing enrollments of minorities, coupled with a shortage of minority teachers, should cause efforts to recruit minority teachers to intensify. Also, the number of non-English-speaking students will continue to grow, creating demand for bilingual teachers and for those who teach English as a second language. Specialties that have an adequate number of qualified teachers include general elementary education, physical education, and social studies. Qualified vocational teachers also are currently in demand in a variety of fields at both the middle school and secondary school levels.

The number of teachers employed is dependent as well on state and local expenditures for education and on the enactment of legislation to increase the quality and scope of public education. At the federal level, there has been a large increase in funding for education, particularly for the hiring of qualified teachers in lower income areas. Also, some states are instituting programs to improve early childhood education, such as offering full day kindergarten and universal preschool. These last two programs, along with projected higher enrollment growth for preschool age children, will create many new jobs for preschool teachers, which are expected to grow much faster than the average for all occupations.

The supply of teachers is expected to increase in response to reports of improved job prospects, better pay, more teacher involvement in school policy, and greater public interest in education. In recent years, the total number of bachelor's and master's degrees granted in education has increased steadily. Because of a shortage of teachers in certain locations, and in anticipation of the loss of a number of teachers to retirement, many States have implemented policies that will encourage more students to become teachers. In addition, more teachers may be drawn from a reserve pool of career changers, substitute teachers, and teachers completing alternative certification programs.

Salary

Median annual earnings of kindergarten, elementary, middle, and secondary school teachers ranged from $41,400 to $45,920 in May 2004; the lowest 10 percent earned $26,730 to $31,180; the top 10 percent earned $66,240 to $71,370. Median earnings for preschool teachers were $20,980.

According to the American Federation of Teachers, beginning teachers with a bachelor's degree earned an average of $31,704 in the 2003–04 school year. The estimated average salary of all public elementary and secondary school teachers in the 2003–04 school year was $46,597. Private school teachers generally earn less than public school teachers, but may be given other benefits, such as free or subsidized housing.

In 2004, more than half of all elementary, middle, and secondary school teachers belonged to unions, such as the American Federation of Teachers and the National Education Association. These unions bargain with school systems over wages, hours, and other terms and conditions of employment. Fewer preschool and kindergarten teachers were union members—about 17 percent in 2004.

Teachers can boost their salary in a number of ways. In some schools, teachers receive extra pay for coaching sports and working with students in extracurricular activities. Getting a master's degree or national certification often results in a raise in pay, as does acting as a mentor. Some teachers earn extra income during the summer by teaching summer school or performing other jobs in the school system.

Alternative Career Paths in Physical Education: Sport Management

KEY CONCEPT

Perhaps the most viable of the alternative career options is sport management.

Perhaps the most viable of the alternative career options is **sport management**. Beginning in 1966 with but a single master's program established at Ohio University, the field has expanded to several hundred institutions that prepare sport managers and administrators on the undergraduate and/or graduate levels.

Current and future job demands on the sport professional necessitate that the individual possess a depth of knowledge and a broad range of specific competencies in business and in sport to be able to deal successfully with ever-changing challenges and problems associated with the business of sport (Figure 18-5).

The initial impetus for sport management developing into a distinct academic discipline can be traced to Walter O'Malley, then president of the Brooklyn Dodgers. In 1957, O'Malley voiced his concern with Dr. James G. Mason about the lack of formal education programs for individuals desiring to work in professional baseball. Almost a decade later, 1966, Dr. Mason, who was then a professor at Ohio University, was instrumental in establishing the first master's degree program in sport management. In 1993 the National Association for Sport and Physical Education (NASPE) and the North American Society for Sport Management (NASSM) approved standards and protocol for accrediting sport management preparation programs.

The basis of most sport-management professional preparation programs revolves around an interdisciplinary or multidisciplinary approach. Fields of study such as physical education, sport, business, computers,

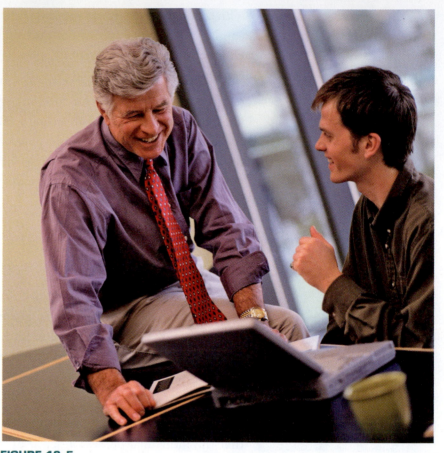

FIGURE 18–5
Sports management is important to the overall success of any program. (Courtesy of Photodisc)

and communications are all intricately intertwined in the preparation of future sport managers and administrators. Sport management programs can include courses in communications, interpersonal relations, business, accounting, finance, economics, statistics, and the historical, sociological, psychological, and philosophical perspectives of sport. Core courses typically include introduction to sport management, sport management theory, sport marketing, fundraising, promotions, public relations, ethics in sport management, legal aspects of sport, facility planning and management, computer applications to sport, research methods, sport management problems and issues, and risk management. Internships are normally included in almost all undergraduate and graduate programs. This experience is usually full time, and the student is expected to provide meaningful assistance to the intern site.

Although there is seemingly a wealth of job opportunities in sport, the competition for these positions has been and will remain severe. In addition, many of these positions involve extremely low pay in comparison to the amount of work expected. Career paths in sport management can include athletic team management, finance, sports medicine/athletic training, journalism, broadcasting, public relations, development and fund raising, sports information, facility management, cardiovascular fitness and wellness administration, and aquatics management, among others.

Alternative Career Paths in Physical Education: Fitness Workers

> **• KEY CONCEPT •**
>
> Some fitness workers may combine the duties of group exercise instructors and personal trainers, and in smaller facilities, the fitness director may teach classes and do personal training.

Fitness workers lead, instruct, and motivate individuals or groups in exercise activities, including cardiovascular exercise, strength training, and stretching. They work in commercial and nonprofit health clubs, country clubs, hospitals, universities, **yoga** and **Pilates** studios, resorts, and clients' homes. Increasingly, fitness workers also are found in workplaces, where they organize and direct health and fitness programs for employees of all ages. Although gyms and health clubs offer a variety of exercise activities such as weightlifting, yoga, cardiovascular training, and karate, fitness workers typically specialize in only a few areas.

Personal trainers work one-on-one with clients either in a gym or in the client's home (Figure 18-6). Trainers help clients assess their level of physical fitness and set and reach fitness goals. Trainers also demonstrate

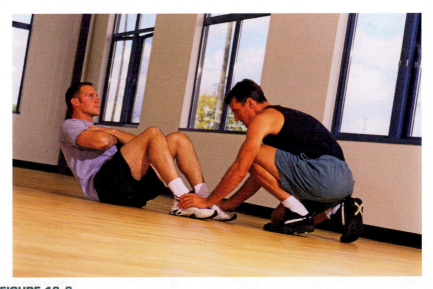

FIGURE 18–6
Fitness trainers are actively involved helping people attain their fitness goals. (Courtesy of Photodisc)

various exercises and help clients improve their exercise techniques. Trainers may keep records of their clients' exercise sessions to assess clients' progress toward physical fitness.

Group exercise instructors conduct group exercise sessions that involve aerobic exercise, stretching, and muscle conditioning. Because cardiovascular conditioning classes often involve movement to music, outside of class, instructors must choose and mix the music and choreograph a corresponding exercise sequence. Pilates and yoga are two increasingly popular conditioning methods taught in exercise classes. Instructors demonstrate the different moves and positions of the particular method; they also observe students and correct those who are doing the exercises improperly. Group exercise instructors are responsible for ensuring that their classes are motivating, safe, and challenging, yet not too difficult for the participants.

Fitness directors oversee the fitness-related aspects of a health club or fitness center. Their work involves creating and maintaining programs that meet the needs of the club's members, including new member orientations, fitness assessments, and workout incentive programs. They also select fitness equipment; coordinate personal training and group exercise programs; hire, train, and supervise fitness staff; and carry out administrative duties.

Fitness workers in smaller facilities with few employees may perform a variety of functions in addition to their fitness duties, such as tending the front desk, signing up new members, giving tours of the fitness center, writing newsletter articles, creating posters and flyers, and supervising the weight training and cardiovascular equipment areas. In larger commercial facilities, personal trainers are often required to sell their services to members and to make a specified number of sales. Some fitness workers may combine the duties of group exercise instructors and personal trainers, and in smaller facilities, the fitness director may teach classes and do personal training.

Most fitness workers spend their time indoors at fitness centers and health clubs. Fitness directors and supervisors, however, typically spend most of their time in an office, planning programs and special events and tending to administrative issues. Those in smaller fitness centers may split their time among the office, personal training, and teaching classes. Directors and supervisors generally engage in less physical activity than do lower-level fitness workers. Nevertheless, workers at all levels risk suffering injuries during physical activities.

• Did You Know? •

Did you know that only 2 percent of health club members actually use the gym?

Since most fitness centers are open long hours, fitness workers often work nights and weekends and even occasional holidays. Some may have to travel from place to place throughout the day, to different gyms or to clients' homes, to maintain a full work schedule. Fitness workers generally enjoy a lot of autonomy. Group exercise instructors choreograph or plan their own classes, and personal trainers have the freedom to design and implement their clients' workout routines.

Education and Certification

Personal trainers must obtain certification in the fitness field to gain employment, while group fitness instructors do not necessarily need certification to begin working. The most important characteristic that an employer looks for in a new group fitness instructor is the ability to plan and lead a class that is motivating and safe. Group fitness instructors often get started by participating in exercise classes, and some become familiar enough to successfully audition and begin teaching class. They also may improve their skills by taking training courses or attending fitness conventions. Most organizations encourage their group instructors to become certified, and many require it.

In the fitness field, there are many organizations that offer certification. Becoming certified by one of the top certification organizations is increasingly important, especially for personal trainers. One way to ensure that a certifying organization is reputable is to see whether it is accredited or seeking accreditation by the National Commission for Certifying Agencies. Most certifying organizations require candidates to have a high school diploma, be certified in cardiopulmonary resuscitation (CPR), and pass an exam. All certification exams have a written component, and some also have a practical component. The exams measure knowledge of human physiology, proper exercise techniques, assessment of client fitness levels, and development of appropriate exercise programs.

There is no particular training program required for certifications; candidates may prepare however they prefer. Certifying organizations do offer study materials, including books, CD-ROMs, other audio and visual materials, and exam-preparation workshops and seminars, but exam candidates are not required to purchase materials to sit for the exams. Certification generally is good for two years, after which workers must become recertified by attending continuing education classes. Some organizations offer more advanced certification, requiring an associate or bachelor's degree in an exercise-related subject for individuals interested in training athletes, working with people who are injured or ill, or advising clients on whole-life health.

Training for Pilates and yoga teachers is changing. Because interest in these forms of exercise has exploded in recent years, the demand for teachers has grown faster than the ability to train them properly. However, because inexperienced teachers have contributed to student injuries, there has been a push toward more standardized, rigorous requirements for teacher training.

Pilates and yoga teachers usually do not need group exercise certifications like the ones described above. It is more important that they have specialized training in their particular method of exercise. For Pilates, training options range from weekend-long workshops to year-long programs, but the trend is toward requiring more training. The Pilates Method Alliance has established training standards that recommend at

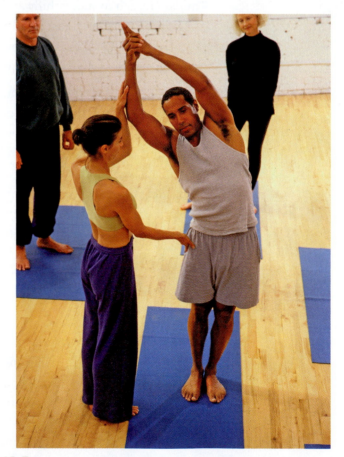

FIGURE 18–7
Instructor helping student with proper stretching technique. (Courtesy of Photodisc)

least 200 hours of training; the group also has standards for training schools and maintains a list of training schools that meet the requirements. However, some Pilates teachers are certified group exercise instructors who go through short Pilates workshops; currently, many fitness centers hire people with minimal Pilates training if the applicants have a fitness certification and group fitness experience.

Training Requirements

Training requirements for yoga teachers are similar to those for Pilates teachers. Training programs range from a few days to more than two years. Many people get their start by taking yoga; eventually, their teachers may consider them suited to assist or to substitute teach. Some students may begin teaching their own classes when their yoga teachers think they are ready; the teachers may even provide letters of recommendation. Those who wish to pursue teaching more seriously usually then pursue formal teacher training. Currently, there are many training programs through the yoga community as well as programs through the fitness industry. The Yoga Alliance has established training standards of at least 200 training hours, with a specified number of hours in areas including techniques, teaching methodology, anatomy, physiology, and philosophy. The Yoga Alliance also registers schools that train students to the standards. Because some schools may meet the standards but not be registered, prospective students should check the requirements and decide if particular schools meet them.

An increasing number of employers require fitness workers to have a bachelor's degree in a field related to health or fitness, such as exercise science or physical education. Some employers allow workers to substitute a college degree for certification, but most employers who require a bachelor's degree require both a degree and certification. People planning fitness careers should be outgoing, good at motivating people, and sensitive to the needs of others. Excellent health and physical fitness are important due to the physical nature of the job. Those who wish to be personal trainers in a large commercial fitness center should have strong sales skills.

Fitness workers usually do not receive much on-the-job training; they are expected to know how to do their jobs when they are hired. The exception is newly-certified personal trainers with no work experience, who sometimes begin by working alongside an experienced trainer before being allowed to train clients alone. Workers may receive some organizational training to learn about the operations of their new employer. They occasionally receive specialized training if they are expected to teach or lead a specific method of exercise or focus on a particular age or ability group.

A bachelor's degree, and in some cases a master's degree, in exercise science, physical education, kinesiology, or a related area, along with experience, usually is required to advance to management positions in a health club or fitness center. As in many fields, managerial skills are needed to advance to supervisory or managerial positions. College courses in management, business administration, accounting, and personnel management may be helpful for advancement to supervisory or managerial jobs, but many fitness companies have corporate universities in which they train employees for management positions.

Personal trainers may advance to head trainer, with responsibility for hiring and overseeing the personal training staff and for bringing in new personal training clients. Group fitness instructors may be promoted to group exercise director, responsible for hiring instructors and coordinating exercise classes. A next possible step is the fitness director, who manages the fitness budget and staff. The general manager's main focus is on the financial aspect of the organization, particularly setting and achieving sales goals in a small fitness center; however, the general manager usually is involved with all aspects of running the facility. Some workers go into business for themselves and open their own fitness centers.

Employment Outlook

Fitness workers held about 205,000 jobs in 2004. Almost all personal trainers and group exercise instructors worked in physical fitness facilities, health clubs, and fitness centers, mainly in the amusement and recreation industry or in civic and social organizations. About 7 percent of fitness workers were self-employed; many of these were personal trainers, while others were group fitness instructors working on a contract basis with fitness centers. Many fitness jobs are part time, and many workers hold multiple jobs, teaching and/or doing personal training at several different fitness centers and at clients' homes.

Opportunities are expected to be good for fitness workers because of rapid growth in the fitness industry. Many job openings also will stem from the need to replace the large numbers of workers who leave these occupations each year. Employment of fitness workers is expected to increase much faster than the average for all occupations through 2014. An increasing number of people spend more time and money on fitness, and more businesses are recognizing the benefits of health and fitness programs, and other services such as wellness programs, for their employees.

Aging baby boomers are concerned with staying healthy, physically fit, and independent. They have become the largest demographic group of health club members. The reduction of physical education programs in schools, combined with parents' growing concern about childhood obesity, has resulted in rapid increases in children's health club membership. Increasingly, athletic youth also are hiring personal trainers, and weight-training gyms for children younger than eighteen are expected to continue to grow. Health club membership among young adults also has grown steadily, driven by concern about physical fitness and by rising incomes.

As health clubs strive to provide more personalized service to keep their members motivated, they will continue to offer personal training and a wide variety of group exercise classes. Participation in yoga and Pilates is expected to continue to grow, driven partly by the aging population demanding low-impact forms of exercise and relief from ailments such as arthritis.

Salary

Median annual earnings of personal trainers and group exercise instructors in May 2004 were $25,470. The middle 50 percent earned between $17,380 and $40,030. The bottom 10 percent earned less than $14,530 while the top 10 percent earned $55,560 or more. Earnings of successful self-employed personal trainers can be much higher. Because many fitness workers work part time, they often do not receive benefits such as health insurance or retirement plans from their employers. They do get the unusual benefit of the use of fitness facilities at no cost.

Alternative Career Paths in Physical Education: Recreation Workers

People spend much of their leisure time participating in a wide variety of organized recreational activities, such as arts and crafts, the performing arts, camping, and sports. **Recreation workers** plan, organize, and direct these activities in local playgrounds and recreation areas, parks, community centers, religious organizations, camps, theme parks, and tourist attractions. Increasingly, recreation workers also are being found in workplaces, where they organize and direct leisure activities for employees.

Recreation workers hold a variety of positions at different levels of responsibility. Recreation leaders, who are responsible for a recreation program's daily operation, primarily organize and direct participants. They may lead and give instruction in dance, drama, crafts, games, and sports; schedule the use of facilities; keep records of equipment use; and ensure that recreation facilities and equipment are used properly. Workers who provide instruction and coach groups in specialties such as art, music, drama, swimming, or tennis may be called activity specialists. Recreation supervisors oversee recreation leaders and plan, organize, and manage recreational activities to meet the needs of a variety of populations. These workers often serve as liaisons between the director of the park or recreation center and the recreation leaders. Recreation supervisors with more specialized responsibilities also may direct special activities or events or oversee a major activity, such as aquatics, gymnastics, or performing arts. Directors of recreation and parks develop and manage comprehensive recreation programs in parks, playgrounds, and other settings (Figure 18-8). Directors usually serve as technical advisors to state and local recreation and park commissions, and may be responsible for recreation and park budgets.

Camp counselors lead and instruct children and teenagers in outdoor-oriented forms of recreation, such as swimming, hiking, horseback riding, and camping. In addition, counselors provide campers with specialized instruction in subjects such as archery, boating, music, drama, gymnastics, tennis, and computers. In resident camps, counselors also provide guidance and supervise daily living and general socialization. Camp directors typically supervise camp counselors, plan camp activities or programs, and perform the various administrative functions of a camp.

Recreation workers may work in a variety of settings; for example, a cruise ship, a woodland recreational park, a summer camp, or a playground in the center of a large urban community. Regardless of the setting, most recreation workers spend much of their time outdoors and may work in a variety of weather conditions. Recreation directors and supervisors, however, typically spend most of their time in an office, planning programs and special events. Directors and supervisors generally engage in less physical activity than do lower level recreation workers. Nevertheless, recreation workers at all levels risk suffering injuries during physical activities.

Many recreation workers work about forty hours a week. People entering this field, especially camp counselors, should expect some night and weekend work and irregular hours. Many recreation jobs are seasonal.

• KEY CONCEPT •

Recreation workers may work in a variety of settings; for example, a cruise ship, a woodland recreational park, a summer camp, or a playground in the center of a large urban community.

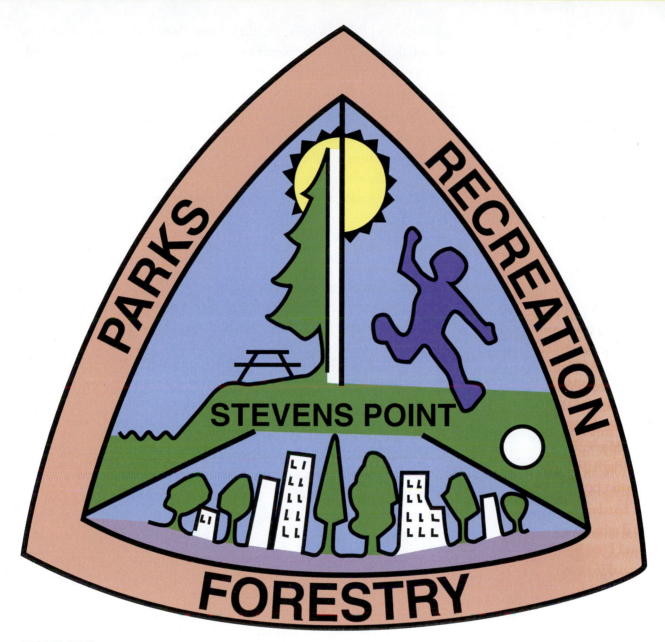

FIGURE 18–8
(Courtesy of City of Stevens Point)

Education Requirements

Educational requirements for recreation workers range from a high school diploma (or sometimes less for many summer jobs) to graduate degrees for some administrative positions in large public recreation systems. Full-time career professional positions usually require a college degree with a major in parks and recreation or leisure studies, but a bachelor's degree in any liberal arts field may be sufficient for some jobs in the private sector. In industrial recreation, or "employee services" as it is more commonly called, companies prefer to hire those with a bachelor's degree in recreation or leisure studies and a background in business administration.

Specialized training or experience in a particular field, such as art, music, drama, or athletics, is an asset for many jobs. Some jobs also require certification. For example, a lifesaving certificate is a prerequisite for teaching or coaching water-related activities. Graduates of associate's degree programs in parks and recreation, social work, and other human services disciplines also enter some career recreation positions. High school graduates occasionally enter career positions, but this is not common. Some college students work part time as recreation workers while earning degrees.

A bachelor's degree in a recreation-related discipline and experience are preferred for most recreation supervisor jobs and are required for higher-level administrative jobs. However, an increasing number of recreation workers who aspire to administrative positions are obtaining master's degrees in parks and recreation, business administration, or public administration. Certification in the recreation field may be helpful for advancement. Also, many persons in other disciplines, including social work, forestry, and resource management, pursue graduate degrees in recreation.

Programs leading to an associate's or bachelor's degree in parks and recreation, leisure studies, or related fields are offered at several hundred colleges and universities. Many also offer master's or doctoral degrees in the field. In 2004, about a hundred bachelor's degree programs in parks and recreation were accredited by the National Recreation and Park Association (NRPA). Accredited programs provide broad exposure to the history, theory, and practice of park and recreation management. Courses offered include community organization; supervision and administration; recreational needs of special populations, such as the elderly or disabled; and supervised fieldwork. Students may specialize in areas such as therapeutic recreation, park management, outdoor recreation, industrial or commercial recreation, or camp management.

The NRPA certifies individuals for professional and technical jobs. Certified Park and Recreation Professionals must pass an exam; earn a bachelor's degree with a major in recreation, park resources, or leisure services from a program accredited by the NRPA and the American Association for Leisure and Recreation; or earn a bachelor's degree and have at least five years of relevant full-time work experience. Continuing education is necessary to remain certified.

Persons planning recreation careers should be outgoing, good at motivating people, and sensitive to the needs of others. Excellent health and physical fitness are often required, due to the physical nature of some jobs. Volunteer experience, part-time work during school, or a summer job can lead to a full-time career as a recreation worker. As in many fields, managerial skills are needed to advance to supervisory or managerial positions.

Job Outlook

Recreation workers held about 310,000 jobs in 2004, and many additional workers held summer jobs in the occupation. Of those with year-round jobs as recreation workers, about 35 percent worked for local governments, primarily in park and recreation departments. Around 11 percent of recreation workers were employed in civic and social organizations, such as the Boy Scouts or Girl Scouts or the Red Cross. Another 15 percent of recreation workers were employed by nursing and other personal care facilities.

The recreation field has an unusually large number of part-time, seasonal, and volunteer jobs, including summer camp counselors, craft specialists, and after-school and weekend recreation program leaders. In addition, many teachers and college students accept jobs as recreation workers when school is not in session. The vast majority of volunteers serve as activity leaders at local day camp programs, or in youth organizations, camps, nursing homes, hospitals, senior centers, and other settings.

Competition will remain strong for career positions as recreation workers because the field attracts many applicants and because the number of career positions is limited in comparison with the number of lower-level seasonal jobs. Opportunities for staff positions should be best for persons with formal training and experience gained in part-time or seasonal recreation jobs. Those with graduate degrees should have the best opportunities for supervisory or administrative positions. Job openings also will stem from the need to replace the large numbers of workers who leave the occupation each year.

Overall employment of recreation workers is expected to grow about as fast as the average for all occupations through 2014. People will spend more time and money on recreation, spurring growth in civic and social organizations and, to a lesser degree, state and local government. Much growth will be driven by retiring baby boomers, who, with more leisure time, high disposable income, and concern for health and fitness, are expected to increase their consumption of recreation services. Job growth also will be driven by rapidly increasing employment in nursing and residential care facilities. Employment growth may be inhibited, however, by budget constraints that local governments may face over the 2004–2014 projection period.

The large numbers of temporary, seasonal jobs in the recreation field typically are filled by high school or college students, generally do not have formal education requirements, and are open to anyone with the desired personal qualities. Employers compete for a share of the vacationing student labor force, and although salaries in recreation often are lower than those in other fields, the nature of the work and the opportunity to work outdoors are attractive to many.

Salary

In May 2004, median annual earnings of recreation workers who worked full time were $19,320. The middle 50 percent earned between $15,640 and $25,380. The lowest paid 10 percent earned less than $13,260, while the highest paid 10 percent earned $34,280 or more. However, earnings of recreation directors and others in supervisory or managerial positions can be substantially higher. Most public and private recreation agencies provide full-time recreation workers with typical benefits; part-time workers receive few, if any, benefits.

Alternative Career Paths in Physical Education: Certified Athletic Trainers

Certified athletic trainers help prevent and treat injuries for people of all ages. Their clients include everyone from professional athletes to industrial workers. Recognized by the American Medical Association as allied health professionals, certified athletic trainers specialize in the prevention, assessment, treatment, and rehabilitation of musculoskeletal injuries. Athletic trainers are often the first health-care providers on the scene when injuries occur, and therefore must be able to recognize, evaluate, and assess injuries and provide immediate care when needed. They also are heavily involved in the rehabilitation and reconditioning of injuries (Figure 18-9).

Athletic trainers often help prevent injuries by advising on the proper use of equipment and applying protective or injury-preventive devices such as tape, bandages, and braces. Injury prevention also often includes

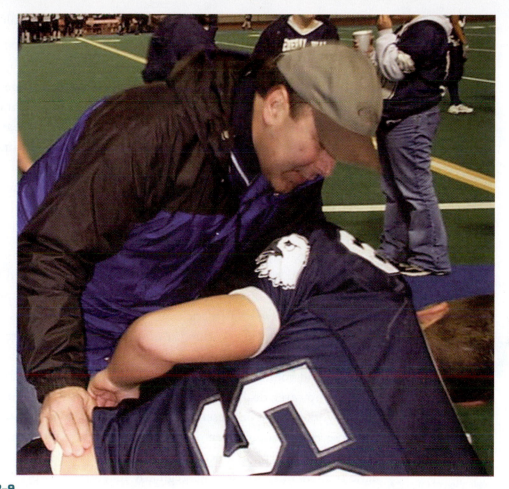

FIGURE 18–9
Certified Athletic Trainers are crucial to the health and well-being of athletes.

educating people on what they should do to avoid putting themselves at risk for injuries. Athletic trainers should not be confused with fitness trainers or personal trainers, who are not health-care workers but rather train people to become physically fit.

Athletic trainers work under the supervision of a licensed physician and in cooperation with other health care providers. The level of medical supervision varies depending upon the setting. Some athletic trainers meet with the team physician or consulting physician once or twice a week; others interact with a physician every day. The extent of the supervision ranges from discussing specific injuries and treatment options with a physician to performing evaluations and treatments as directed by a physician.

Athletic trainers also may have administrative responsibilities. These may include regular meetings with an athletic director or other administrative officer to deal with budgets, purchasing, policy implementation, and other business-related issues.

The work of athletic trainers requires frequent interaction with others. This includes consulting with physicians as well as frequent contact with athletes and patients to discuss and administer treatments, rehabilitation programs, injury-prevention practices, and other health-related issues. Many athletic trainers work indoors most of the time; others, especially those in some sports-related jobs, spend much of their time working outdoors. The job also might require standing for long periods, working with medical equipment or machinery, and being able to walk, run, kneel, crouch, stoop, or crawl. Some travel may be required.

Schedules vary by work setting. Athletic trainers in non-sports settings generally have an established schedule with nights and weekends off; the number of hours differs by employer, but usually are about forty to fifty hours per week. Athletic trainers working in hospitals and clinics spend part of their time working at other locations on an outreach basis. Most commonly, those outreach programs include secondary schools, colleges, and commercial business locations. Athletic trainers in sports settings, however, deal with schedules that are longer and more variable. These workers must be present for team practices and games, which often are on evenings and weekends, and their schedules can change on short notice when games and practices have to be rescheduled. As a result, athletic trainers in sports settings regularly may have to work six or seven days per week, including late hours. In high schools, athletic trainers who also teach may work at least sixty to seventy hours a week.

In NCAA Division I colleges and universities, athletic trainers generally work with one team; when that team's sport is in season, working at least fifty to sixty hours a week is common. Athletic trainers in smaller colleges and universities often work with several teams and have teaching responsibilities. During the off-season, a forty-hour to fifty-hour work week may be normal in most settings. Athletic trainers for professional sports teams generally work the most hours per week. During training camps, practices, and competitions, they may be required to work up to twelve hours a day.

There is some stress involved with being an athletic trainer, as there is with most health-related occupations. Athletic trainers are responsible for their clients' health, and sometimes have to make quick decisions that could affect the health or career of their clients. Athletics trainers also can be affected by the pressure to win that is typical of competitive sports teams.

> ● **KEY CONCEPT** ●
>
> Recognized by the American Medical Association as allied health professionals, certified athletic trainers specialize in the prevention, assessment, treatment, and rehabilitation of musculoskeletal injuries.

Education

A bachelor's degree from an accredited college or university is required for almost all jobs as an athletic trainer. In 2004, there were more than three hundred accredited programs nationwide. Students in these programs are educated both in the classroom and in clinical settings. Formal education includes many science and health-related courses, such as human anatomy, physiology, nutrition, and biomechanics.

A bachelor's degree with a major in athletic training from an accredited program is part of the requirement for becoming certified by the National Athletic Trainers Association Board of Certification. In addition, a successful candidate for board certification must pass an examination that includes written questions and practical applications. To retain certification, credential holders must continue taking medicine-related courses and adhere to standards of practice. In the forty-three states with athletic trainer licensure or registration or both in 2004, NATA certification was required.

According to the National Athletic Trainers' Association, 70 percent of athletic trainers have a master's or doctoral degree. Athletic trainers may need a master's degree or higher to be eligible for some positions, especially those in colleges and universities, and to increase their advancement opportunities. Because some positions in high schools involve teaching along with athletic training responsibilities, a teaching certificate or license could be required.

There are a number ways in which athletic trainers can advance or move into related positions. Assistant athletic trainers may become head athletic trainers and, eventually, athletic directors. Athletic trainers might also enter a physician group practice and assume a management role. Some athletic trainers move into sales and marketing positions, using their athletic trainer expertise to sell medical and athletic equipment. Because all athletic trainers deal directly with a variety of people, they need good social and communication skills. They should be able to manage difficult situations and the stress associated with them; for example, when disagreements arise with coaches, clients, or parents regarding suggested treatment. Athletic trainers also should be organized, be able to manage time wisely, be inquisitive, and have a strong desire to help people.

Job Outlook

Athletic trainers held about 15,000 jobs in 2004 and are found in every part of the country. Most athletic-trainer jobs are related to sports, although many also work in non-sports settings. About one-third of athletic trainers worked in health care settings, including hospitals, offices of physicians, and offices of other health practitioners. Another one-third were found in public and private educational services, primarily in colleges, universities, and high schools. About 20 percent worked in fitness and recreational sports centers.

Employment of athletic trainers is expected to grow much faster than the average for all occupations through 2014. Job growth will be concentrated in health-care industry settings, such as ambulatory heath care services and hospitals. Growth in sports-related positions will be somewhat slower, as most professional sports clubs and colleges, universities, and professional schools already have complete athletic training staffs. Job prospects should be good for people looking for a position in the health care industry. Athletic trainers looking for a position with a sports team, however, may face stiff competition.

The demand for health care should grow dramatically as the result of advances in technology, increasing emphasis on preventive care, and an increasing number of older people who are more likely to need medical care. Athletic trainers will benefit from this expansion, because they provide a cost-effective way to increase the number of health professionals in an office or other setting. Also, employers increasingly emphasize sports medicine, in which an immediate responder, such as an athletic trainer, is on site to help prevent injuries and provide immediate treatment for any injuries that do occur. Athletic trainers' increased licensure requirements and regulation has led to a greater acceptance of their role as qualified health care providers. As a result, third-party reimbursement is expected to continue to grow for athletic training services. As athletic trainers continue to expand their services, more employers are expected to use these workers to realize the cost savings that can be achieved by providing health care in-house. Settings outside the sports world, especially those that focus on health care, are expected to experience fast employment growth among athletic trainers over the next decade. Continuing efforts to have an athletic trainer in every high school reflect concern for student-athletes' health as well as efforts to provide more funding for schools, and may lead to growth in the number of athletic trainers employed in high schools.

Turnover among athletic trainers is limited. When dealing with sports teams, there is a tendency to want to continue to work with the same coaches, administrators, and players when a good working relationship already exists. Because of relatively low worker turnover, the settings with the best job prospects will be the ones that are expected to grow most quickly, primarily positions in heath care settings. There will also be opportunities in elementary and secondary schools as more positions are created. Some of these positions also will require teaching responsibilities. There will be more competition for positions within colleges, universities, and professional schools as well as professional sports clubs. The occupation is expected to continue to change over the next decade including more administrative responsibilities, adapting to new technology, and working with larger populations, and job seekers must be able to adapt to these changes.

Salary

Most athletic trainers work in full-time positions and typically receive benefits. The salary of an athletic trainer depends on experience and job responsibilities, and varies by job setting. Median annual earnings of athletic trainers were $33,940 in May 2004. The middle 50 percent earned between $27,140 and $42,380. The lowest 10 percent earned less than $20,770, while the top 10 percent earned more than $53,760. Also, many employers pay for some of the continuing education required of certified athletic trainers, although the amount covered varies from employer to employer.

Alternative Career Paths in Physical Education: Sport Psychology

Sport psychology can be considered a subdiscipline of psychology as well as sport and exercise science. It is presumed to be an applied field whereby the principles of psychology are transferred to settings including exercise programs and organized sport. As an academic discipline, sport and exercise psychology is the scientific study of people and their behavior in sport and exercise contexts and involves such topics as personality, motivation, attributions, leadership, and goal-setting. In essence, the field is concerned with the psychological determinants of behavior in movement situations, as well as with the psychological effects of sport engagement and physical activity.

Some opportunities in the sport psychology field are available in the private sector for people with masters' degrees. However, not only are these opportunities limited, but there is stiff competition from individuals holding doctorate degrees. Many people who want to work as a sport psychologist aim to work for a sports team. The few individuals asked to do so almost always have doctorates or post-doctoral training, and are employed at the university or professional level. Full-time positions in sport psychology at any level, university or private sector, are limited.

Sport and Exercise Researcher

This requires a PhD in either psychology or kinesiology. Job opportunities center on universities, teaching, and doing research. These individuals, with the proper training, may also consult with college or professional teams as applied or clinical sport psychologists.

Applied Sport Psychologist

This specialty requires a masters' degree or PhD, usually in kinesiology. These specialists work with individual athletes or teams as a mental skills coach. Job opportunities are limited because many teams and universities want someone who can also do clinical work.

Clinical Sport Psychologist

This requires a PhD in psychology and an APA-approved internship. These individuals are qualified to do mental-skills training, but are also qualified to deal with clinical disorders such as anorexia, depression, and drug abuse. Job opportunities include work at universities in the athletic department or counseling center, high schools in the guidance department, consulting with professional teams, or in an independent practice.

Job Outlook

Job placement is very difficult in sport psychology, especially if one wants to develop an independent practice that focuses solely on mental-skills training. Most of the jobs are at universities and centers on research and teaching, or require clinical training. Thus, many individuals are left looking for other opportunities, such as coaching, athletic training, or guidance counseling, that allows them to simultaneously pursue their interest in sport psychology.

Chapter Summary

Physical education majors will have many different options for employment once they have obtained their degree. Options are not limited to traditional physical education teaching roles. Career opportunities include, but are not limited to, teaching, sport management, fitness workers (personal trainers, group exercise instructors, fitness directors, managers and supervisors), recreation workers, certified athletic trainers, and sport psychologists. Employment, advancement, and salary are dependant upon education, experience, and geographical location.

Chapter Review Questions

1. List the different career options available to the physical education major.

2. What certifications and licenses are required to become a teacher?

3. What is the job outlook for physical education teachers in the near future?

4. What are the advantages and disadvantages of teaching in a private school?

5. Explain the salary range for a teaching career.

6. Summarize the career options of sport management as described in this chapter.

7. Summarize the career options of fitness trainers as described in this chapter.

8. Summarize the career options of recreation workers as described in this chapter.

9. Summarize the career options of certified athletic trainers as described in this chapter.

10. What career choice explained in this chapter most closely fits your career objectives? Why?

Projects and Activities

1. Choose one of the career options explained in this chapter, and write a research paper on the career that you are most interested in entering.

2. After you have decided on a career option, meet with someone in this career field. Your interview should include education requirements, entry requirements, job responsibilities, hours per week, salary, and job advancement. You will also want to ask what they feel are the best and worst aspects of their job. Report your findings.

Website Resources

American Association for Leisure and Recreation (AALR): http://www.aahperd.org/aapar/

American Federation of Teachers (AFT): http://www.aft.org

National American Society for Sport Management (NASSM): http://www.nassm.org/

National Association for Sport and Physical Education (NASPE): http://www.aahperd.org/naspe/

National Athletic Trainers Association (NATA): http://www.nata.org

National Education Association: http://www.nea.org

National Recreation and Park Association (NRPA): http://www.nrpa.org/

Pilates Method Alliance: http://www.pilatesmethodalliance.org/

This site, sponsored by Ohio State University School of Physical Activity and Education Services, has a wealth of information available for job searching.: http://education.osu.edu/

Fitness after Retirement

Objectives

Upon completion of this chapter, the reader should be able to:

- Restate the fitness objectives for healthy living after retirement.
- Describe the objectives of *The National Blueprint*.
- Explain the *Healthy People 2010* objectives.
- Describe what public policy and advocacy strategies can be carried out at the local, state, and national level.
- Explain what the basic exercise requirements are for seniors.

Key Terms

Healthy People 2010

The National Blueprint: Increasing Physical Activity Among Adults Age 50 and Older

Fitness after Retirement

On May 1, 2001 in Washington, D.C., a coalition of national organizations released a major national planning document in the area of aging and physical activity. *The National Blueprint: Increasing Physical Activity Among Adults Aged 50 and Older* (the *Blueprint*) was developed to serve as a guide for multiple organizations, associations, and agencies, to inform and support their planning work related to increasing physical activity among America's aging population. This document is intended to outline broad strategies that will lead to increasing physical activity among older Americans (Figure 19-1). The plan was developed with input from more than sixty individuals, representing forty-six organizations with expertise in health, medicine, social and behavioral sciences, epidemiology, gerontology/geriatrics, clinical science, public policy, marketing, medical systems, community organization, and environmental issues.

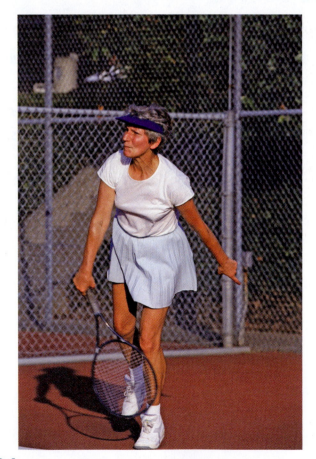

FIGURE 19–1
Fitness should be an important part of the retirement lifestyle. (Courtesy of Photodisc)

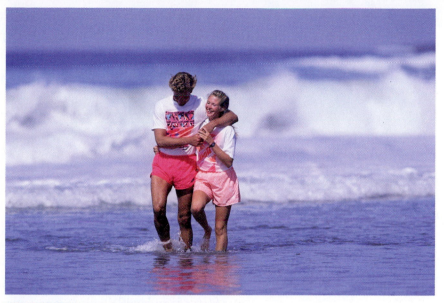

FIGURE 19-2
Staying active is a major goal as adults get older. (Courtesy of Photodisc)

The *Blueprint* concludes that there is a substantial body of scientific evidence which indicates that regular physical activity can bring dramatic health benefits to people of all ages and abilities, and that this benefit extends over the entire lifespan. Increasingly, evidence indicates that physical activity offers one of the greatest opportunities to extend years of active independent life, reduce disability, and improve the quality of life for older persons (Figure 19-2).

Major goals of the *Blueprint* are to identify the principal barriers to physical activity participation in older adults and to outline strategies for increasing physical activity levels throughout the population. The *Blueprint* identifies specific needs in the areas of research, home and community programs, workplace settings, medical systems, public policy and advocacy, and crosscutting issues.

The *Blueprint* recognizes that there is significant interest and enthusiasm among health care organizations, health providers, aging service organizations, the private sector, government, nonprofit, and philanthropic organizations in working collaboratively to support increased physical activity in older Americans. Effective efforts to increase physical activity among older adults will require an integrated and collaborative approach across delivery channels and among areas of professional expertise.

● **KEY CONCEPT** ●

The *Blueprint* concludes that there is a substantial body of scientific evidence which indicates that regular physical activity can bring dramatic health benefits to people of all ages and abilities, and that this benefit extends over the entire life span.

On April 4 and 5, 2000, the Robert Wood Johnson Foundation hosted a meeting titled "Technical Experts Working Group Meeting on Physical Activity and Mid Life and Older Adults" in Nashville, Tennessee. The twenty-three participants (representing science and medicine, public health, aging services, communications, academia, government, and the Robert Wood Johnson Foundation) reviewed the current situation related to increasing physical activity among mid life and older adults, discussed some of the most important gaps and opportunities for program development, and considered elements of effective interventions.

Discussion at the Nashville meeting highlighted the fact that the issue of physical activity and the fifty and older population is currently under-addressed, is complex, is a difficult issue to undertake, and lacks adequate leadership. In addition, it is an issue that is poorly understood and widely unrecognized. Those organizations that have been working in the area of physical activity and the fifty-and-older population are often working in isolation. Efforts to address the issue have been diffuse, lacking adequate resources and communications channels.

Participants recommended that a national "blueprint" be developed to help guide and focus the work of the organizations that are involved, or interested in, physical activity among people age fifty and older, as well as to engage additional groups.

As an outcome of the Nashville meeting, representatives of the American Association of Retired People (AARP), the American College of Sports Medicine, American Geriatrics Society, Centers for Disease Control and Prevention, National Institute on Aging, and the Robert Wood Johnson Foundation formed a steering committee and developed an agenda for the Blueprint Conference, which was held in October 2001. The conference provided a forum for the participating organizations to discuss and strategize ways to increase physical activity among the age fifty-and-older population. This document is the outcome report of that conference, and represents the work of the steering committee as well as the conference participants and expert reviewers.

The National Blueprint: Increasing Physical Activity Among Adults Age 50 and Older was developed as a guide for organizations, associations and agencies to plan strategies to help people age fifty and older increase their physical activity. This plan synthesizes input from more than sixty individuals, representing forty-seven organizations with expertise in health, medicine, social and behavioral sciences, epidemiology, gerontology/geriatrics, clinical science, public policy, marketing, medical systems, community organization, and environmental issues.

It states:

Regular physical activity can bring dramatic health benefits to people of all ages and abilities, according to a substantial body of scientific evidence. Media and medical professionals often tout the benefits of exercise for younger and middle-aged people. But scientific evidence increasingly indicates that physical activity can extend years of active independent life, reduce disability, and improve the quality of life for older persons as well. Although the evidence is clear, it has not yet been translated into national action. That is the aim of this Blueprint.

This Blueprint outlines steps to achieve this vision. The first section provides background on physical activity and health of Americans age fifty and older. The second section addresses the barriers to increasing physical activity among the aging population. It outlines suggested strategies related to research, home and community, workplace, medical systems, public policy and advocacy, and crosscutting issues to overcome these barriers.

Organizations are already working together to encourage physical activity among older Americans. These groups include health care organizations, health providers, aging service organizations, the private sector, government, nonprofit, and philanthropic organizations. These efforts aim to help people maintain their health, reduce chronic illness and disability and enhance their well-being and functional abilities as they age.

*The National Institute of Aging has laid excellent groundwork to support a national initiative to increase physical activity among mid life and older adults. In addition this document aligns with the United States Department of Health and Human Services **Healthy People 2010** objectives.*

However, no national organization or coalition is systemically addressing physical activity and older Americans. No organization is taking into account the comprehensive health issues, medical systems and reimbursement, marketing, environmental issues, education, and research that are involved in helping older Americans become physically active. Not enough visible, physically active older role models exist at the community and national level. This document is intended to encourage more aggressive action, facilitate collaboration, and enhance development of additional ideas.

• KEY CONCEPT •

Regular physical activity can bring dramatic health benefits to people of all ages and abilities, according to a substantial body of scientific evidence.

To translate this plan into action, organizations will have to reach beyond their comfort zone. For example, many mid life and older people are not likely to walk if they live in neighborhoods that have no sidewalks, or are dangerous. Public health professionals will have to learn about local transportation planning and how to work with elected officials to encourage exercise friendly neighborhoods. Effective efforts to increase physical activity among older adults will require an integrated and collaborative approach that will involve community health professionals, health associations and agencies, planners, health care providers, employers, community centers, senior living facilities, transportation experts, community planners, and other diverse groups and organizations and areas of professional expertise.

This document outlines a variety of approaches to address barriers to physical activity among the age fifty and older population and suggests strategies to increase physical activity. The strategies are divided into five categories: research, home/community, workplace, medical systems and public policy. In addition, there is a category of "cross-cutting" strategies that relate to more than one of these areas. Marketing and communications strategies are integrated throughout the recommendations. Research strategies identify steps needed in research, including medical, social, behavioral, policy and marketing research. In many cases, integrating program development, implementation and evaluation will be the most effective way to implement these strategies.

The home/community strategies take into account the nature of how people live and carry out the normal tasks of daily life.

Workplace strategies recognize that people generally work in or near the community in which they live, and worksites can often operate as a community resource or center. Medical systems are broadly defined to include health care delivery centers, such as clinicians' offices, clinics, medical centers, hospitals, and health-care reimbursement organizations. Professional education and continuing education are covered in these strategies.

Public policy and advocacy strategies can be carried out at the local, state and national level. Effective policy and advocacy initiatives should include coordination and collaboration among organizations and associations that share priorities and objectives. The effective implementation of the strategies outlined in this Blueprint hinge on a number of factors:

- *Organizations will need to identify clearly which strategies they wish to address, and collaborate with other groups that share an interest in that (those) strategy(ies).*

- *Organizations should develop formal coalitions and partnerships with other like-minded organizations.*

- *Organizations should establish systems to facilitate communication and exchange information on best practices.*

This Blueprint is designed to support an increase in physical activity among aging adults, and to improve the health and well being of all Americans. The key to success lies in developing and channeling resources, and in working collaboratively to move the evidence about the benefits of physical activity into national action.

This Blueprint is designed to support an increase in physical activity among adults age fifty and older, and ultimately to improve the health and well being of all Americans. The key to success lies in developing and channeling resources and working collaboratively to move the evidence about the benefits of physical activity into national action. The following action steps can help mobilize use of this document:

- *Organizations should identify which of the strategies they are already addressing or will address, and collaborate with other groups that share an interest in that (those) strategy(ies). Organizations should make efforts to work with existing coalitions and coordinate with other groups and organizations. Participating organizations should also identify and involve other organizations that are not working on this issue, but that can play a major supportive role.*

- *Organizations, associations and agencies working collaboratively should focus on activities that they can reasonably expect to accomplish.*

- *Organizations need to undertake detailed tactical planning to delineate the specific actions that are needed to achieve the strategies.*

- *Organizations will need to allocate money and people to help support coalition and collaborative efforts.*

- *Health organizations and government agencies must encourage the exchange and dissemination of best practices. These groups must establish systems to enable this approach.*

- *Evaluation should be a key tool in all implementation steps. In some cases evaluation can be objective, based on set measurable objectives. In other cases, evaluation will be process or formative.*

Until recently, promotion of exercise programs for seniors was rather nonexistent. From the results of prolonged bed rest and exercise studies involving older individuals, research has concluded with regular exercise, the elderly can expect to receive most of the benefits enjoyed by younger people as a result of physical fitness. Some of the benefits of regular exercise include:

- *improvement and maintenance of cardiorespiratory fitness.*
- *improvement and maintenance of muscle strength, endurance and flexibility.*
- *regulation of metabolism and weight gain (maintain lean body mass).*
- *regulation of blood pressure.*
- *prevention of loss of bone mass.*
- *lowered concentration of fatty substances in the blood, thereby preventing or reducing the effects of heart disease.*
- *improved psychological health (improved self-image).*
- *thinner and more elastic (younger) blood vessels.*
- *maintenance and improvement of maximal oxygen uptake.*
- *maintenance of glucose regulation.*

(National Blue print, 2001)

Heart Rate and Aging

Maximal heart rate is age-related. This means as we get older, our maximal heart rate declines. The main reason for the decline is reduced elasticity of the heart wall and a decrease in the time it takes the heart to fill with blood. The maximal heart rate is usually represented by 220 minus one's age in years. Other factors that affect maximal heart rate include certain types of medication, as well as known or suspected cardiovascular disease. Ideally, anyone over the age of forty wishing to start an exercise program should be evaluated on a treadmill to obtain an accurate maximal heart rate. The accuracy of estimating training intensity based on heart rate diminishes when working with the elderly.

Maximal Oxygen Uptake and Aging

Maximal oxygen uptake is the single best predictor of aerobic fitness. It represents the greatest amount of oxygen that can be utilized by the body. From the normal aging process, maximal oxygen uptake declines about 8 to 10

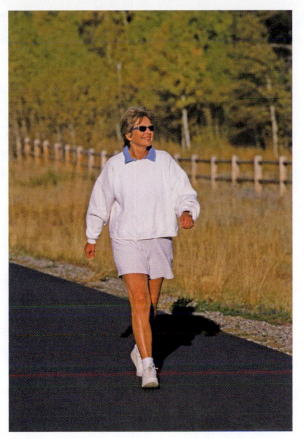

FIGURE 19–3
Regular aerobic exercise will have numerous health benefits as we get older. (Courtesy of Photodisc)

percent per decade after age thirty. This decline is partly due to the decrease in maximal heart rate and the subsequent decrease in heart function.

There is growing evidence that regular aerobic exercise may delay the normal decline in maximal oxygen uptake. Studies have shown improvements in aerobic fitness over the years. Older participants can enjoy most of the benefits of increased cardiovascular conditioning as well as lowered submaximal heart rate at any given workload, a faster recovery heart rate, and decreased systolic blood pressure at rest and during exercise (Figure 19-3).

Bone Health and Aging

Osteoporosis is a serious problem in older people, particularly women. An estimated 40 million people suffer from bone deterioration. As bones lose minerals, they become fragile, and fractures from falls become more likely. Osteoporosis results in bone with less density and strength. Exercise has been shown to play a role in the prevention and treatment of osteoporosis. Exercise places stress on the bones, which causes bones to adapt to the stress and become stronger by increasing bone mineral composition.

Muscle, Strength, and Aging

Skeletal muscle mass declines with age, which results in decreased strength. Each decade after twenty-five, we lose 3 to 5 percent of our muscle mass. Older individuals have the capacity to increase muscle size and strength. Studies have shown the natural decline in muscle mass can be altered by maintaining a mild strength and conditioning program throughout one's lifetime.

Flexibility and Aging

Age causes connective tissue to become stiffer, and joints to become less mobile. Loss of flexibility with age may also be the result of certain disease processes such as arthritis. An active range-of-motion and flexibility program should be part of any exercise program, regardless of age. Loss of flexibility can be reduced through regular exercise and an active lifestyle.

Body Composition and Aging

With age, body weight generally increases and height gradually decreases. When muscle mass is lost with age, it is usually replaced with fat. In addition to loss of muscle mass and an increase in fat supplies, the human body uses fewer calories with age. Resting basal metabolism uses less energy (fewer calories) to keep the human body running. This decrease in basal metabolism often leads to gradual weight gain. Regular exercise can enable older people to consume more calories while maintaining their ideal or desired body weight.

Exercise Recommendations for Seniors

Regular exercise has been shown to improve the quality of life and may delay some of the normal physiological changes that take place with age (Figure 19-4). Before starting a fitness program, seniors should consult a physician. While the principles of an exercise prescription apply to people of any age, greater care must be given when setting up a fitness program for older participants.

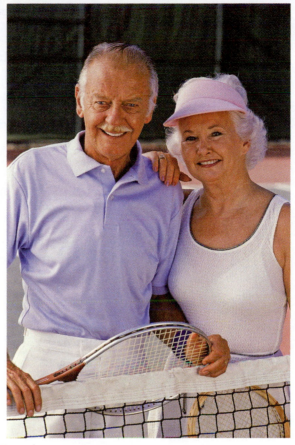

FIGURE 19–4
Regular exercise helps seniors to maintain an active lifestyle. (Courtesy of Photodisc)

The following are recommendations for developing an exercise prescription for seniors:

- Encourage individuals to start slowly and progress gradually from a low intensity, working up to a mild-to-moderate level.

- The warm-up should be thorough. A good warm-up should take five to ten minutes. Care should be given so that local muscle groups are not suddenly overloaded.

- Physician clearance should be obtained for individuals with medical conditions, including diabetes, arthritis, heart disease, and orthopedic problems.

- Care should be given when prescribing weight-lifting exercises to those with high blood pressure, heart disease, or arthritis. Routines using high repetitions with low weights are recommended.

- Encourage an extended cool-down period, approximately ten to fifteen minutes.

- Elderly individuals often have a more difficult time when exercising in the heat and cold. Avoid exercising in these conditions if possible.

- Encourage plenty of water and rest breaks.

- Some elderly individuals with arthritis or poor joint mobility may have to participate in non-weight-bearing activities, such as cycling, swimming, and chair and floor exercises.

- Seniors should be encouraged to exercise frequently (five to seven days per week). Exercising more frequently will help improve flexibility and cardio-respiratory fitness as well as exercise compliance.

Chapter Summary

Americans are living longer; this is partly due to the fact people are taking better care of themselves: eating right, exercising, and leading active lifestyles. As aging baby boomers take their quest for fitness immortality seriously, there will be a marked increase in seniors utilizing health clubs and fitness facilities.

Chapter Review Questions

1. Create an outline of the major points of the *National Blueprint: Increasing Physical Activity Among Adults Aged 50 and Older*.

2. It is stated in this chapter that the physical activity of the fifty-and-older population is under-addressed; why?

3. What are the health benefits of regular exercise for older adults?

4. What implementation strategies are outlined in the *Blueprint*?

5. What are the exercise recommendations for seniors?

Projects and Activities

1. Visit the Robert Wood Johnson Foundation's website (www.rwjf.org), and write a paper detailing its work, objectives, and outcomes.

2. Visit a local retirement home or community. Write a detailed report showing what activities are available to enhance the fitness of the elderly. What evidence is there that shows that seniors utilize the activities offered? Interview several seniors about their fitness program.

Website Resources

Aerobics and Fitness Association of America: http://www.afaa.com/

American Association of Retired People: http://www.aarp.org

American College of Sports Medicine: http://www.acsm.org

American Geriatrics Society: http://www.americangeriatrics.org

Centers for Disease Control and Prevention: http://www.cdc.gov/

Lifelong Fitness Alliance: http://www.50plus.org/

MedlinePlus: http://www.medlineplus.gov

National Blueprint: Increasing Physical Activity among Adults Aged 50 and Over:
http://www.agingblueprint.org

National Institute on Aging: http://www.nia.nih.gov/

The Robert Wood Johnson Foundation: http://www.rwjf.org/

United States Department of Health and Human Services: http://www.hhs.gov/

Dimensions of Athletic Facilities and Arenas

BASKETBALL
HIGH SCHOOL & COLLEGE COURT

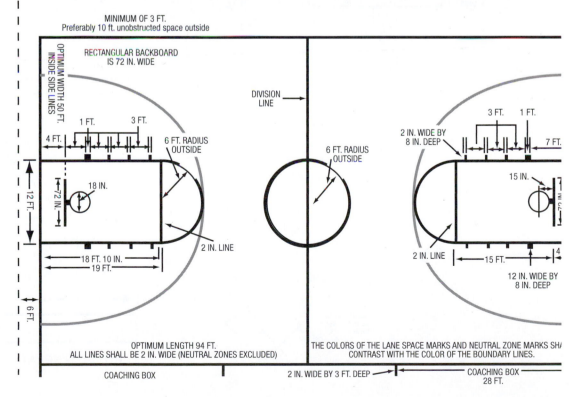

MINIMUM OF 3 FT.
Preferably 10 ft. unobstructed space outside

OPTIMUM WIDTH 50 FT.
INSIDE SIDE LINES

RECTANGULAR BACKBOARD IS 72 IN. WIDE

DIVISION LINE

1 FT.   3 FT.

4 FT.

6 FT. RADIUS OUTSIDE

6 FT. RADIUS OUTSIDE

3 FT.   1 FT.

2 IN. WIDE BY 8 IN. DEEP

7 FT.

12 FT.

72 IN.

18 IN.

15 IN.

2 IN. LINE

18 FT. 10 IN.
19 FT.

2 IN. LINE

15 FT.

6 FT.

12 IN. WIDE BY 8 IN. DEEP

OPTIMUM LENGTH 94 FT.
ALL LINES SHALL BE 2 IN. WIDE (NEUTRAL ZONES EXCLUDED)

THE COLORS OF THE LANE SPACE MARKS AND NEUTRAL ZONE MARKS SHALL CONTRAST WITH THE COLOR OF THE BOUNDARY LINES.

COACHING BOX

2 IN. WIDE BY 3 FT. DEEP

COACHING BOX
28 FT.

BASEBALL

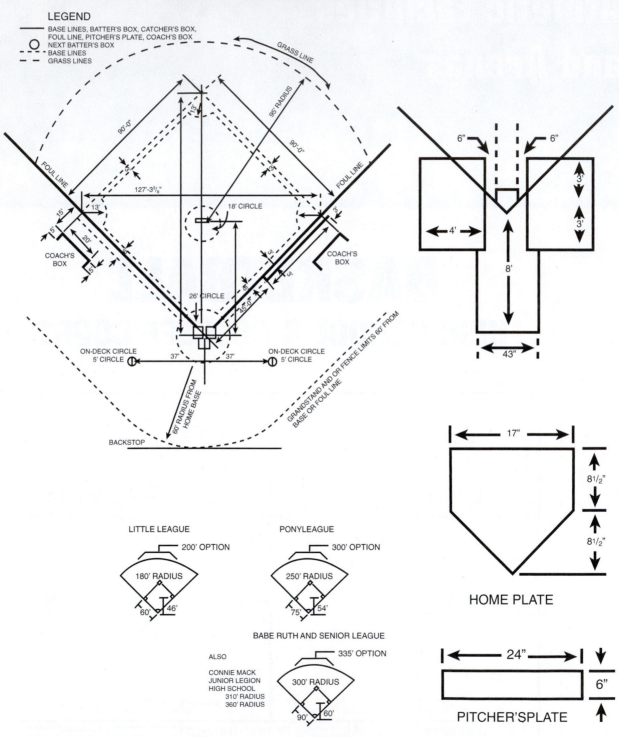

LEGEND
BASE LINES, BATTER'S BOX, CATCHER'S BOX,
FOUL LINE, PITCHER'S PLATE, COACH'S BOX
NEXT BATTER'S BOX
BASE LINES
GRASS LINES

GRASS LINE

90'-0"

95 RADIUS

90'-0"

FOUL LINE

FOUL LINE

127'-3³/₈"

18' CIRCLE

13'

15'

5'

20'

COACH'S BOX

COACH'S BOX

3'

26' CIRCLE

45'-0"

ON-DECK CIRCLE
5' CIRCLE

37'   37'

ON-DECK CIRCLE
5' CIRCLE

60' RADIUS FROM HOME BASE

GRANDSTAND AND OR FENCE LIMITS 60' FROM BASE OR FOUL LINE

BACKSTOP

6"   6"

3'

4'

3'

8'

43"

17"

8¹/₂"

8¹/₂"

HOME PLATE

24"

6"

PITCHER'S PLATE

LITTLE LEAGUE
200' OPTION
180' RADIUS
60'   46'

PONYLEAGUE
300' OPTION
250' RADIUS
75'   54'

BABE RUTH AND SENIOR LEAGUE
335' OPTION

ALSO

CONNIE MACK
JUNIOR LEGION
HIGH SCHOOL
    310' RADIUS
    360' RADIUS

300' RADIUS

90'   60'

RACQUETBALL/ HANDBALL

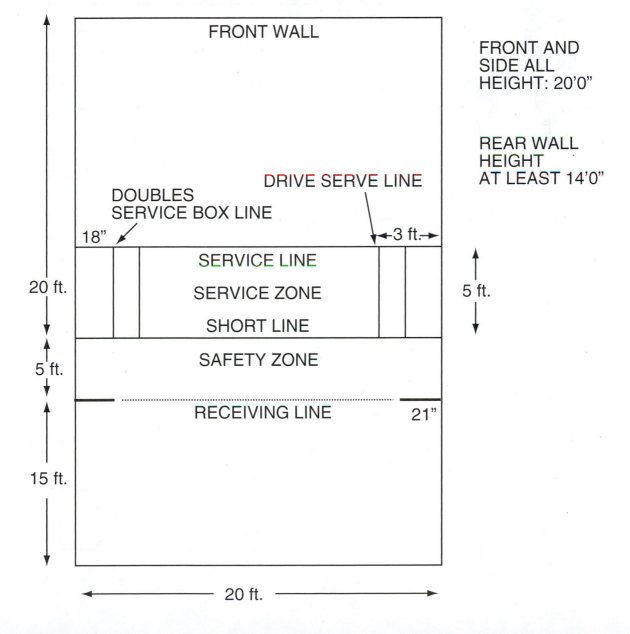

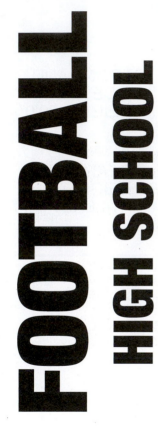

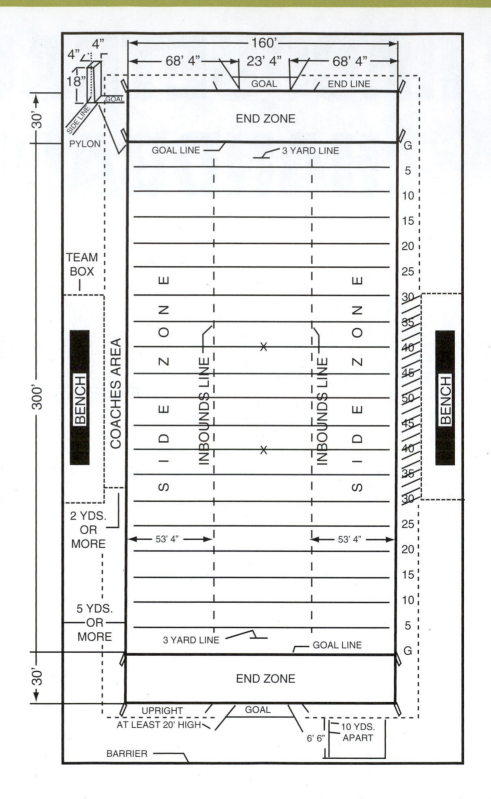

VOLLEYBALL

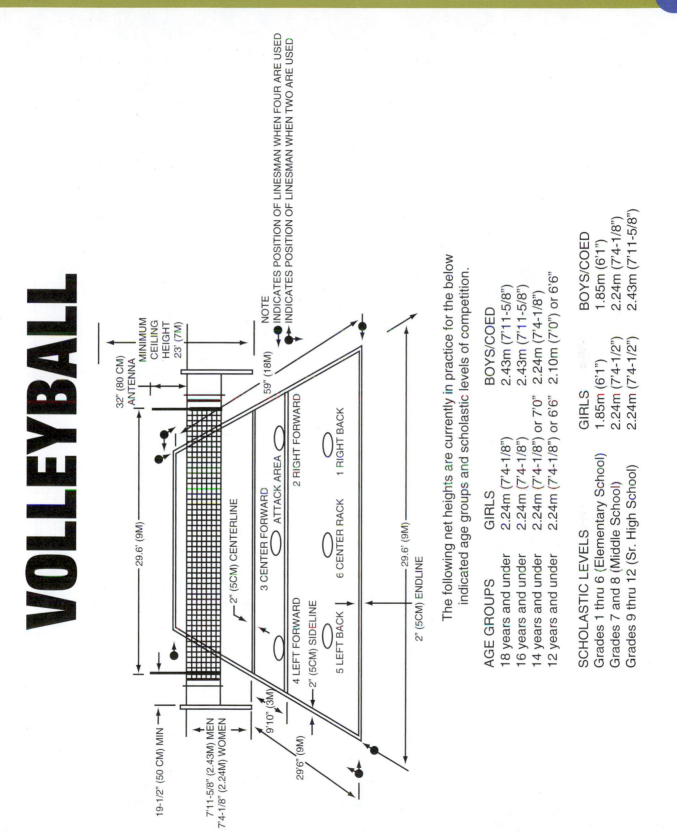

MINIMUM CEILING HEIGHT 23' (7M)

ANTENNA

32" (80 CM)

59' (18M)

29.6' (9M)

19-1/2" (50 CM) MIN

7'11-5/8" (2.43M) MEN
7'4-1/8" (2.24M) WOMEN

9'10" (3M)

29'6" (9M)

2" (5CM) SIDELINE

2" (5CM) CENTERLINE

2" (5CM) ENDLINE

3 CENTER FORWARD

ATTACK AREA

2 RIGHT FORWARD

1 RIGHT BACK

6 CENTER BACK

4 LEFT FORWARD

5 LEFT BACK

29.6' (9M)

NOTE

● INDICATES POSITION OF LINESMAN WHEN FOUR ARE USED

● INDICATES POSITION OF LINESMAN WHEN TWO ARE USED

The following net heights are currently in practice for the below indicated age groups and scholastic levels of competition.

AGE GROUPS	GIRLS	BOYS/COED
18 years and under	2.24m (7'4-1/8")	2.43m (7'11-5/8")
16 years and under	2.24m (7'4-1/8")	2.43m (7'11-5/8")
14 years and under	2.24m (7'4-1/8") or 7'0"	2.24m (7'4-1/8")
12 years and under	2.24m (7'4-1/8") or 6'6"	2.10m (7'0") or 6'6"

SCHOLASTIC LEVELS	GIRLS	BOYS/COED
Grades 1 thru 6 (Elementary School)	1.85m (6'1")	1.85m (6'1")
Grades 7 and 8 (Middle School)	2.24m (7'4-1/2")	2.24m (7'4-1/8")
Grades 9 thru 12 (Sr. High School)	2.24m (7'4-1/2")	2.43m (7'11-5/8")

SOFTBALL
OFFICIAL DIMENSIONS FOR SOFTBALL DIAMONDS

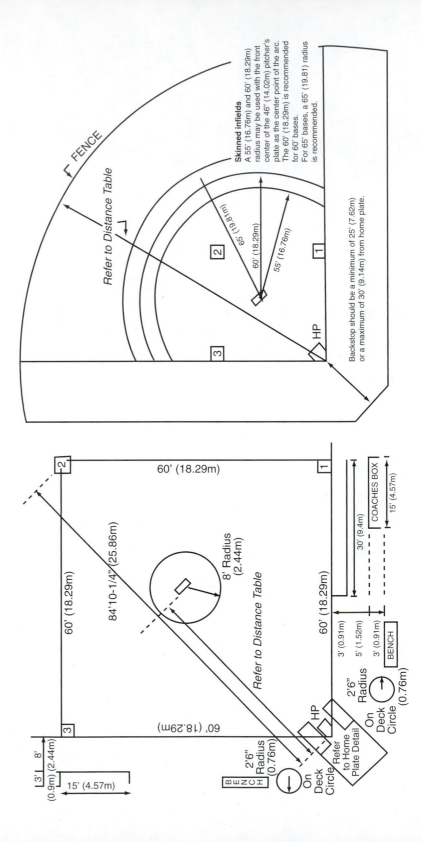

FENCE

Refer to Distance Table

Skinned infields
A 55' (16.76m) and 60' (18.29m) radius may be used with the front center of the 46" (14.02m) pitcher's plate as the center point of the arc. The 60' (18.29m) is recommended for 60' bases.
For 65' bases, a 65' (19.81) radius is recommended.

65' (19.81m)
60' (18.29m)
55' (16.76m)

2

1

3

HP

Backstop should be a minimum of 25' (7.62m) or a maximum of 30' (9.14m) from home plate.

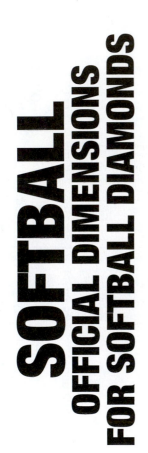

2

1

60' (18.29m)

60' (18.29m)

60' (18.29m)

60' (18.29m)

3

84'10-1/4" (25.86m)

8' Radius (2.44m)

Refer to Distance Table

COACHES BOX

15' (4.57m)

30' (9.4m)

3' (0.91m)

5' (1.52m)

3' (0.91m)

BENCH

2'6" Radius
On Deck Circle
(0.76m)

HP

On Deck Circle

Refer to Home Plate Detail

BENCH

2'6" Radius
(0.76m)

On Deck Circle

3'
8'
(0.9m) (2.44m)

15' (4.57m)

DISTANCE TABLE

ADULT

GAME	DIVISION	BASES	PITCHING	FENCES Minimum	Maximum
Fast Pitch	Women	60' (18.29m)	40' (12.19m)	200' (60.96m)	250' (76.20m)
	Men	60' (18.29m)	46' (14.02m)	225' (68.58m)	250' (76.20m)
	Jr. Men	60' (18.29m)	46' (14.02m)	225' (68.58m)	250' (76.20m)
Modified	Women	60' (18.29m)	40' (12.19m)	200' (60.96m)	
	Men	60' (18.29m)	46' (14.02m)	265' (80.80m)	
Slow Pitch	Women	65' (19.81m)	50' (15.24m)	265' (80.80m)	275' (83.82m)
	Men	65' (19.81m)	50' (15.24m)	275' (83.82m)	315' (96.01m)*
	Co-Ed	65' (19.81m)	50' (15.24m)	275' (83.82m)	300' (91.44m)
	Super	65' (19.81m)	50' (15.24m)	325' (99.06m)	No Max
16 Inch Slow Pitch	Women	55' (16.76m)	38' (11.58m)	200' (60.96m)	
	Men	55' (16.76m)	38' (11.58m)	250' (76.20m)	
14 Inch Slow Pitch	Women	60' (18.29m)	46' (14.02m)		
	Men	60' (18.29m)	46' (14.02m)		

YOUTH

GAME	DIVISION	BASES	PITCHING	FENCES Minimum	Maximum
Slow Pitch	Girls 10-under	55' (16.76m)	35' (10.67m)	150' (45.72m)	175' (53.34m)
	Boys 10-under	55' (16.76m)	35' (10.67m)	150' (45.72m)	175' (53.34m)
	Girls 12-under	60' (18.29m)	40' (12.19m)	175' (53.34m)	200' (60.96m)
	Boys 12-under	60' (18.29m)	40' (12.19m)	175' (53.34m)	200' (60.96m)
	Girls 14-under	65' (19.81m)	46' (14.02m)	225' (68.58m)	250' (76.20m)
	Boys 14-under	65' (19.81m)	46' (14.02m)	250' (76.20m)	275' (83.82m)
	Girls 16-under	65' (19.81m)	50' (15.24m)	225' (68.58m)	250' (76.20m)
	Boys 16-under	65' (19.81m)	50' (15.24m)	275' (83.82m)	300' (91.44m)
	Girls 18-under	65' (19.81m)	50' (15.24m)	225' (68.58m)	250' (76.20m)
	Boys 18-under	65' (19.81m)	50' (15.24m)	275' (83.82m)	300' (91.44m)
Fast Pitch	Girls 10-under	55' (16.76m)	35' (10.67m)	150' (45.72m)	175' (53.34m)
	Boys 10-under	55' (16.76m)	35' (10.67m)	150' (45.72m)	175' (53.34m)
	Girls 12-under	60' (18.29m)	35' (10.67m)	175' (53.34m)	200' (60.96m)
	Boys 12-under	60' (18.29m)	40' (12.19m)	175' (53.34m)	200' (60.96m)
	Girls 14-under	60' (18.29m)	40' (12.19m)	175' (53.34m)	200' (60.96m)
	Boys 14-under	60' (18.29m)	46' (14.02m)	175' (53.34m)	200' (60.96m)
	Girls 16-under	60' (18.29m)	40' (12.19m)	200' (60.96m)	225' (68.58m)
	Boys 16-under	60' (18.29m)	46' (14.02m)	200' (60.96m)	225' (68.58m)
	Girls 18-under	60' (18.29m)	40' (12.19m)	200' (60.96m)	225' (68.58m)
	Boys 18-under	60' (18.29m)	46' (14.02m)	200' (60.96m)	225' (68.58m)

Note: The only difference between college and high school is the pitching distance.

high school fast pitch..............46'
             slow pitch...........46'
             slow pitch female.....46'
             fast pitch female.......40'

college..................43'

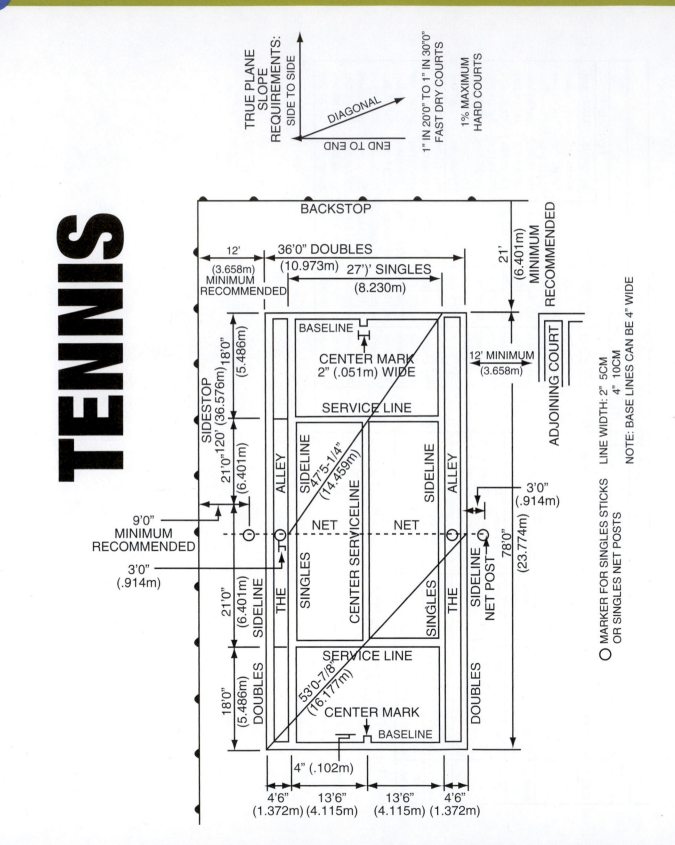

BADMINTUN

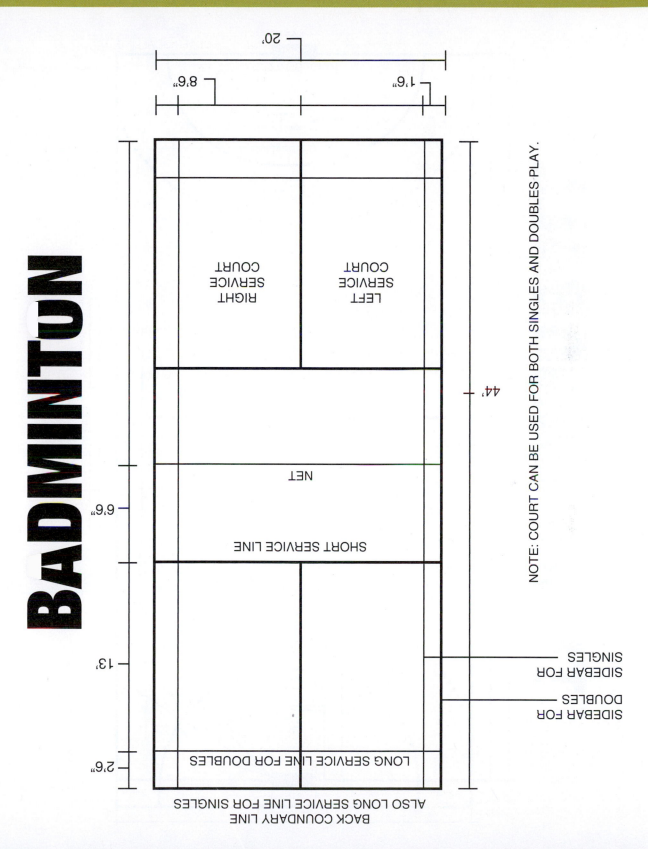

20'

8'6"

1'6"

RIGHT SERVICE COURT

LEFT SERVICE COURT

44'

NET

SHORT SERVICE LINE

6'6"

13'

NOTE: COURT CAN BE USED FOR BOTH SINGLES AND DOUBLES PLAY.

SIDEBAR FOR SINGLES

SIDEBAR FOR DOUBLES

2'6"

LONG SERVICE LINE FOR DOUBLES

BACK COUNDARY LINE
ALSO LONG SERVICE LINE FOR SINGLES

TEAM HANDBALL

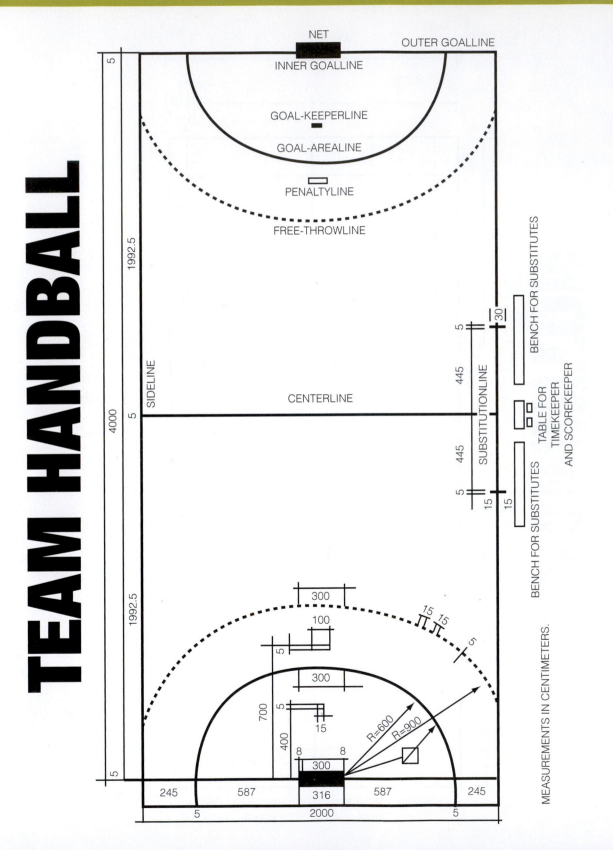

NET

INNER GOALLINE

OUTER GOALLINE

GOAL-KEEPERLINE

GOAL-AREALINE

PENALTYLINE

FREE-THROWLINE

SIDELINE

CENTERLINE

BENCH FOR SUBSTITUTES

SUBSTITUTIONLINE

TABLE FOR TIMEKEEPER AND SCOREKEEPER

BENCH FOR SUBSTITUTES

MEASUREMENTS IN CENTIMETERS.

5

1992.5

4000

5

1992.5

5

30

5

445

445

5

15

15

300

100

5

300

5

15

700

400

8

8

300

R=600

R=900

245

587

316

587

245

5

2000

5

15 15

5

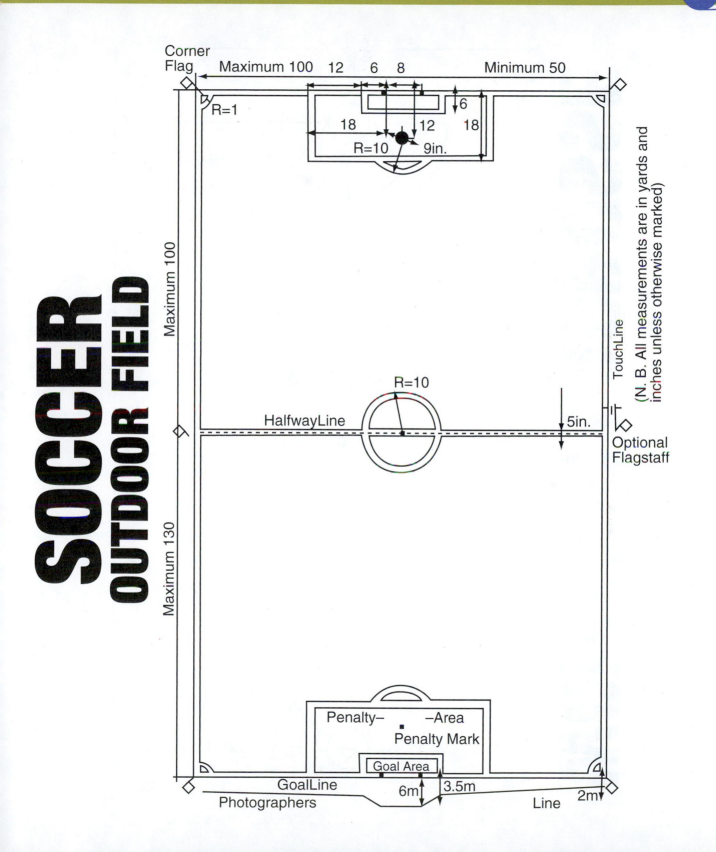

SOCCER
OUTDOOR FIELD

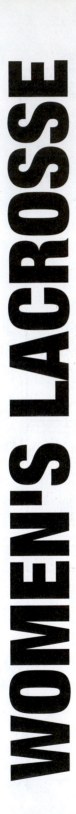

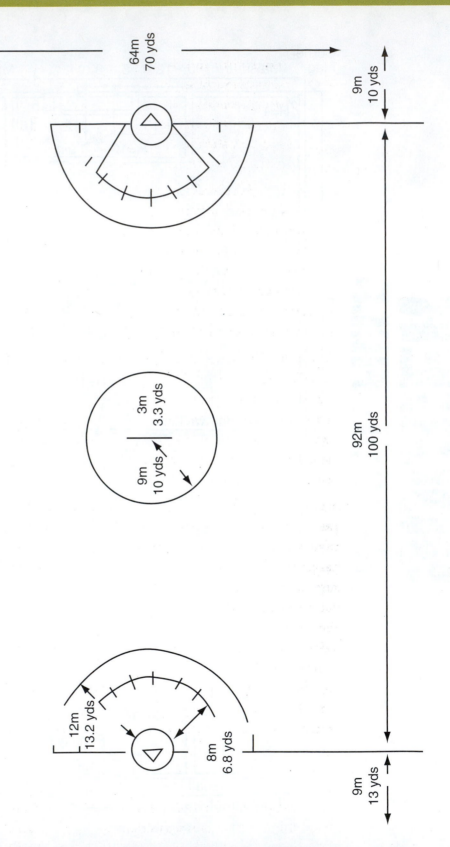

MEN'S LACROSSE
THE LACROSSE FIELD OF PLAY

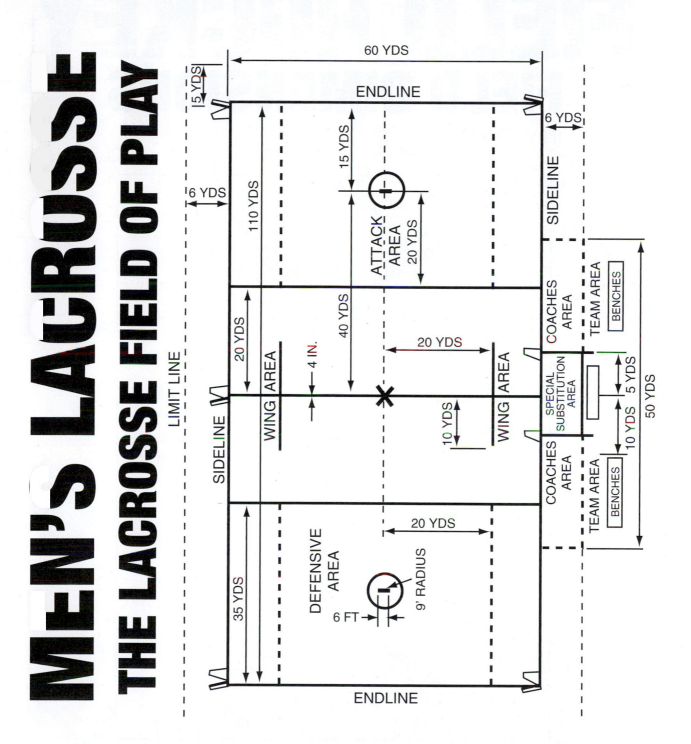

FIELD HOCKEY
FIELD DIMENSIONS

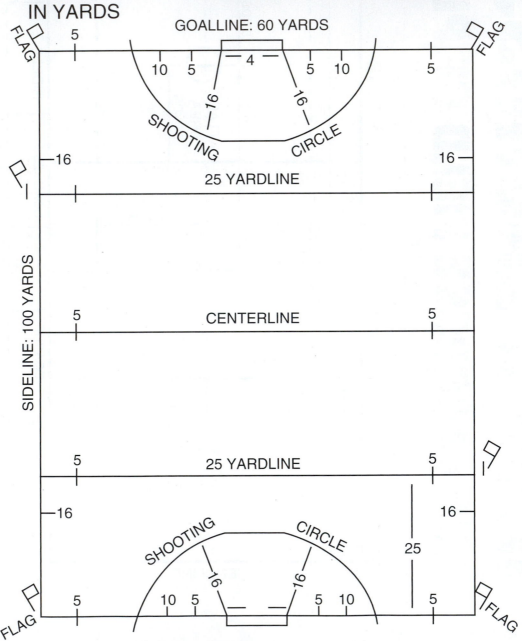

IN YARDS

GOALLINE: 60 YARDS

FLAG

5

10 5 4 5 10 5

SHOOTING   CIRCLE

16 16

FLAG

16 16

25 YARDLINE

SIDELINE: 100 YARDS

5 CENTERLINE 5

5 25 YARDLINE 5

16 16

SHOOTING CIRCLE

16 16

25

FLAG 5 10 5 5 10 5 FLAG

Organizations, Periodicals, and the Internet

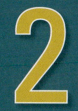
DISABILITY ISSUES

Access to Recreation
http://www.accesstr.com/

Internet Resource for Special Children (IRSC)
http://www.joeant.com/DIR/info/get/1249/47728

National Center on Accessibility
http://www.indiana.edu/

Parent Special Needs
http://specialchildren.about.com/

We Media Sports
http://www.wemedia.com

Yahoo Society & Culture Disability
http://dir.yahoo.com/society_and_culture/disabilities

Adapted Physical Education National Standards
http://www.cortland.edu/APENS

APE Aerobics
http://www.turnstep.com/

California State Council on Adapted Physical
Education (SCAPE) *http://sc-ape.org/*

Center on Motor Behavior in Down syndrome
http://www.umich.edu/

Disability Resources.org
http://www.disabilityresources.org

IFAPA - International Federation of Adapted Physical
Activity *http://www.ifapa.biz/*

ISBE regulations are available at
http://www.isbe.net/

National Center on Physical Activity and Disability
(NCPAD) *http://www.ncpad.org*

National Consortium on Physical Education and Recreation
for Individuals with Disabilities *http://ncperid.usf.edu*

World Association of Persons with Disabilities
http://www.wapd.org

PHYSICAL EDUCATION ASSOCIATIONS

AAHPERD (AALF/APAC)
http://www.aahperd.org/

American Fitness Alliance
http://www.americanfitness.net/

CAHPERD
http://www.cahperd.org/

California State Council APE go to links on CAPHERD site
and ESCAPE *http://sc-ape.org/*

Cooper Institute Fitnessgram and Activitygram
http://www.cooperinst.org/

The President's Council on Physical Fitness and Sport
http://www.fitness.gov/

National Association for Sport and Physical Education
(NASPE) *http://www.naspeinfo.org*

Aerobics and Fitness Association of America
http://www.afaa.com/

American Alliance for Health, Physical Activity, Recreation
and Dance *http://www.aahperd.org*

American Association for Leisure and Recreation (AALR) *http://www.aahperd.org/*

International Association of Athletics Federations *http://www.iaaf.org*

National Association for Sport and Physical Education (NASPE) *http://www.aahperd.org/*

National Recreation and Park Association (NRPA) *http://www.nrpa.org/*

PHYSICAL EDUCATION RESOURCES

California Physical Education Resources *http://www.stan-co.k12.ca.us/*

Games Kids Play *http://www.gameskidsplay.net/*

KidsRunning.com *http://www.kidsrunning.com*

Physical Education Model Content Standards for California Public Schools *http://www.cde.ca.gov/*

Physical Education Technology Newsletter *http://www.pesoftware.com/*

Sport for All: training, equipment, activities for sport skill development *http://www.sportforall.net/*

P.E. Central: The Premier Web Site for Health and PE Teachers *http://www.pecentral.org*

P.E. Links 4-U *http://www.pelinks4u.org*

Teachnology: The Web Portal for Educators *http://www.teach-nology.com/*

American Sports Education Program *http://www.asep.com*

Institute for International Sport *http://www.internationalsport.com/*

President's Council on Physical Fitness and Sports *http://www.fitness.gov*

IDEA97 regulations are available at *http://www.ed.gov/*

Pilates Method Alliance *http://www.pilatesmethodalliance.org/*

SPECIAL EDUCATION

California Department of Education Special Education Division *http://www.cde.ca.gov/*

Council Exceptional Children *http://www.cec.sped.org*

Professions in special education *http://www.special-ed-careers.org/*

The National Information Center for Children and Youth with Disabilities *http://www.nichcy.org/*

OTHER PROFESSIONAL ASSOCIATIONS

Occupational therapy *http://www.aota.org/*

Physical therapy *http://www.apta.org/*

Therapeutic recreation *http://www.recreationtherapy.com*

National Assn. of Collegiate Directors of Athletics *http://nacda.cstv.com/*

National Assn. of Collegiate Women Athletic Administrators *http://www.nacwaa.org/*

Missouri State High School Activities Association *http://www.mshaa.org*

National Education Association *http://www.nea.org*

National Collegiate Athletic Association (NCAA) *http://www.ncaa.org*

American Federation of Teachers (AFT) *http://www.aft.org*

PROFESSIONAL JOURNALS

Human Kinetics *http://www.humankinetics.com/*

PALAESTRA Journal *http://www.palaestra.com/*

Sports on Spoke Magazine (Paralyzed Vets of America) *http://www.pva.org*

EQUIPMENT COMPANIES

Flaghouse *http://www.flaghouse.com/*

Sportime *http://www.Sportime.com*

Sportime Adapt Talk *http://www.lyris.sportime.com/*

Gatorade Sports Science Institute *http://www.gssiweb.com/*

Fieldhouse *http://www.fieldhouse.com*

Summit Sports Medicine Products *http://www.summitsmp.com*

MEDICAL INFORMATION

Mayo Health Clinic (Go to Library/Disease & Conditions)
http://www.mayoclinic.com/

Neuromuscular Disease Center
http://www.neuro.wustl.edu/

AllRefer.com: References to health topics/news/medical encyclopedia, etc. *http://health.allrefer.com/*

PubMed (Index to medical) resources
http://www.ncbi.nlm.nih.gov/

American College of Sports Medicine
http://www.acsm.org

Centers for Disease Control and Prevention
http://www.cdc.gov/

Medline Plus
http://www.medlineplus.gov

National Athletic Trainers Association (NATA)
http://www.nata.org

DISABLED SPORT ORGANIZATIONS

America's Athletes with Disabilities
http://www.americasathletes.org

American Association of Adapted Sports Programs
http://www.aaasp.org

Blaze Sports
http://www.blazesports.com/

Challenged Athletes Foundation
http://www.challengedathletes.org/

National Disability Sport Alliance
http://www.ndsaonline.org/

Disabled Sports USA
http://www.dsusa.org

Dwarf Athletic Association of America
http://www.daaa.org

International Paralympic Committee
http://www.paralympic.org

National Disability Sport Alliance
http://www.uscpaa.org/main.htm

Paralyzed Veterans of America
http://www.pva.org

Special Olympics
http://www.specialolympics.org

United States Association for Blind Athletes (USABA)
http://www.usaba.org

United States Paralympics
http://www.usparalympics.org

US Olympic Committee on Sport for the Disabled
http://www.olympic-usa.org

USA Deaf Sports Federation
http://www.usdeafsports.org/

Wheelchair Sport USA (WSUSA)
http://www.wsusa.org

FITNESS AND AGING

American Association of Retired People
http://www.aarp.org

American Association of School Administrators
http://www.aasa.org

Coalition for Active Living (Canada)
http://www.activeliving.ca/

Fifty Plus Life-Long Fitness
http://www.50plus.org/

National Blueprint: Increasing Physical Activity among Adults Aged 50 and Older *http://www.nationalblueprint.org*

National Institute on Aging
http://www.nia.nih.gov/

United States Department of Health and Human Services
http://www.hhs.gov/

The Robert Wood Johnson Foundation
http://www.rwjf.org/

COACHING ASSOCIATIONS AND SITES

American Geriatrics Society
http://www.americangeriatrics.org

Coaching Tips on Dealing with Parents
http://www.boosterclubs.org

Guide to Coaching Youth Sports
http://www.guidetocoachingsports.com

National Federation of State High Schools
http://www.nfhs.org

National High School Coaches Association
http://nhsca.com

Positive Coaching Alliance
http://www.positivecoach.org/

The North American Booster Club Association, Inc.
http://www.boosterclubs.org

TITLE IX, EQUITY, ETHICS

Equity Education, Office of Superintendent of Public Instruction, Washington State *http://www.k12.wa.us/*

Law and Exceptional Students
http://www.unc.edu/

Josephson Institute of Ethics
http://www.josephsoninstitute.org

SPORT MANAGEMENT

National American Society for Sport Management (NASSM) *http://www.nassm.org/*

School Planning & Management magazine *http://www.peterli.com/*

JOB SEARCHING

This site, sponsored by Ohio State University School of Physical Activity and Education Services, has a wealth of information available for job searching *http://education.osu.edu/*

MISCELLANEOUS SITES OF INTEREST

National Alliance for Youth Sports *http://www.nays.org*

Pursuing Victory with Honor program *http://www.aiaonline.org/*

Sport Rage *http://www.dsr.nsw.gov.au/sportrage*

SportsKids *http://www.SportsKids.com*

References

This list supplements the Website Resources at the end of each chapter.

Allensworth, D., & Kolbe, L. (1987). The comprehensive school health program: Exploring an expanded concept. *Journal of School Health, 57*, 409–412.

American Alliance for Health, Physical Education, Recreation, and Dance. (2004). National standards for physical education. Reston, VA: American Alliance for Health, Physical Education, Recreation, and Dance.

"Balancing Booster Budgets." *Athletic Management, 13.2.* (2001, February/March), retrieved (2008) from http://www.momentummedia.com/articles/am/am1302/booster.htm

Bassett, S. (2002, March 17). Equality in sports is vital for both sexes. *Finger Lakes Times.*

Beginning Teacher Standards Task Force of the National Association for Sport and Physical Education. (1995). *National standards for beginning physical education teachers.* Reston, VA: National Association for Sport and Physical Education.

Berry, L. (2001, February/March). Balancing booster budgets. *Athletic Management,* 1–11.

Berryman. J. W. (1992). Exercise and the medical tradition from Hippocrates through antebellum America: A review essay. In Berryman, J. W. & Park, R. J. (Eds.), *Sport and exercise science: Essays in the history of sports medicine* (1–56). Urbana, IL: University of Illinois Press.

Bryant, K. M. (2006). Athletic directors have a big impact on high schools. Confederation of Oregon School Administrators.

Burns, C. R. (1976). The nonnaturals: A paradox in the western concept of health. *Journal of Medicine and Philosophy, 1,* 202–211.

Bylebyl, J. J. (1979). The school of Padua: humanistic medicine in the sixteenth century. In Webster C. (Ed.), *Health, medicine, and mortality in the sixteenth century,* 335–370. Manhattan, NY: Cambridge University Press.

California Department of Education, Standards and Assessment Division. (1999). *California physical fitness test 1999: Report to the governor and legislature.* Sacramento: California Department of Education.

Carnegie Council on Adolescent Development. (1994). *A matter of time: Risk and opportunity in the out-of-school hours. Recommendations for strengthening community programs for youth.* New York: Carnegie Corporation of New York.

Catalano, R. F., Loeber, R., & McKinney, K. C. (1999, October). School and community interventions to prevent serious and violent offending. *Juvenile Justice Bulletin,* 1–12.

Centers for Disease Control and Prevention. (1996). CDC surveillance summaries, 1995. *Morbidity and Mortality Weekly Report, 45(SS-4),* 1–83.

Centers for Disease Control and Prevention. (1997). Guidelines for school and community health programs to promote physical activity among youth. *Morbidity and Mortality Weekly Report, 46(RR-6),* 1–36.

Centers for Disease Control and Prevention. (1999). Neighborhood safety and the prevalence of physical inactivity—selected states, 1996. *Morbidity & Mortality Weekly Report, 48(7),* 143–146.

Centers for Disease Control and Prevention. (1999). Physical education. From CDC's 1994 School Health Policies and Programs Study [fact sheet]. Atlanta: Centers for Disease Control and Prevention.

Centers for Disease Control and Prevention. (2000). *Promoting better health for young people through physical activity and sports.* Atlanta: Centers for Disease Control and Prevention.

Centers for Disease Control and Prevention. (2001). *Risk behaviors overview.* Atlanta: Centers for Disease Control and Prevention.

Centers for Disease Control and Prevention. (2001, December). *Preventing unintentional injuries and violence: guidelines for school health programs.* Atlanta: Centers for Disease Control and Prevention.

Centers for Disease Control and Prevention. (2000). *School health index for physical activity and healthy eating: A self-assessment and planning guide.* Atlanta: Centers for Disease Control and Prevention.

Centers for Disease Control and Prevention. (2000). Youth risk behavior surveillance—United States, 1999. *Morbidity & Mortality Weekly Report, 49(SS-5),* 1–94.

Centers for Disease Control and Prevention. (2001). *School health programs: An investment in our schools.* Atlanta: Centers for Disease Control and Prevention.

Centers for Disease Control and Prevention. (2001, December). *Unintentional injuries, violence, and the health of young people:* [fact sheet]. Atlanta: Centers for Disease Control and Prevention.

Centers for Disease Control and Prevention. (2002). *Physical activity and good nutrition: Essential elements to prevent chronic diseases and obesity.* Atlanta: Centers for Disease Control and Prevention, pp. 1, 7, 21.

Centers for Disease Control and Prevention. (2002). *Surveillance summaries. Morbidity and Mortality Weekly Report, 51(SS-4),* pp. 1–4, 6.

Christensen, E. H. (1960). Intervallarbeit und intervalltraining. *Arbeitsphysiologie, 18,* 345–356.

Coakley, J. (2004). Sports in society: Issues and controversies (8th ed.). New York: McGraw-Hill.

Cooper K. H. (1968). A means of assessing maximal oxygen intake: correlation between field and treadmill testing. *Journal of the American Medical Association, 203,* 135–138.

Corbin C. B., & Pangrazi, R. P. (1998). *Physical activity for children: A statement of guidelines.* Reston, VA: National Association for Sport and Physical Education.

Cureton, T. K. (1947). *Physical fitness workbook: A manual of conditioning exercises and standards, tests, and rating scales for evaluating physical fitness* (3rd ed.). St. Louis: C. S. Mosby.

DeAngelis, K., & Rossi, R. (1997). *Schools serving family needs: extended-day programs in public and private schools.* Washington, DC: National Center for Education Statistics.

Eaton, S. B., Shostak, M., & Konner, M. (1988). *The paleolithic prescription: A program of diet and exercise and a design for living.* New York: Harper and Row.

Epstein, A. (2003). *Sports law.* Clifton Park, NY: Delmar Learning.

Escobedo, L. G., Marcus, S. E., Holtzman, D., & Giovino, G. A. (1993). Sports participation, age at smoking initiation and the risk of smoking among US high school students. *Journal of the American Medical Association, 269,* 1391–5.

Finley, P. S. (2006). Title IX and booster club management: Experts' suggestions for managing challenging scenarios. Fort Lauderdale, FL: Nova Southeastern University.

Fishbein, M. (1947). A history of the American Medical Association, 1847 to 1947. Philadelphia: W.B. Saunders.

Flegal, K. M., Carroll, M. D., Kuczmarski, R. J., & Johnson, C. L. (1998). Overweight and obesity in the United States: Prevalence and trends, 1960–1994. *International Journal of Obesity, 22(1),* 39–47.

Foster, W. L. (1914). A test of physical efficiency. *American Physical Education Review, 19,* 632–636.

Freedman, D. S., Dietz, W. H., Srinivasan, S. R., & Berenson, G. S. (1999). The relation of overweight to cardiovascular risk factors among children and adolescents: The Bogalusa heart study. *Pediatrics, 103,* 1175–82.

Gender and Sports Participation. (1998): European Federation of Sport Psychology.

Georgia Tech Sports Medicine and Performance Newsletter. (2000, November)

Gruman, G. J. (1961). The rise and fall of prolongevity hygiene, 1558–1873. *Bulletin of the History of Medicine, 35,* 221–229.

Gunn, J. C. (1830/1986). *Gunn's domestic medicine, or poor man's friend.* Reprinted, with an introduction by C. E. Rosenberg. Knoxville, TN: University of Tennessee Press.

Ham, S. Calculations from the 1995 Nationwide Personal Transportation Survey. (Unpublished data, 2000).

Hippocrates. (1953). *Regimen I.* (W. H. Jones, Trans.). Cambridge, MA: Harvard University Press.

Huang, Ti. (1951). *Nei Ching Su Wen: The Yellow Emperor's classic of internal medicine.* (I. Veith, Trans.). Baltimore: Williams and Wilkins.

Huard, P., & Wong, M. (1968). *Chinese medicine.* (B. Fielding, Trans.). London: Weidenfeld and Nicolson.

Insurance 101: As a coach, supervision means more than just watching the kids. (2004, July/August). *Lacrosse,* 1–2.

Johnson, J., & Deshpande, C. (2000). Health education and physical education: Disciplines preparing students as productive, healthy citizens for the challenges of the 21st century. *Journal of School Health, 70(2),* 66–8.

Joint Committee on National Health Education Standards. (1995). *National health education standards.* Atlanta: American Cancer Society.

Kaiser Family Foundation. (1999, November). *Kids & media @ the new millenium.* Menlo Park, CA: Kaiser Family Foundation.

Kaiserman, K. (2008). *Coaching Youth Sports.* Retrieved July 22, 2008, from http://www.sportskids.com.

Kanaby, R. (1984). Athletics & academics: Accept the challenge . . . change the perception . . . promote the truth. *Interscholastic Athletic Administration, 11(1),* 4–7, 9.

Karvonen, M. J., Kentala, E., & Mustala, O. (1957). The effects of training on heart rate. *Acta Medica Exp Fenn, 35,* 308–315.

Kleinginna, P. R., & Kleinginna, A. M. (1981). A Categorized List of Emotion Definitions, with Suggestions for a Consensual Definition. *Motivation and Emotion, 5(4),* 345–359.

Knitt, D. (n/d). *Case study: Disability awareness in physical activity.* Winter Haven, FL: Hewett Academy Middle School.

Larson, L. A., & Yocom, R. D. (1951). *Measurement and evaluation in physical, health, and recreation education.* St. Louis: C.V. Mosby.

Leonard, F. E., & Affleck, G. B. (1947). *A guide to the history of physical education* (3rd ed.). Philadelphia: Lea and Febiger.

Mair, D. (n/d). *Risk Management Essentials for Local Sports Programs.* Colorado Springs: USOC Risk and Insurance Management.

Marx, E., Wooley, S., & Northrup, D. (Eds.). (1998). *Health is academic: A guide to coordinated school health programs.* New York: Teachers College Press.

McCurdy, J. H. (1901). The effect of maximum muscular effort on blood pressure. *American Journal of Physiology, 5*, 95–103.

McFarland, A. (2001, July). Altering the Evaluation Process of Interscholastic Coaches Based on Alternative Classroom Teacher Appraisal Methods. 1-19. Retrieved 11/15/2005, from ERIC database (ED 465737)

McGinnis, J. M., & Foege, W. H. (1993). Actual causes of death in the United States. *Journal of the American Medical Association, 270*(18), 2207–12.

McKenzie, R. T. (1913). The influence of exercise on the heart. *American Journal of the Medical Sciences, 145*, 69–74.

Meade, L. K. (2005, June 23). Gifts can throw teams off balance. *The Boston Globe*, p. 1.

Mendez C. (1553/1960). *Book of bodily exercise.* (F. Guerra, Trans.). New Haven: Elizabeth Licht.

Mohnsen, B. (ed.). Concepts of physical education: What every student needs to know. Reston, VA: National Association for Sport and Physical Education, 1998.

Mokdad, A., Serdula, M., Dietz, W., Bowman, B., Marks, J., & Koplan, J. (1999). The spread of the obesity epidemic in the United States, 1991–1998. *Journal of the American Medical Association, 282*, 1519–22.

Montoye, H. J., Van Huss, W. D., Brewer, W. D., Jones, E. M., Ohlson, M. A., Maloney, E, et al. (1959). The effects of exercise on blood cholesterol of middle-aged men. *American Journal of Clinical Nutrition, 7*, 139–145.

Mumford, V., & Gergley, G. (2005). Loser or legend: Beginning considerations for interscholastic coaches. *The Sport Journal.* Retrieved June 1, 2007, from http://www.thesportjournal.org/.

Nabokov, P. (1981). *Indian running: Native American history and tradition.* Santa Barbara: Capra Press.

National Association for Sport and Physical Education. (1995). *Moving into the future: National standards for physical education.* Reston, VA: National Association for Sport and Physical Education.

National Association for Sport and Physical Education. (1995). *Quality coaches, quality sports: National standards for athletic coaches.* Reston, VA: National Association for Sport and Physical Education.

National Association for Sport and Physical Education. (1998). *Shape of the nation report: A survey of state physical education requirements.* Reston, VA: National Association for Sport and Physical Education, 1998.

National Association of State Boards of Education. (2000). *Physical activity, healthy eating and tobacco-use prevention.* Part I of *Fit, healthy and ready to learn: A school health policy guide.* Alexandria, VA. National Association of State Boards of Education.

National Center for Chronic Disease Prevention and Health Promotion. (Winter 2000). *Chronic disease notes and reports.*

Atlanta: National Center for Chronic Disease Prevention and Health Promotion, Centers for Disease Control and Prevention.

National Center for Health Statistics. (2000). *Health, United States, 2000. With adolescent health chartbook.* Hyattsville, MD: National Center for Health Statistics.

National Collegiate Athletic Association. (1993). *Gender Equity.* Overland Park, KS: National Collegiate Athletic Association.

National Consortium for Physical Education and Recreation for Individuals with Disabilities. (1995). *Adapted physical education national standards.* Champaign, IL: Human Kinetics.

National Federation of State High Schools. (2006). *Coaching Code of Ethics.* Indianapolis, IN: National Federation of State High Schools. Retrieved October 12, 2007, from http://www.nfhs.org.

National Intramural Sports Council. (1995). *Guidelines for school intramural programs.* Reston, VA: National Association for Sport and Physical Education.

National School-Age Care Alliance. (1998). *The NSACA standards for quality school-age care.* Boston: National School-Age Care Alliance.

Newman, T. (2005). Coaches' roles in the academic success of male student athletes. *The Sport Journal, 8*(2), 2.

Obernauer, M. The rising price of victory; Fundraising for athletic

Obernauer, M. (2005, July 16). The rising price of victory; Fundraising for athletic programs incites cries of inequity. *The Austin-American Statesman*, p. A1.

Pavlovic, S. (2002). *Coaching Tips on Dealing with Parents* (e-book). Blacksburg, VA: P. E. Central.

Pennington, B. (2004, June 29). Title IX trickles down to girls of generation z. *New York Times*, p. D1.

Pollock, M. L. (1973). The quantification of endurance training programs. *Exercise and Sport Sciences Reviews, 1*, 155–188.

President's Council on Physical Fitness and Sports. (1997). *Physical activity and sport in the lives of girls: Physical and mental health dimensions from an interdisciplinary approach.* Washington, DC: President's Council on Physical Fitness and Sports.

Rampmeyer, K. (2000). *Developmentally appropriate practice in movement programs for young children ages 3–5.* Reston, VA: National Association for Sport and Physical Education.

Reed, J. A. (2006, March 4). Separating teacher, coach roles would improve physical education, *Greenville News* (SC), retrieved (December 2, 2007) from http://www.greenvilleonline.com.

Reiser, S. J. (1985). Responsibility for personal health: A historical perspective. *Journal of Medicine and Philosophy, 10*, 7–17.

Roberts, D. (1990, March/April). Active aging; exercise and the older athlete. Retrieved March 17, 2007, from http://www.afaa.com/

Robert Wood Foundation. (2001). *The National Blueprint: Increasing Physical Activity among Adults 50 and Older.* Princeton, NJ.

Rutherford, G. S., McCormack, E., & Wilkinson, M. (1998). *Travel aspects of urban form: Implications from an analysis of two Seattle area travel diaries.* Paper presented at the TMIP Conference on Urban Design, Telecommunications and Travel Forecasting.

Sallis, J. F., & McKenzie, T. (1991). Physical education's role in public health. *Research Quarterly for Exercise and Sport, 62,* 124–137.

Sallis, J. F., McKenzie, T. L., Alcaraz, J. E., Kolody, B., Faucette, N., & Hovell, M. (1997). The effects of a 2-year physical education program (SPARK) on physical activity and fitness in elementary school students. *American Journal of Public Health, 87,* 1328–34.

Sallis, J. F., McKenzie, T. L., Kolody, B., Lewis, M., Marshall, S., & Rosengard, P. (1999). Effects of health-related physical education on academic achievement: Project SPARK. *Research Quarterly for Exercise and Sport, 70(2),* 127–34.

Sallis, J. F., & Patrick, K. (1994). Physical activity guidelines for adolescents: Consensus statement. *Pediatric Exercise Science, 6,* 302–14.

Sallis, J. F., Prochaska, J. J., Taylor, W. C., Hill, J. O., and Geraci, J. C. (1999). Correlates of physical activity in a national sample of girls and boys in grades 4 through 12. *Health Psychology, 18,* 410–5.

Sanchez, R. (2003, November 10). Holding back boosters: Districts worry that funding could result in Title IX challenge. *Rocky Mountain News,* p. 20A.

Schneider, E. C., & Ring, G. C. (1929). The influence of a moderate amount of physical training on respiratory exchange and breathing during physical exercise. *American Journal of Physiology, 91,* 103–114.

Seefeldt, V. D., & Ewing, M. E. (1997). Youth sports in America: An overview. *President's Council on Physical Fitness and Sports Research Digest, 2(11),* 1–12.

Shampo, M. A., & Kyle, R. A. (1989), Nei Ching, oldest known medical book. *Mayo Clinic Proceedings, 64,* 134.

Simons-Morton, B., Eitel, P., & Small, M. (1999). School physical education: Secondary analyses of the school health policies and programs study. *Journal of School Health, 30(5),* 558–564.

Lambert, L. T. (2000, March.) The new physical education. *Educational Leadership, 57(6),* 1–2.

Smith, E. (1857). The influence of the labour of the tread-wheel over respiration and pulsation, and its relation to the waste of the system, and the diet of the prisoners. *Medical Times and Gazette, 14,* 601–603.

Smith, G. (1985). Prescribing the rules of health: Self-help and advice in the late eighteenth century. In Porter R., (Ed.), *Patients and practitioners: Lay perceptions of medicine in pre-industrial society* (249–282). Cambridge, UK: Cambridge University Press.

Smith, J. W., Jr. (1994, February). Interscholastic athletic programs: A positive factor in school reform. *NASSP Bulletin,* 93–97.

Soltz, D. F. (1986, October). Athletics and academic achievement: What is the relationship? *NASSP Bulletin,* 20–24.

Souza, L. M. (1990, December). A model program of preventive academic support. *NASSP Bulletin,* 24–27.

Storey, T. A. (1903). The influence of fatigue upon the speed of voluntary contraction of human muscle. *American Journal of Physiology, 8,* 355–375.

Taylor, H. L., Anderson, J. T., & Keys, A. (1957). Physical activity, serum cholesterol and other lipids in man. *Proceedings of the Society for Experimental Biology and Medicine, 95,* 383–388.

Throop, R. K., & Castelluci, M. B. (1999). *Reaching your potential: Personal and professional development* (2nd ed.). Clifton Park, NY: Delmar Learning.

U.S. Bureau of the Census. (1998) March 1998 CPS, P20-514, Table 6. Washington, DC: U.S. Bureau of the Census.

U.S. Department of Agriculture and U.S. Department of Health and Human Services. (2000). *Nutrition and your health: Dietary guidelines for Americans* (5th ed.). Washington, DC: U.S. Department of Agriculture and U.S. Department of Health and Human Services, Government Printing Office.

U.S. Department of Health and Human Services. (2001). *The Surgeon General's call to action to prevent and decrease overweight and obesity.* Rockville, MD: U.S. Department of Health and Human Services.

U.S. Department of Health and Human Services. (2000). *Healthy people 2010: Understanding and improving health.* Washington, DC: U.S. Department of Health and Human Services, Government Printing Office.

U.S. Department of Health and Human Services. (1985). National children and youth fitness study. *Journal of Physical Education, Recreation, and Dance, 56,* 44–90.

U.S. Department of Health and Human Services. (1987). National children and youth fitness study II. *Journal of Physical Education, Recreation, and Dance, 58,* 49–96.

U.S. Department of Health and Human Services. (1996). *Physical activity and health: A report of the Surgeon General.* Atlanta: U.S. Department of Health and Human Services, Centers for Disease Control and Prevention, National Center for Chronic Disease Prevention and Health Promotion.

U. S. Department of Education. (2000). *A guide to the individualized education program.* Retrieved February 22, 2008, from http://www.ed.gov/parents/needs/speced/iepguide/index.html.

U. S. Department of Education. (2004). *Special education and rehabilitative services.* Retrieved December 11, 2007, from http://idea.ed.gov/

U.S. Department of Transportation, Federal Highway Administration, Research and Technical Support Center. (1997). *Nationwide Personal Transportation Survey.* Lanham, MD: Federal Highway Administration.

Whorton, J. C. (1982). *Crusaders for fitness: The history of American health reformers.* Princeton, NJ: Princeton University Press.

Winnick, J. P. (Ed.). (2005). *Adapted physical education and sport.* Champaign, IL: Human Kinetics.

Wolf, A. M., & Colditz, G. A. (1998). Current estimates of the economic cost of obesity in the United States. *Obesity Research, 6(2),* 97–106.

Yakovlev, N. N., Kaledin, S. V., Krasnova, A. F., Leshkevich, L. G., Popova, N. K., Rogozkin, V. A., et al. (1961). Physiological and chemical adaptation to muscular activity in relation to length of rest periods between exertions during training. *Sechenov-Physiological Journal of the USSR, 47,* 56–59.

Zill, N., Nord, C. W., & Loomis, L. S. (1995). *Adolescent time use, risky behavior and outcomes: An analysis of national data.* Rockville, MD: Westat.

Glossary

A

Abduction Movement of a limb away from the midline of the body

Academic eligibility Successful completion of all requirements imposed by a school to participate in an athletic contest and/or athletic program

Accelerated pairings A tournament system in which players are seeded from highest to lowest based on their ratings. In the first round, players seeded in the top quarter of the draw are paired against those in the second quarter and those in the third quarter are paired against those in the fourth quarter. The next-round winners in the top half of the tournament play each other, as do losers in the bottom half. However, nonwinners in the top half play winners in the bottom half. Thus, it is possible to have a first-round winner play a first-round loser. The idea is to try to avoid having anyone in the bottom half of the draw among the tournament leaders after the second round.

Adaptation The systematic application of exercise stress sufficient to stimulate muscle fatigue, but not so severe that breakdown and injury occur

Adapted Physical Education National Standards Standards developed in 1995 to guide the certification of physical education professionals in adaptive physical education

Adaptive physical education Physical education that is adapted or modified to address the individualized needs of children and youth who have gross motor developmental delays

Adduction Movement of a limb toward the midline of the body

Algorithm A procedure for assigning competitors into tournament formats

Americans with Disabilities Act This law gives civil rights protection to individuals with disabilities. The ADA also guarantees equal opportunity for individuals with disabilities in the areas of employment, state and local government services, public transportation, privately operated transportation available to the public, places of public accommodation, and telephone services offered to the public.

Amphiarthroses (singular: **amphiarthrosis**) Slightly movable joints connected by fibrocartilage

Arthrology The study of joints

Articular cartilage The layer of connective tissue covering the ends of long bones

Athletic administration The decision-making body for athletics in a school or other institution

Athletic booster clubs Private, nonprofit organizations created to help and financially support an athletic team or program

Atrophy Weakness and wasting away of muscle tissue

Axial plane A horizontal flat surface dividing the body into upper and lower parts; also known as the transverse plane

B

Ball-and-socket joint A freely movable joint in which a rounded end of one bone fits into an indented end of another bone; allows the widest range of motion

Ballistic stretching A rhythmical, bouncing action that stretches the muscles a little further each time.

Body composition A calculation that determines the amount of body fat present in a person

Burnout Mental and physical exhaustion; specifically, exhaustion that causes an athlete to drop out of a sport or quit an activity that was once enjoyable

C

Camp counselor An individual that is responsible for managing camps and camp activities

Cardiorespiratory conditioning Engaging in activity that puts an increased demand on the lungs, heart, and other body systems; also known as aerobic or endurance training

Cardiorespiratory endurance The ability of the body's circulatory and respiratory systems to supply fuel during sustained physical activity

Centers for Disease Control and Prevention (CDC) Public health organization that promotes health and quality of life by preventing and controlling disease, injury, and disability

Certified athletic administrator (CAA) An athletic administrator who has passed the certification exam of the National Interscholastic Athletic Administrators Association

Certified Athletic Trainers An athletic trainer that has successfully passed all requirements for certification of the National Athletic Trainers Association

Certified master athletic administrator (CMAA) A greater level of recognition awarded to certified athletic trainers who go beyond normal levels of certification

Circuit training The use of six to ten strength exercises completed one right after another; each exercise is done for a specific number of repetitions or for a specific period of time before the athlete moves to the next exercise

Circumduction Circular movement of a limb around an axis

Civil Rights Restoration Act of 1987 Legislation that ensured that any federally funded program must comply with laws outlawing discriminatory practices based upon race, religion, color, national origin, gender, age, or disability

Closed kinematic chain A sequence of actions in which the body part farthest from the trunk is fixed during movement

Coaches Individuals that lead or direct people in specific activities

Coaching code of ethics A set of agreed-upon rules and procedures for coaches that governs their dealings with athletes

Coaching evaluation A process by which coaches are evaluated for effectiveness in a variety of categories

Coaching philosophy A set of beliefs or ideas that coaches adhere to so that their athletes can meet their personal and performance goals

Coaching standards Criteria set by local, state, and national organizations to hold coaches accountable

Communication skill Developed method for communicating effectively with others

Concave Having a half-circle–shaped indentation

Condyloid (ellipsoidal) joint Freely movable joint that allows bones to move in many different directions, but not to rotate

Conflict resolution A method to resolve conflicts in a professional, knowledgeable manner

Convex A half-circle–shaped protrusion

Coronal plane A vertical flat surface running from side to side of the body; also known as the frontal plane

Corporate sponsorship To give financial support at the business level; may be given to local school districts as well as professional sports teams

D

Decisiveness The ability to make a decision quickly

Defined medical emergency An illness or traumatic injury that has the potential to be life-threatening or progress to a life-threatening event in the absence of treatment

Delegation Assignment of responsibilities to a person or entity

Depression Movement of a body part downward in a frontal plane

Diarthroses (singular: **diarthrosis**) Freely movable joints; also known as synovial joints

Dorsiflexion Movement that flexes the foot

Double-elimination tournament A tournament in which one must lose two contests before being eliminated from play

Dynamic (isotonic) exercise An activity that causes the muscle to contract and shorten

E

Education for All Handicapped Children Act (Public Law 94-142) Legislation passed on 1975 that was intended to support states and localities in protecting the rights and individual needs of children and youths with disabilities, as well as their families

Elevation Movement of a body part upward in a frontal plane

Emergency action plan (EAP) A formal document outlining the steps that should be taken in the event of a medical crisis or disaster

Emergency preparedness Condition of being properly equipped and trained for any medical crisis or disaster.

EMS system The response system in a particular area that is called upon in the event of a medical crisis or traumatic injury. This usually consists of personnel trained in basic or advanced life support and an ambulance or equipped emergency vehicle capable of transporting an injured victim to a hospital emergency room.

Equity in Athletics Disclosure Act Legislation requiring coeducational colleges and universities to prepare a yearly report detailing athletic participation by gender

Ethical responsibilities A set of moral principles that create a framework for working with others

Eversion Movement of the sole of the foot outward

Exercise physiology Procedures used to study the metabolic responses to exercise

Exercise science Exercise science examines the effects of exercise and physical activity on people so they may optimize their fitness routine to provide a greater physical and mental health benefit.

Extension Movement that increases the angle between two bones

F

Fast twitch fiber Fiber in a motor unit that produces quick and forceful contractions; these fibers are easily fatigued

Fibrocartilage Specialized connective tissue containing thick collagen fibers

Field house A large building designed as a site for a number of different sports activities

Fitness directors Individuals whose responsibilities involve the direction and success of fitness programs

Fitness facilities Areas where various exercise programs can be conducted

Fitness workers People who are employed in the fitness industry

Flexibility The ability of a joint to move freely through its full range of motion

Flexion Movement that decreases the angle between two bones

G

Galen Second-century Greek physician who wrote numerous works of great importance to medical history

Gender discrimination Discrimination based on someone's gender (sex)

Gender equity Equal treatment of each person despite his or her gender (sex)

Gliding joint A freely movable joint that allows bones to make a sliding motion

Goal setting Identifying clearly defined, specific objectives that are measurable

Goal statement A statement describing what can reasonably be accomplished within a certain time

Gomphosis An immovable joint in which a conical process fits into a socket held in place by ligaments

Gout An accumulation of uric acid crystals in the joint at the base of the large toe and other joints of the feet

Ground fault interrupter Outlets designed to prevent electrical shock by interrupting the circuit when there is a wiring problem

Gymnasium A facility for athletics and exercise

H

Healthy People 2010 The national health objective signed by President Clinton in 2000 that promotes physical activity and sports among the nation's youth

Herodicus A Greek physician who was the first to study therapeutic gymnastics

Hinge joint A freely movable joint that allows flexion and extension

Hippocrates A Greek physician known as the father of preventive medicine

Hua T'o Famous Chinese surgeon (c. 145–208) credited with the invention of anesthetic drugs as well as other medical practices

Hyperextension Movement beyond the natural range of motion

Hypertrophy An increase in the size of muscle tissue

I

Imagery The process of reviewing a training process in the mind only, using visualization

Individualized Education Program (IEP) A specific education program designed around a disabled individual's specific, identifiable needs.

Individuals with Disabilities Act Legislation that requires states to provide special services to students with disabilities

Individuals with Disabilities Education Act (IDEA) A law ensuring provision of services to children with disabilities throughout the nation

Influence To impose one's opinion on others

Initiative A beginning act or step

Inversion Movement of the sole of the foot inward

Isokinetic exercise A type of exercise in which a machine is used to control the speed of contraction within the range of motion

Isometric exercise An activity that causes tension in the muscle to increase but does not cause the muscle to shorten

Isotonic exercise An activity that causes tension in the muscle to increase and also causes the muscle to shorten

J

Joint articulation The connecting point of two bones

K

Kinesiology The multidisciplinary study of physical activity or movement; encompasses anatomy, biomechanics, physiology, psychomotor behavior; and social and cultural factors

Konrad system A flexible tournament system that may last for an extended period of time

L

Least restricted environment The result of adapting or modifying the physical education curriculum and/or instruction to address the abilities of each child. Adaptations are made to ensure that each student will experience success in a safe environment.

Liability Risk of bearing the cost of injury sustained by another when one fails to meet one's legal responsibilities

M

Manual resistance training A form of dynamic exercise in which one works with a training partner

McMahon system tournament A tournament system in which players start at different levels; named after Lee McMahon

Medical kit A portable container that contains medical supplies used to treat injuries

Mission statement A collection of beliefs or doctrines that are used as guiding principles

Motivation An internal state or condition (need or desire) that serves to activate or energize behavior and give it direction

Motor unit A motor nerve plus all the muscle fibers it stimulates

Muscular endurance The ability for muscles to sustain work for an extended period of time

Muscular strength The ability of muscles to exert the power necessary to complete a certain task goal

N

National Association for Sport and Physical Education (NASPE) A national organization tasked with enhancing knowledge, improving professional practice, and increasing support for high-quality physical education, sport, and physical activity programs

National Blueprint Popular name of a major national planning document regarding aging and physical activity released in 2001 by a coalition of national organizations

National standards Criteria set forth by national organizations

No Child Left Behind Act of 2001 (NCLB) Legislation that makes schools accountable for students' achievement of high standards

Non-emergency Any medical illness or injury that does not pose a serious threat to life or limb

O

Occupational Safety and Health Administration (OSHA) Federal agency charged with the enforcement of safety and health legislation

Office of Civil Rights (OCR) Federal entity that ensures equal access to education and promotes educational excellence through vigorous enforcement of civil rights

Olympic Games International amateur sporting event, held every four years, whose mission is to bring the world together through sport

Open kinematic chain A sequence of actions in which the body part farthest from the trunk is free during movement

Opposition Movement of the thumb enabling it to touch each finger

Osteoarthritis A degenerative joint disease

Overload Progressive overwork of muscles at a controlled, increased rate; intended to achieve consistent gains in strength

P

Personal trainers Professionals who use exercise to enhance their clients' physical conditioning level in a safe and effective way

Physical education Instruction in the development and care of the body

Pilates A form of exercise developed in the early twentieth century by Joseph Pilates.

Pivot joint A freely movable joint in which a bone moves around a central axis, creating rotational movement

Plantarflexion Movement that extends the foot

Prehabilitation Use of a preventative management program to reduce the likelihood of injury

Preseason conditioning A program, typically begun six to eight weeks prior to sports participation, that allows the body to adapt gradually to the demands the sport will place on it

President's Council on Physical Fitness and Sports (PCPFS) A committee of volunteers who advise the president, through the Department of Health and Human Services, about physical activity, fitness, and sports in America

Primary fibrositis An inflammation of the fibrous connective tissue in a joint

Progressive resistance exercise A type of training in which muscles are worked until they reach their capacity. Once the athlete is able to maintain that capacity, the workload on the muscle is increased to build additional strength and endurance.

Pronation Movement of the radius and ulna posteriorly or inferiorly

Proprioceptive neuromuscular facilitation (PNF) A combination of relaxing and contracting of the muscles in which an initial isometric contraction against maximum resistance is held at the end of the range of motion, followed by relaxation and passive stretching

Protraction Movement of a body part forward in a transverse plane

R

Rating A method of determining which athletes should be seeded higher in tournament play

Recreation workers Individuals that work in the recreation field

Registered athletic administrator (RAA) Athletic administrator that has registered with the National Interscholastic Athletic Administrators Association

Rehabilitation The process of restoring function through programmed exercise to enable a return to competition or other accustomed activity

Retraction Movement of a body part backward in a transverse plane

Reversibility Process of muscle atrophy due to disuse, immobilization, or starvation; leads to decreased strength and muscle mass.

Risk management Management of the risks associated with physical education, sports, and athletic competition

Rotation Movement of a bone toward or away from the body on an axis

Round-robin tournament Type of group tournament in which each participant plays each other participant an equal number of times

S

Saddle joint A freely movable joint between two bones that have complementary shapes; allows a wide range of motion

Sagittal plane A vertical flat surface running from front to back of the body

Section 504 of the Rehabilitation Act of 1973 National law that protects qualified individuals from discrimination based on their disability

Seeding A drawing for positions in a tournament; structured so that the more skilled contestants meet in the later rounds

Shape of the Nation Report A national report providing current information on the status of physical education in each of the states and the District of Columbia

Sharps container Provides safe storage for contaminated material that will be transported to a proper disposal site

Simulation A training environment designed to be as similar as possible to actual competition

Single-elimination tournament A tournament in which a contestant is eliminated from further competition after the first loss

Slow twitch fiber Fiber in a motor unit that requires a long time to generate force. These fibers are resistant to fatigue.

Specificity The ability of particular muscle groups to respond to targeted training of those muscles so that increased strength is gained in that muscle group only

Sport management Career in which one specializes in the care and management of sports and athletic venues

Sports psychology The study of sport, exercise, and the mental (psychological) factors that influence athletic performance

Sportsmanship The practice and belief that fair play and proper conduct are paramount to the well-being of contestants

Static stretching A gradual, slow stretching of a muscle through the entire range of motion, followed by holding the stretched position for 20–30 seconds

Stress A factor that causes awareness, anxiety, focus, or fear; stress can be either good or bad and can have both positive and negative effects

Stretching Moving the joints beyond their normal range of motion

Student-athlete A person who competes in school athletics

Supervision Management and oversight of the performance or operation of a person or group

Supination Movement of the radius and ulna anteriorly or superiorly

Sutures Immovable joints composed of dense fibrous connective tissue; located in the skull at the junction of the cranial bones

Swiss-system tournament A tournament format that combines elements of the round-robin and elimination formats; typically identifies a champion within fewer rounds than a round-robin, while allowing draws and losses

Synarthroses (singular **synarthrosis**) Immovable joints that lack a synovial cavity and are held together by fibrous connective tissue

Syndesmoses (singular **syndesmosis**) Slightly movable joints at which bones are connected by ligaments

Synovial fluid A lubricating substance produced by the synovial membrane; found in joints

Synovial joint Freely movable joint; also known as a *diarthrosis*

Synovial membrane Layer of tissue that lines joint cavities and produces synovial fluid

T

Tai chi chu'an A Chinese exercise system that teaches graceful movements

Teamwork Coordinated effort on the part of a group; effort toward achieving a common goal

Title IX A law guaranteeing that no person in the United States shall, on the basis of sex, be excluded from participation in, be denied the benefits of, or be subjected to discrimination under any education program or activity receiving federal financial assistance

Training room A dedicated facility where athletes can be treated for various injuries or conditions

W

Weight rooms A dedicated facility designed for weight training activities

Y

Yoga A system of ancient spiritual practices that originated in India; said to promote healing and the feeling of well being

Youth Risk Behavior Surveillance System (YRBSS) Survey system established by the Centers for Disease Control (CDC) to monitor the prevalence in youth of certain behaviors that influence health

Index